IMMUNOLOGY FOR THE MEDICAL SCIENCES

REVISED PRINTING

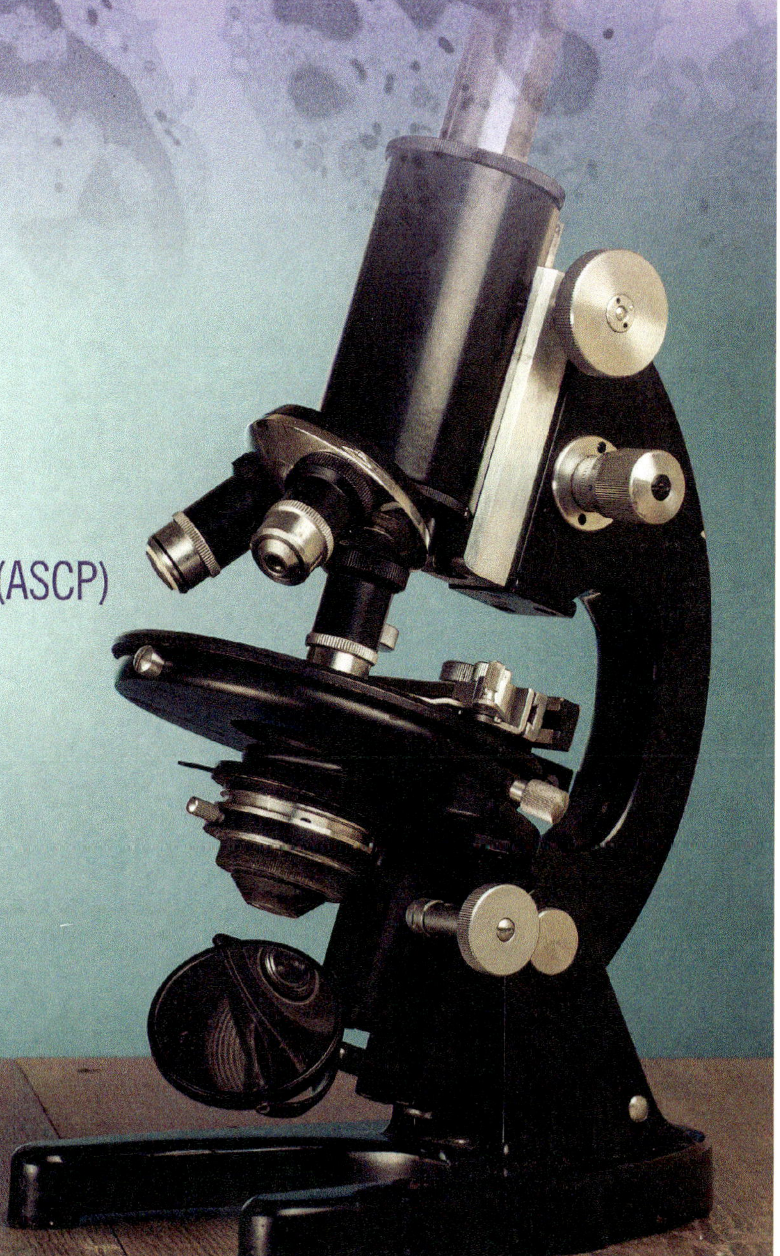

Anthony Azenabor Ph.D., C.S (ASCP)

Kendall Hunt
publishing company

Cover image © Shutterstock.com

Kendall Hunt
publishing company
www.kendallhunt.com
Send all inquiries to:
4050 Westmark Drive
Dubuque, IA 52004-1840

ISBN 978-1-4652-9516-3

Printed in the United States of America

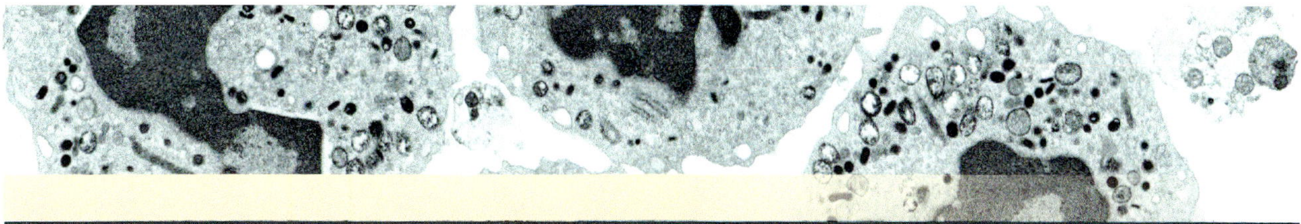

CONTENTS

ACKNOWLEDGEMENTS

I will like to thank my ever-dependable students who have listened year in year out to my lectures in Clinical Immunology and Case Studies in Immunology, for they constituted the initial audience through whom the lectures in this book matured to fruition. I must specially thank Jenniffer Citron Cuevas, Julia Alba, Anthony Matsche, and Afsaneh Hemmat for their roles in recording my lectures, helping with figures and editorials and ensuring that my research laboratory did not suffer when I became so focused on writing and other international engagements. The wonderful ring of colleagues I have at the University of Wisconsin-Milwaukee also deserve mention: I thank them.

I must remember to thank staffs of Kendall Hunt Publishing Co. for their consistent kind words and sometimes a little subtle pressure; I guess it finally paid off. I must say it was a good experience working with them. My unreserved thanks go to my wife, Okwuchi, who is an expert in reminding me of the need to meet my commitments in terms of this book contract.

PREFACE

Immunology is a subject that cuts across the frontiers of biomedical sciences and for this reason has emerged to be a subject that requires diverse approaches depending on the interest of the student and profession. In the past 30 years, the subject has incorporated the needs of these diverse parties such that new books need to lay emphasis on the area of interest of their intended users. The rapid progress in molecular biology has necessitated that each professional area with interest in immunology adopts an approach to the subject that incorporates molecular sciences to the extent needed.

This book has been written to address the needs of students of medical sciences bias studying a one-semester course in immunology. The contents have been selected to correspond with what I have used over the past decade of teaching the subject. It satisfies the required fundamentals both in immunologic concepts and in molecular biochemistry that constitute the part of the knowledge required by a student of medical sciences. It is written, therefore, mainly for undergraduate-level students in medical laboratory sciences, medicine, dentistry, and nursing. It can also serve as a textbook for general health sciences majors, including those interested in public health microbiology, medical microbiology, and continuing education in laboratory medicine.

The overall design of the book, therefore, has incorporated a format that includes helpful pedagogical features such intermittent outlines and summaries, numerous illustrations that simplify more complex concepts, and mechanisms. In this regard, colorful boxes provide information at a glance, making reviews faster and easy. Since this book is not a laboratory manual, at the end of each chapter is some suggested laboratory practical topics.

The organization of this text is such that one topic leads to the other, thereby filling all gaps. In this regard, the text starts with an introduction which details the meaning of immunology and the development of the subject. It presents in a chronological fashion the historical background of the subject. The next sets of chapters treat topics such as innate immunity, nature of antibodies, lymphoid tissues, and cellular interactions, among others, terminating with immunity to infections.

Immunology is a fast-growing area and as such readers are encouraged to feel free to offer constructive criticisms, more so since this is the first edition of this book.

Anthony A. Azenabor
Ph.D, C.S (ASCP)
Department of Biomedical Sciences
University of Wisconsin-Milwaukee, WI
aazenabo@uwm.edu

CHAPTER 1

INTRODUCTION TO IMMUNOLOGY

WELCOME TO THE EXCITING WORLD OF IMMUNOLOGY!

This book addresses the fundamentals of the body's protective mechanisms in a way that is suited for students of medical sciences in general and those training to become medical laboratory professionals in particular. The term *immunology* was crafted from the Latin word *immunis* meaning to *exempt*, the *logy* is from Greek *logos*, meaning *science*. Therefore, immunology is the science of how the body is exempted from diseases. Immunology is a broad branch of biomedical science that spans the aspects of the body systems that help to mount a defense against challenges in the state of health or disease.

It also addresses the diseases that afflict the immune system; these are the immunological disorders such as hypersensitivities, autoimmune diseases, immune deficiency, and transplant rejection. Immunology cuts across the frontiers of biomedical sciences and, therefore, has continued to develop with new areas emerging. The goal of this book is to provide those principles in immunology required by the medical science student, fashioning it in a practical way that it will be understood by one being introduced to the subject without compromising the essential science.

THE HISTORICAL BACKGROUND

- Recovery from illness was accompanied by the ability to resist reinfection.
- The knowledge of immunology preceded the knowledge of organized bacteriology.
- Chinese physicians in 11th century observed that inhalation of smallpox crusts prevented the subsequent occurrence of the disease.

TYPE OF PATHOGENS	EXAMPLES OF PATHOGENS	ASSOCIATED DISEASES
Viruses	*Varicella zoster*	Chicken pox
	Ebola	Hemorrhagic fever
	Rubeola	Measles
Bacteria	*Shigella sonnei*	Dysentery
	Haemophilus influenza type B	Respiratory infection
	Neisseria meningitidis	Meningitis/Sepsis
Fungi	*Candida albicans*	Urogenital tract infections
	Pneumocystis carinii	Pneumonia
	Microsporum canis	Ringworm (Tinea capitis)
Parasites: Protozoans	*Trichomonas vaginalis*	STD
	Trypanosoma gambiense	Sleeping sickness
	Plasmodium falciparum	Malaria
Helminths (worms)	*Ancylostoma duodenale*	Hookworm
	Enterobius vermicularis	Pinworm infection

The pattern of development of immunology is as natural as the subject. So, human beings have always been smart enough to know that those who survive infectious diseases are able to resist subsequent infections. This observation superseded the establishment of the germ theory of disease, in which Louis Pasteur and Robert Koch defined microorganisms as the etiologic agent of a large number of diseases.

HISTORICAL TREND OF THE DEVELOPMENT OF IMMUNOLOGY	
1000 A.D.	Chinese: prophylactic infection to prevent smallpox
1718	Lady Mary Wortley Montagu (wife of British ambassador to Constantinople): observed positive effects of variolation on the native population and her own children
1798	Jenner: cowpox vaccination
1837	Schwann: first description of the role of microbes in putrefaction and fermentation
1838	Charles Cagniard de la Tour: confirmation of the role of yeast in fermentation of sugar to alcohol
1840	Henle: first to propose the germ theory of disease
1850	Semmelweis: demonstration of the contagious nature of puerperal fever
1857–70	Pasteur: confirmation of the role of microbes in fermentation
1862	Haeckel: phagocytosis
1867	Lister: first aseptic practice in surgery
1878	Pasteur: confirmation of the germ theory of disease
1880	Koch: discovered delayed hypersensitivity to tuberculosis (cell-mediated immunity)

Source of historical trend of development in Immunology (tabulation of year and discovery only): Wikipedia,http://en.wikipedia.org/wiki/Timeline_of_immunology

1881	Pasteur: developed killed and attenuated vaccines
1885	Roux and Yersin: first described bacterial toxins
1885	Pasteur: introduction of the concept of therapeutic vaccination; live attenuated vaccine for rabies
1888	Nuttall: bactericidal action of blood
1890	von Behring and Kitasato: first described antibody activity against diphtheria and tetanus toxins
1893	Buchner: discovered complement (alexine)
1893	Coley: use of live bacteria and bacterial lysates (Coley's toxins) to treat tumors
1894	Pfeiffer: elucidated action of complement and antibody in cell lysis
1896	Durham and von Gruber: described agglutination test for bacteria
1896	Bordet: description of an antibacterial, heat-labile serum component (complement)
1896	Widal: described test for diagnosis of typhoid fever
1883	Metchnikoff: Cellular theory of immunity via phagocytosis
1905	Ehrlich: Humoral theory of immunity via antibody formation (side chain theory)
TISSUE INJURY	
1902	Richet and Portier: anaphylaxis
1903	Arthus: intermediate hypersensitivity—"Arthus reaction"
1905	von Pirquet and Schick: "serum sickness" allergy
1921	Prausnitz and Kustner: cutaneous allergic reactions
1924–38	Sanarelli-Shwartzman: necrotic reactions—endotoxin
1945	Landsteiner and Chase: cellular transfer of "delayed hypersensitivity"
CELLULAR	
1924	Aschoff : reticuloendothelial system named
1942	Landsteiner and Chase: anaphylaxis—cellular transfer of sensitivity
1942	Freund and McDermott: adjuvants
1944	Medawar and Burnet: tolerance; "self" versus "nonself"
1945	Owen: chimerism
1947	Levine and Stetson: discovered Rh blood system
1949	Burnet and Fenner: immunological tolerance hypothesis
1952	Bruton: first description of agammaglobulinemia
1957	Jerne and Burnet: clonal selection theory
1957	Isaacs and Lindenmann: discovery of interferon
1959	Gowans: discovery of lymphocyte circulation

1960	Nowell: discovery of lymphocyte "blastogenic transformation" and proliferation in response to mitogenic lectins—phytohemagglutinin (PHA)
1961–62	Miller and Good: role of thymus
1961	Nowell: demonstration that glucocorticoids inhibit PHA-induced lymphocyte proliferation
1963	Jerne and Nordin: development of the plaque assay for enumeration of antibody forming cell in vitro
1964–68	Davis: T- and B-cell cooperation in immune response
1965	Kamakura, Lowenstein, Gordon, and MacLean: discovery of the first lymphocyte monogenic activity, called "blastogenic factor"
1965	Wheelock: discovery of "immune interferon" (gamma)
1968	Elkins and Guttmann: passenger leukocytes identified as significant immunogens in allograft rejection
1969	Brunner and Certottini: lymphocyte cytolysis Cr51 release assay
1973	Steinman: dendritic cells described
1974	Zinkernagel and Doherty: T-cell restriction to major histocompatibility complex
1979	Smith: generation of the first monoclonal T-cells
1980–83	Smith: discovery and characterization of the first interleukins (IL-1 and IL-2)
1983	Smith: discovery of IL-2 receptor IL2R
1983	Reinherz, Marrack, Kappler, and Allison: discovery of the T-cell antigen receptor TCR
1983	Montagnier: discovery of HIV
1984	Cantrell and Smith: first single cell analysis of lymphocyte proliferation
1985–87	Identification of the genes for the T-cell receptor
1986	Mosmann: Th1 vs. Th2 model of T-helper cell function
1988	Rudd: discovery of biochemical initiators of T-cell activation—CD4 and CD8-p56Ick
1990	Gene therapy for SCID
1992	Allmanman Cancro: discovery of transitional B-cells
1994	Matzinger: "Danger" model of immunological tolerance
1995	Sakaguchi: regulatory T-cells
1995	Mukherji: first dendritic cell vaccine trial
2001	Discovery of FOXP3: the gene directing regulatory T-cell development

HUMORAL	
1900	Landsteiner: ABO blood groups
1903	Write and Douglas: opsonization
1909	Ehrlich: "immune surveillance" hypothesis of tumor recognition and eradication
1917	Rous: demonstration of filterable agent that caused tumors
1930	Landsteiner: hapten
1934	Heidelberger: quantitative precipitin reaction
1939	Marrack: antigen—antibody binding theory—"lattice theory"
1940	Kabat and Tiselius: demonstration that antibodies are gamma globulins
1940	Landsteiner and Weiner: identification of Rh antigen sensitization
1944	Pauling: primary structure of protein
1945	Medwar: hypothesis of allograft rejection
1946	Coombs: antiglobulin test developed—"Coombs' test"
1948	Snell and Gorer: identification of mouse MHC
1949	Fagraeus: antibody production in plasma B-cells Enders, Weller, and Robbins: growth of polio virus in tissue culture, neutralization with immune sera and demonstration of attenuation of neurovirulence with repeated passage
1951	Theiler: vaccine against yellow fever
1953	Simonsen and Dempster: Graft vs. host disease
1958–62	Dausset: discovery of human leukocyte antigens of the first monoclonal antibodies
1959–62	Porter: structure and formation of antibody (gamma globulin)
1960	Edelman: continued identification of structure and formation of gamma globulin
1967	Tomasi: Secretory immunoglobulins
1971	Ishizaka: Identification of IgE as the reaginic antibody
1972	Perlmann and Engvall: invent ELISA
1975	Defined structure of antibody molecules
1976	Kohler and Milstein: generation Tonegawa: identification of somatic recombination of immunoglobulin genes
1986	Blumberg and Millman: Hepatitis B vaccine produced by genetic engineering
1991	Sadegh-Nasseri and Germain: role of peptide for MHC Class II structure defined
1996–98	Identification of Toll-like receptors
2005	Frazer: development of human papillomavirus vaccine

In terms of very highly organized awareness, it is reasonable to think that the Chinese physicians in the 11th century already knew how to protect against smallpox by encouraging the inhalation of smallpox crust. So, they were vaccinating themselves (although they didn't call it vaccination then), thus greatly reducing the incidence of the disease. Around the 15th century, the practice of applying powdered smallpox "crusts" and inserting them with a pin or "poking" device into the skin became commonplace. This was described as variolation.

The Middle-Easterners copied what the Chinese were doing. The proximity of the Middle East to Egypt, which was a great place of learning, led to the modification of the practice in China, so the technique of variolation became intradermal inoculation instead of intranasal sniffing. It was dangerous, and it killed some individuals. It killed them because some of the individuals who had survived an infection before would develop such a serious response to the intradermal inoculation that it would result in the death of the individual. This is because when the powder from the scrapings was introduced under the skin, it would find cells that were already in the state of preparedness to fight infectious agents in the powder, this kind of response is more aggressive. This is a hypersensitivity reaction. The cells were primed; they had become so aware of the nature of the challenge such that an additional repeat of the same challenge would produce a serious effect that could cause death. We would delve more into the topic of hypersensitivity in this text. It is important to note that the type of hypersensitivity that would cause this kind of reaction would be the type 4, mediated by lymphocytes.

Figure 1.1 illustrates the effect of repeated exposure to a challenge on antibody elaboration.

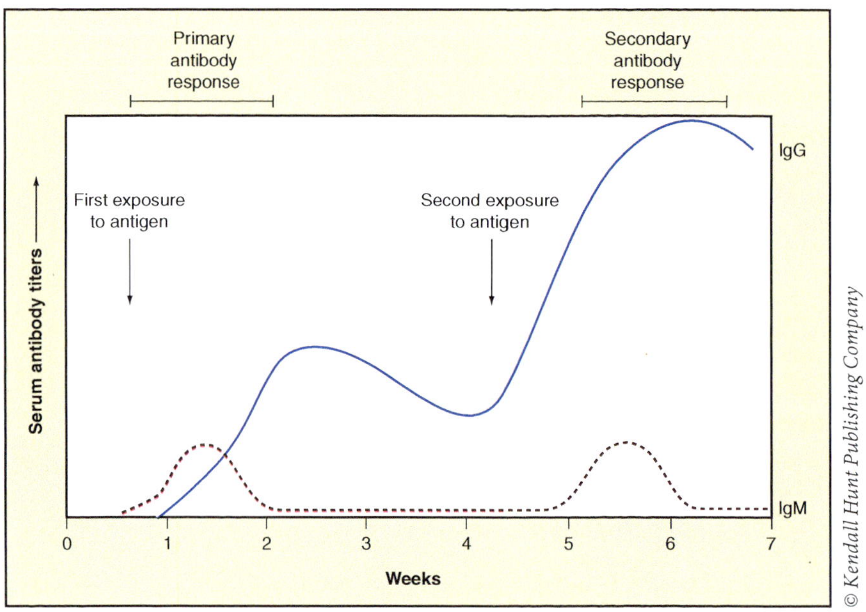

Figure 1.1 *Comparison of a primary and secondary immune response.*

In Europe, the first major contributor to the field of immunology was Edward Jenner, a medical student. He observed that women and girls who milked cows that had been exposed to the cowpox virus, the cattle smallpox (it is not exactly Variola, it is Vaccinia virus, its cousin), did not have problems with smallpox. Since this cowpox does not infect human beings in a deadly way, he decided to give cowpox scrapings to individuals in the community. The wisdom in this act will become obvious when we deal with the topic, vaccines and vaccination. Jenner's observation is very historic. It may not be very mechanistic, but the reasoning was very smart, and it is in part the foundation of many of our designs of vaccines today.

The chart given in Figure 1.2 shows the relationship between cowpox and smallpox.

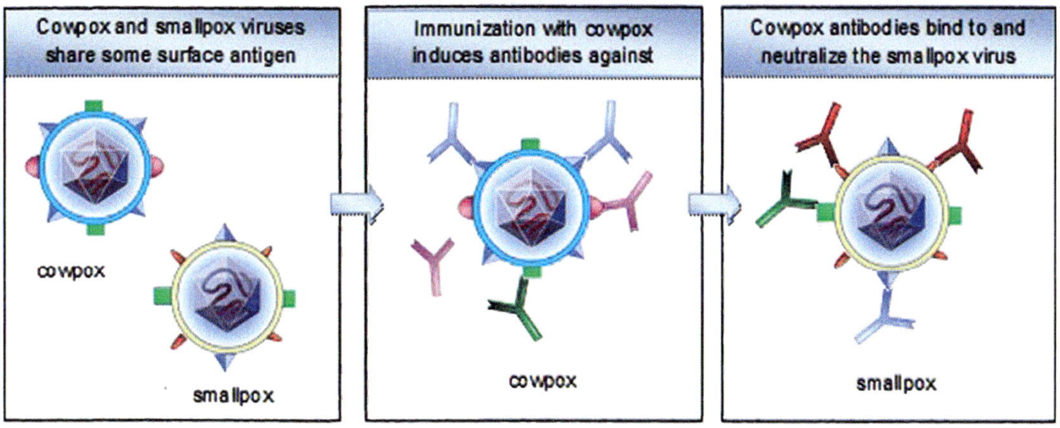

Figure 1.2 *Relationship between cowpox and smallpox.*

One of the central dogmas of immunity is that, if immunity has to be efficient, then it must be able to protect and prevent infection. The body's way of doing it is to wait for the onset of infection and confront the infection using the innate immune system. This is the form of protection that is part and parcel of the body, it is nonspecific. It is important to note that the acquired arm of immune response is specific against agents of infection, against challenges. It is elicited later during the infection cycle. The element of delay in specific response to a challenge is dangerous because the individual concerned may not be able to adequately respond or may be overwhelmed by more than one infectious agent. It is against this background that preventive immunization is of enormous importance. It is a form of efficacious preemptive protection of a community by immunizing individuals.

- The enhancement and further development of preventive immunization was made by Louis Pasteur.
- Louis Pasteur coined the word vaccine (from *vacca*: Latin for cow) in honor of Jenner's contribution.
- What did Pasteur do?

  He produced materials that could be used as vaccines: Living, heat-killed, and attenuated (living but with reduced virulence).
- How Pasteur did it?
  1. Old culture (attenuated) of fowl cholera organism inoculated into fowl produced no disease.
  2. Surprisingly, these fowl were resistant to subsequent infection with the organism and were solidly immunized.

Among the earliest workers in the area of fashioning preemptive protection against specific infection was Louis Pasteur, a French chemist, who became so vast in various areas of science that he is regarded as the father of immunology and microbiology today. Among his most impressive discoveries were the novel accidental findings he made in 1881. He was working on fowl cholera, which caused serious devastation in the poultry industry. The infectious agent was the bacterium *Vibrio cholera*. First of all, the emphasis at that time was not to design a vaccine for vibrio, but to understand the bacterial etiology of cholera. How does *Vibrio cholera* cause this problem? In order to answer this question, he needed to grow vibrio and use them on fowl, and he found out that he was having good results when he infected birds with his culture, as they came down with cholera. Then, he went on vacation and due to improper storage of their old stock, this could not be used to establish infection in birds. Also, he observed that a new stock could not cause disease in birds previously inoculated with the old stock but caused disease in uninoculated birds. He thought "maybe those old cultures did something to the birds," because that was the only difference. Today, we know that is how we are all protected from various infections. When infectious agents in culture are kept for so long (attenuation), they lose their capacity to cause disease, but they still retain the ability to protect against disease. This is a big tool in immunology and various means of achieving attenuation have now emerged.

Pasteur called the method of giving the attenuated infectious agent to an animal or human "vaccination," from the Latin word *vacca*, meaning cow in memory of Edward Jenner, whose work made the reasoning of Louis Pasteur's findings easier. Robert Koch showed that living organisms could be the one obtained from continuous culture as in the case of vaccine against tuberculosis, BCG (bacillus calmette-guerin). This involves the continuous culture of bovine tuberculosis agent for 13 years in bile salt medium. This act renders the bacterium incapable of causing disease but capable of protecting against disease by being immunogenic.

Before 1955, smallpox was a big problem, but through the act of vaccination, there was a drastic decline leading to the total eradication of the virus. For viral vaccines, despite attenuation, there can be reversion to virulence. The precautions taken to avoid indiscriminate vaccination will be addressed under the topic vaccines and vaccination. Although smallpox has been eradicated, some ampoules of the live virus were left in the Center for Disease Control and Prevention in USA and Russia. The fear now is that it can find its way into the hands of individuals who can weaponize them for use as bioterrorism agents. The danger of previous exposure of an animal to specific immune response is hypersensitivity: heightened immune response in an adverse manner.

- At about the same period, Robert Koch discovered tubercle bacillus during his studies of the bacterial etiology of infectious diseases.
- While he was trying to develop a vaccine for tuberculosis, he observed the phenomenon known today as delayed hypersensitivity or cell-mediated immunity.
- Following the isolation of diphtheria bacillus, Roux and Yersin demonstrated the existence of potent soluble exotoxin elaborated by the organism.
- This toxin was used by von Behring and Kitasato to inoculate animals that produced in their serum a toxin-neutralizing substance called antitoxin.
- This toxin-neutralizing capability could be transferred by giving the serum to uninoculated animals, a process called passive immunization.
- Pfeiffer and Bordet's work differentiated a substance distinct from antibody in serum, called complement, which participated in destruction of bacteria.
- Durham and von Gruber found that serum could clump or agglutinate bacteria. This forms the basis of tests for diagnosis of infection-specific agglutination reaction, such as the test described by Widal for the diagnosis of typhoid fever (Widal test).

The bacterium that causes diphtheria was described by Roux and Yersin (Yersinia organism is well known), and the most interesting finding from their work was the capacity of the bacterium to produce toxins. Organisms don't necessarily destroy the system by attacking it physically, but some of their metabolic products called toxins can be destructive. They are called exotoxins when these toxins are expressed to the environment, and they are endotoxins when they are not expressed to the environment. When these toxins are rendered nontoxic (toxoid) and given to animals, they produce antitoxins which can be purified and used as agents for passive immunization against the toxins in the blood. The antitoxin is commonly called serum. So, it was when Yersin had made this discovery about exotoxin that von Behring and Kitasato working together came to find that it was possible to attenuate them and inoculate them into animals to produce serum that can neutralize toxin.

Pfeiffer and Bordet were the ones who discovered the group of proteins that we call complement which also destroys bacteria. These complements are part of nonspecific immune system.

Durham and von Gruber were able to observe a unique process called agglutination which has application widely in the laboratory. The body's way of taking care of microorganisms is to produce antibodies that can attack or react with proteins on the organized cell system in a way that they will finally clump the cell system together. We take advantage of it in the lab to observe reactions today; it is used in blood typing reactions and in microbiology area for Widal test.

- The animal body is suitable for microbial incubation because it is warm, has moisture, has cells and is rich in nutrients. There is, therefore, need for protection.
- The immune system *offers protection* and corrects *changes in steady state* arising from assault from microbes and environmental challenges and *mount surveillance* against future attacks.
- Since there is absolute need to eradicate any invader, *redundancy is often built into the immune system* (more than one approach is utilized), thus ensuring *adequate protection.*

It is important to note that infectious agents have a propensity to colonize animals and humans. The colonization processes do not only cause protracted infection but may finally result in the formation of neoplastic changes, making the infected cells cancerous. Infections, therefore, bring about a disturbance in the constancy of the internal environment in a way that there is structural or functional derangement (disease). What is it about the animal or human body that allows it? It is because of the simple fact that pathogenic microbes on their own want to live their lives with minimum exertion and they do not have all the facilities for more complex subsistence, so wherever they find the facilities for it becomes their habitat. The cells of human and animal bodies consist of is 60% water, a very important source of moisture for microbes. The luxuriant propagation of microbes requires carbon, nitrogen, minerals, and vitamins, all of which are available in the human body, thus making the human body a very attractive place for microbial incubation. It is also for this reason that our quest to expand our knowledge in the area of infectious diseases is continuous, without an end. It is this attractiveness of the animal physiology as a habitat for microbes that makes the animal system develop means of protecting itself over evolutionary period against microbial assaults and challenges. That is the reason for the development of an immune system that is useful, effective, and efficacious at disease prevention and protection of the animal host.

INTERACTION BETWEEN MICROBES AND THE ANIMAL SYSTEM

The microbe's intent in this interaction is the need to survive in an environment that is rendered unconducive by the host immune system and so there is a level of metabolic conflict. The immune system usually gains the upper hand. Sometimes, this happens after we have medically intervened; however, it is the efficient immune system and not the intervention that causes lasting restoration to good health. In the absence of a good immune system, no therapeutic intervention would bring about lasting recovery. This fact is more apparent in the acquired immune deficiency syndrome (AIDS) patient. During the conflict arising from microbe–animal system interaction, the body physiology and the system itself experience a level of disorder resulting in homeostatic changes. An efficient immune system, therefore, should not only protect but should also immediately address bringing about a restoration to normalcy. Now, apart from protecting the body from infectious agents and restoring normalcy to the disturbed host physiology, there's a third component of an efficient immune system: it is the capacity to mount adequate surveillance by endowment with a remarkable memory of a previous experience. The three components, namely, protection, restoration to normalcy, and memory, are the hallmarks of an efficient and effective immune system (see Figure 1.3). The efficiency of the system to carryout protection and absolutely eradicate an invader is ensured by an inbuilt redundancy.

Immunology can be defined as the study of defense mechanisms that *afford protection*, *restore steady state* and *mount surveillance*.

- Through cellular attacks and antibody production, protection occurs by producing soluble substances and a return to steady state is ensured. And by having remarkable memory, adequate surveillance is maintained.
- Immune system does not always offer lasting protection, for example, malaria and common cold.

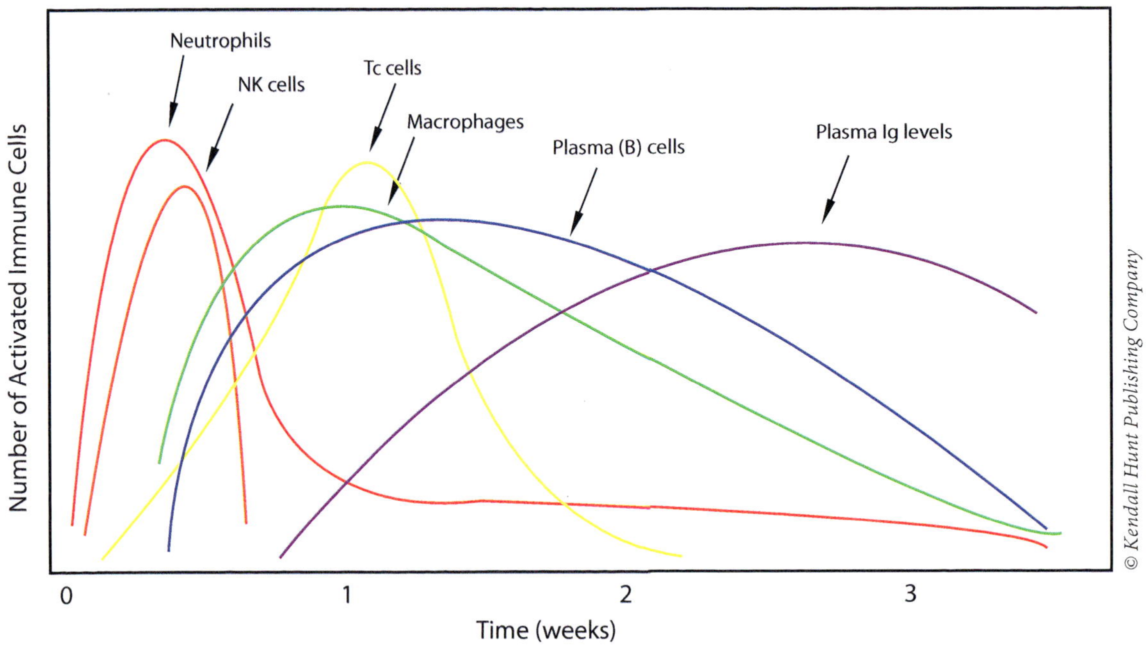

Figure 1.3 *Three components of immunity. Protective immunity consists of both preformed antibodies and immunological memory.*

Discussed next are some common features of immune response.

Immune response could be specific or nonspecific.

- **Antibodies**: Proteins that appear in serum following exposure to foreign substances. They are specific.
- **Antigens**: Foreign substances that can provoke the production of antibodies. Antigens can react specifically with antibodies.
- **Toxoid**: Bacterial toxin that has been rendered nonpoisonous by chemical treatment (formaldehyde treatment) for safe delivery as protection against bacterial toxin. In the host system, they produce an antitoxin.
- **Neutralization**: The rendering of antigen (Ag) nontoxic by antibody (Ab). For instance, tetanus toxoid injected into an animal produces Abs (antitetanus toxoid Abs). If the animal serum is mixed with tetanus toxin, a cloudy solution emerges which renders the toxin ineffective.
- **Cell-Mediated Immunity**: Abs alone cannot provide protection because intracellular agents of infection escape Abs; thus, cellular components of the immune system such as special lymphocytes destroy these invading agents of infection. They are also involved in tissue rejection and killing of tumor cells.
- **First Set Reaction**: This is the reaction of an unsensitized person. It is slow.
- **Second Set Reaction**: This is the rejection by a sensitized person. It is fast.
- **Lag Period**: The period following inoculation of an animal with an Ag. The length of period depends on Ab detection method, but it is not less than 3–4 days.

- **Primary Response**: In 10–14 days, the Ab production reaches its peak, but only a small response is achieved, because this is the first exposure and then decline sets in.
- **Secondary Response**: After a primary response, a subsequent dose of toxoid produces a rapid response in 2–3 days to a very high level before a slow decline in months.
- **Anamnestic or Memory Response**: Because secondary response is rapid and high, it follows that the immune system has memory. This response is called anamnestic (anamnesis = memory).
- **Tumor Rejection**: It is by the same mechanism as tissue rejection, thus immunosuppressive agents used may promote cancer, viral infection, etc.
- **Tolerance**: This is the failure to elicit an immune response. This mechanism has an advantage which is evident in self-tolerance—failure to produce an immune response against self. Tolerance may be created by giving very small or very large doses of Ag.
- **Signal Transduction**: Conversion of an extracellular interaction (signals) into series of intracellular events is called transduction.

DEFINING IMMUNOLOGY

This must encompass the three functional components stated above. Therefore, immunology is the study the animal's capacity to protect itself from infections or challenges, restore a steady state (the disturbance of which must have arisen from host–pathogen interactions), and mount adequate surveillance.

How does the immune system satisfy these functional components? Through the collective effects of the innate immune system and the acquired immune system including antibody production, protection is ensured. The cells of the immune system produce some soluble substances (proteins), these proteins in their function exert effects on cell systems in the body to bring about the restoration to normalcy. What of surveillance? This is anchored in the capacity of a subpopulation of thymus-dependent lymphocytes to exhibit remarkable memory. It is important to note that the elaboration of antibodies will not always result in protective immunity, for instance, the production of antibodies against malaria, influenza, etc., be they natural or through vaccination will not result in lasting protection; so, there is repeated need to immunize.

The sequence of immune response is complex; it depends on the state of the animal system. If the system is naïve, then it is in the order—innate immune response (nonspecific) and then acquired immune response (specific). In this sequence, the naïve animal responds in a nonspecific fashion by using a profile of cells such as neutrophils, macrophages/monocytes, and chemical substances such as interferon and complement components to impair the challenge. The more effective and specific response is the acquired response, which is delayed. The delay is due to a lag phase within which the acquired immune system switches on. In nonnaïve animals, the onset of this phase is faster. Apart from the innate response, the gap in protection during acquired immune response (lag phase) could be prevented by passive immunization, involving the administration of preformed antibodies. The problem with this is that the antibodies delivered starts waning early. After the lag phase, antibody buildup in acquired immune response occurs for a short while and wanes unless there is a secondary exposure. During a secondary exposure, there is then a rapid response and there would no longer be a lag phase because the cells of the acquired immune system carry the memory of the previous exposure. This is the anamnestic response, so called because it is a heightened response. There are organisms that have ways of quickly evading memory response by changing their surface molecular content.

The cellular components of immune response are very important. They are involved in the production of various proteins, including the antibodies produced by B cells. B cells, like the thymus-dependent lymphocytes (T cells), also produce a profile of cytokines that can best be described as immune mediators. There is also the aspect of T cells that carry the memory, and reside close to various portals of entry. This is associated with the cause of hypersensitivity referred to previously. There are also some groups of cells that are involved in the killing of cancerous cells. A very healthy immune system will not allow any cancerous growth. The killing and destruction of tumor cells by healthy immune system requires cell-mediated immunity.

Tumor rejection. It is by the same mechanism as tissue rejection. The immune system is required to reject tumor. It is, therefore, understandable that during transplant, the administration of immunosuppressants to prevent rejection could give rise to sufficiently suppressed immune system resulting in toleration of tumor development.

Tolerance. In the simplest sense, it means lack of response to challenge. The implication of this physiologically can be very beneficial; it means one does not respond to one's own cells (self-tolerance). The failure of this system accounts for autoimmune disorders.

Signal transduction. Is another important aspect of the immune system that will be treated, which explains the generation and transformation of molecular chemical signals. Usually, it arises from ligand—receptor interactions. The binding of a biomolecular component of the challenge or infectious agent and the host cell system brings about the reactions that result in production of various effective chemicals and immune mediators. This has been described under cell–cell interactions and signal transduction.

- **Cytokines**: Soluble chemical substances which are mediators of immune responses. They are hormone-like, that is, produced by cells, and may act on the cells or on other cells distances away.
- **Natural Killer Cells (NK Cells)**: They are non-T, non-B cells. They are large granular lymphocytes that are capable of killing tumor cells and virus-infected cells.
- **Anaphylaxis**: Sudden systemic severe reaction arising from exposure to Ag. It involves mast cells rapid degranulation response and histamine production.

The scope of the book shall also include the topic: the functions of various immune mediators (cytokines). These chemicals are produced by cells—*cyto* means cell and *kines* means proteins; therefore, cytokines mean proteins produced by cells in response to challenges. The cells secrete them into the system and they either have effect on the cells that produce them (autocrine) or effect cells distances away (paracrine). There are some groups of cells that are lymphocyte-related in genealogy, but they are not T cells or B cells; they are the natural killer (NK cells), they are large lymphocytes, and they are granular.

Anaphylaxis is the sudden reaction, resembling hypersensitivity, usually due to mast cells production of histamine. It occurs due to antigen-mediated stimulation leading to copious release of histamine which induces smooth muscle spasms.

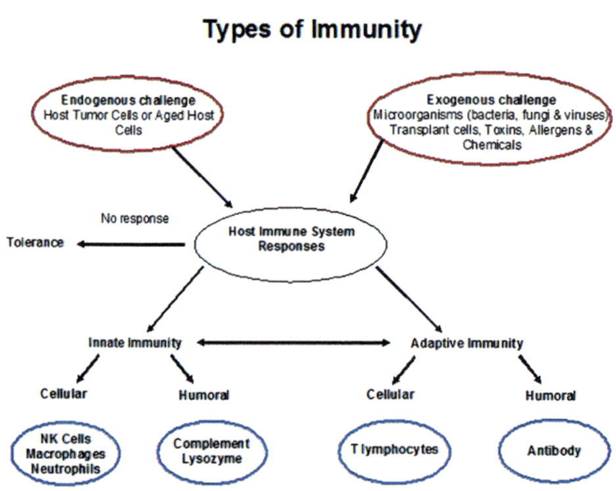

Courtesy of Zainab Ashkanani

Figure 1.4 *Types of immunity: Innate and adaptive immunity.*

TABLE 1.1 COMPARISON OF INNATE AND ADAPTIVE IMMUNITY

	INNATE	ADAPTIVE
Evolution	Throughout vertebrates	Mammals only
Response	General	Specific (antigens)
Properties	Unchanging; first line of defense	Adaptable and has memory
Components	Skin, tears, stomach acid, complement, natural killer cells, inflammation interferon, and macrophages	Antibodies, T lymphocytes, B lymphocytes, complement

Innate immunity is

i. nonspecific (once activated, the same mechanism occurs independent of the challenge).
ii. present at birth (congenital).

Facilities of the host used to mount innate immunity include *physical* (barrier: skin and mucus membrane), *physiological* (unfavorable environment: acidity of stomach, tearing actions of the eyes, flow of urine, cilia and mucus of the respiratory tract, phagocytosis, and inflammation), and *chemicals* (lysozymes, lactic acid, saturated fatty acid, mucoproteins, and interferon).

Adaptive immunity

i. is *specific* against a specific challenge.
ii. it involves *immunologic memory.*
iii. it is *time* requiring.
iv. it is *marked* by *antibody* production (diverse) and *cytokine* elaboration.

There are the following types of adaptive immunity:

1. **Active** immunity: Immune products from immunocompetent cells, for example, *antibodies* production, *sensitization* of lymphocytes, and *cytokines* elaboration.
2. **Passive** immunity: Administration of *preformed immune products*, for example, tetanus serum and hepatitis B serum.
3. **Adoptive** immunity: *Transplantation* of *immunocompetent* cells to an *immunocompetent* host.

ANTIGENS AND ANTIBODIES

- Antigens stimulate nonspecific immune response, specific immune response, or both; they also initiate immune mechanisms that result in products that react with the antigen.
- Haptens react with products of immune response without being able to initiate such response.
- Antibodies are proteins found in plasma and secretions. Structurally, they are bifunctional—Fab end is antigen binding and Fc end defines antibody differences such as IgG, IgM, IgA, IgD, and IgE. All antibodies of the same class share common properties such as placenta crossing and complement binding.

EVALUATION OF SPECIFIC (ADAPTIVE) IMMUNITY

1. Evaluation of *humoral* immunity by measurement of (i) *quantity* of *antibodies* secreted.
   (ii) Antibodies expressed on B-cell and plasma-cell surfaces.
2. Evaluation of **cellular** immunity by *measurement* of (i) the number and types of cells of the *immune* system present.
   (ii) Cytokines elaborated.

Suggested Laboratory Practicals

- Laboratory Tour
- Universal Safety Standards
- Blood borne pathogens
- Quiz on safety

CHAPTER 2

THE INNATE IMMUNE SYSTEM

NATURAL IMMUNITY

This aspect of immunity explores immune response that is not specific and doesn't depend on memory of previous exposure; it is needed because there is a continuous modification of the environment and of challenges (Figure 2.1). It is also described as natural immunity. Natural immune system over millennia has been regarded as first in the line of defense. No matter how efficient and effective adaptive immune response is, it is usually a little bit delayed.

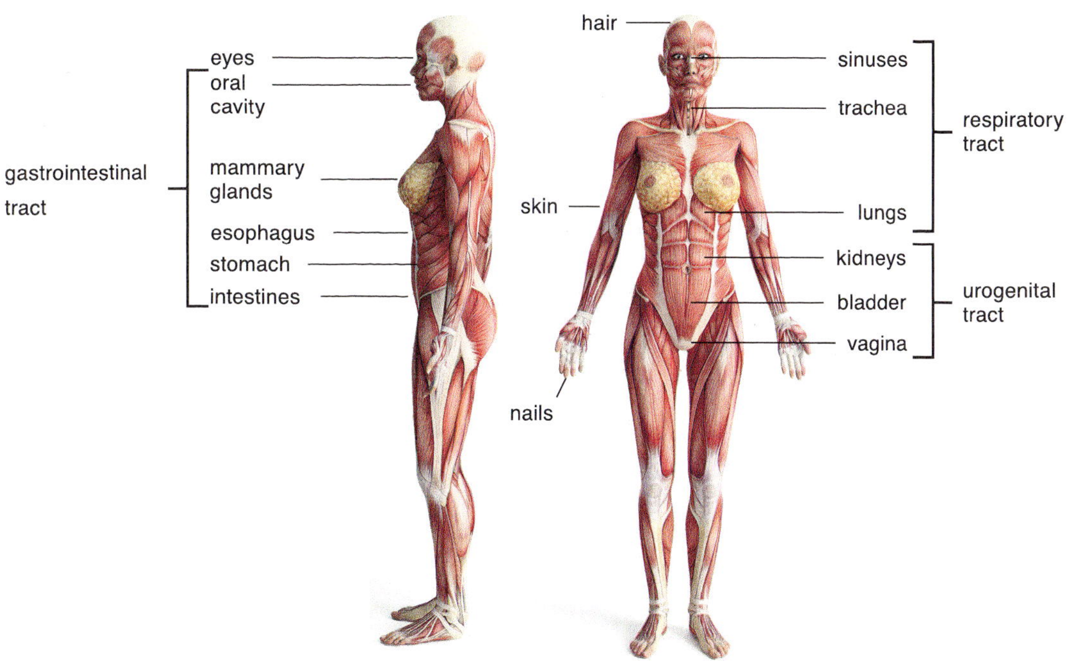

Figure 2.1 *Physical barriers separating the body from the external environment. Physical defenses include skin, mucus membrane, nails, and hair.*

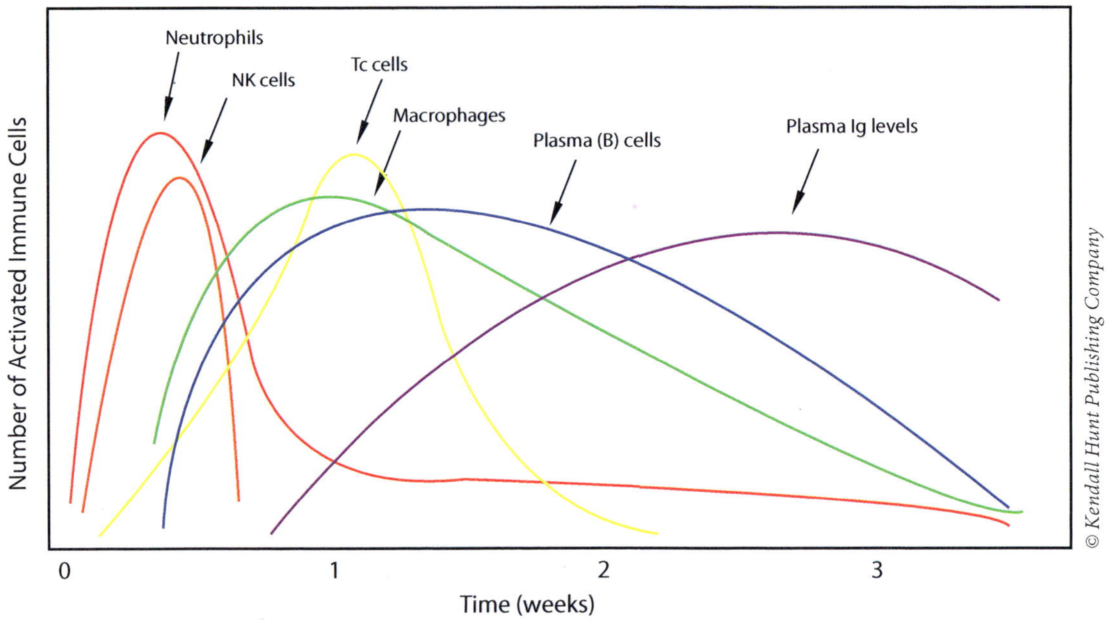

Figure 2.2 *Protective immunity consists of preformed antibodies and immunologic memory.*

Figure 2.2 illustrates how a naive animal, when inoculated with an antigen, exhibits primary immune responses which wanes within a short time. The host's way of defense during this phase is by the actions of the natural immune system. This topic (natural immune system) provides a detailed knowledge of how this system works. We shall examine the cells of the natural immune system and chemical substances elaborated by them. The basic phenomenon that is evident among the cells of the innate immune system is phagocytosis, a process by which cells engulf particles, infectious agents, or challenges. Cells that are capable of this function are endowed with the capacity to destroy engulfed entities. There are some factors that impair engulfment process in biological environment. A prominent factor is the presence of ionic cloud around cells in biological milieu, thus barring cell-to-cell contact. The ionic cloud generates a potential (zeta potential) that must be overcome for the necessary cell—cell contact. The ionic cloud effect is annulled by the opsonization of a bacterial target by molecules such as specific antibodies, complement components, etc., for which cells of the innate immune system have receptors. These molecules are called opsonins. The engulfed infectious agent is encircled in a membrane derived from the plasma membrane of the cell of the immune system, forming the phagosome. The phagosome that is formed quickly fuses with a component of the cell, the lysosome, to form a phagolysosome. The organelle, lysosome, is endowed with a profile of enzymes that can degrade connective tissues, for example, elastase and collagenase. The attachment of opsonins to the surface of infectious agents and to receptors on innate immune cell generates signals that result in the elaboration of enzymes involved in the production of oxygen-derived toxic radicals (superoxide, hypochlorite, and hydroxyl ion) which have lethal effects on the infectious agents. The inflammatory process following the interactions described causes the generation of protein fragments and peptides often described as acute phase proteins or c-reactive proteins which can help clear unfavorable substances that have been elaborated following the confrontation between challenges, infectious agents, and the cells of natural immune system. This is the body's way of quickly restoring normalcy through this kind of reaction that neutralizes mediators and proteolytic enzymes, which if not controlled will continue and become lethal to the host system.

It is important to note that the first aspect of innate immune response is the physical protection including all the external covering of the body; otherwise, infectious agents could secure access to the internal environment effortlessly. Such physical protections are found covering free surfaces in the body. The physical linings are modified depending on the functions of the surface. In the case of surfaces lining the openings into various cavities in the body, the epithelial or endothelial linings have modified linings that contain goblet cells (mucus producing cells), providing a level of protection that makes it difficult for bacteria to establish themselves.

It is logical that the first line of defense is a nonspecific natural immune response; in this way, the body is provided a more general protection irrespective of the infectious agent assailing the body. Other structural barriers of nonspecific nature are skin, hair, cilia, etc. (Figure 2.1).

The internal defenses of nonspecific nature are mainly cells of phagocytic types including white blood cells (neutrophils, monocytes, eosinophils, and basophils), macrophages, and dendritic cells. The macrophage and dendritic cells are unique in their functions which exceed just phagocytosis and degradation of infectious agents but play a nearly central role in the selection of conserved peptides and presenting them as antigens. This phenomenon which will be dealt with later is an important connecting point between innate (nonspecific) and acquired (specific) immune response.

When infectious agents mount challenges, the cells of the immune system are drafted to the site of the challenge by the phenomenon of chemotaxis; chemical movement of cells in response to specialized proteins such as interleukin-8.

CELLS OF THE IMMUNE SYSTEM

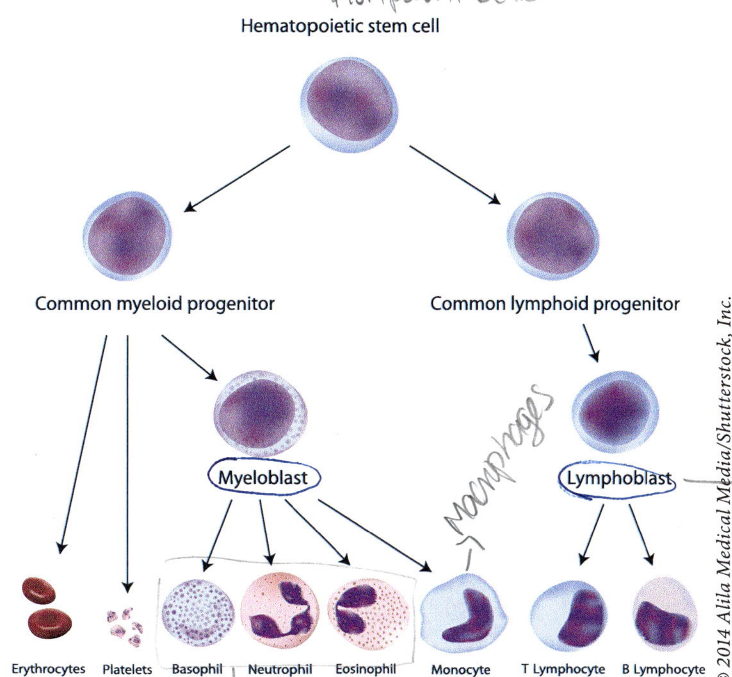

Figure 2.3 *All phagocytic cells originate from myeloid stem cell precursors in the bone marrow.*

These cells are derived from a very primitive cell within the bone marrow (Figure 2.3). The primitive cell is called "hemocytoblast," simply meaning "primitive cell of the blood system." It is this cell that differentiates into the ones known as myeloid stem cells, myeloid standing for "bone"; they are therefore also called bone marrow stem cells. They have the capacity to differentiate into various cells of the blood. The primitive cell, hemocytoblast, is pluripotent; it can differentiate in many directions; and it can go into the erythroid series (becoming red blood cells), megakaryocyte series (becoming platelets), myeloblast series (becoming granulocytes and agranulocytes), or lymphoid series (becoming the lymphocytes or the lymphocytes related cells).

The myeloid cells are of immediate concern here because the cell population of the innate immune system is of this origin. These cells either have granules or don't have granules. Those cells that finally become neutrophils, basophils, eosinophils, and mast cells have granules, so we call them granulocytes. Those cells that become monocytes and may finally differentiate into macrophages are agranulocytes as they do not have granules. The cells called lymphocytes, derived from the lymphoid series, will be discussed under the adaptive (acquired) immune response. The granulocytes usually have a nuclear shape that initially was thought to be more than one nucleus. They were described as "polymorphonuclear" leukocytes as if they have more than one nucleus but it is known that they do not have more than one nucleus. Instead, the single nucleus has lobes. But the old description is retained for convenience; a more correct terminology would be multilobulated. The naming of the granulocytes is in relation to the staining characteristics of their granules. Hematoxylin, a dye with blue color, is a base; it therefore stains the basic components of cells. Those cell contents that stain with hematoxylin are impacted with blue color and are, therefore, described as basophilic. In making cell content observable, a counterstain is often used after an initial stain; in this instance, eosin is used. Eosin, a red stain, is an acid stain which impacts the acidic components of cells with red color. Such components are described as eosinophilic or eosinophils. There are cell populations among the leucocytes that have granules with acid and base staining reactions. Hematoxylin and eosin stains impact them with a purple color, thus they are described as neutral in their staining reactions. These cells are described as neutrophils (Figure 2.4).

Neutrophils. They are the first line of defense in the body. They migrate from the **bone marrow** to the **bloodstream** and **tissue** and their life span is about 24–36 hours. They are of two types:

i. The **primary type**, which is electron **dense** and **dark**. These are rich in bactericidal enzymes.

ii. The **secondary type** are nonelectron **dense** and **pale**. They contain collagenase and iron binding protein **lactoferin**, they also have some **lysozyme**.

Neutrophils are rich in **glycogen**, a source of **glucose**, and have the **capability** of **anaerobic glycolysis** (breakdown of glucose to generate energy, ATP, without oxygen).

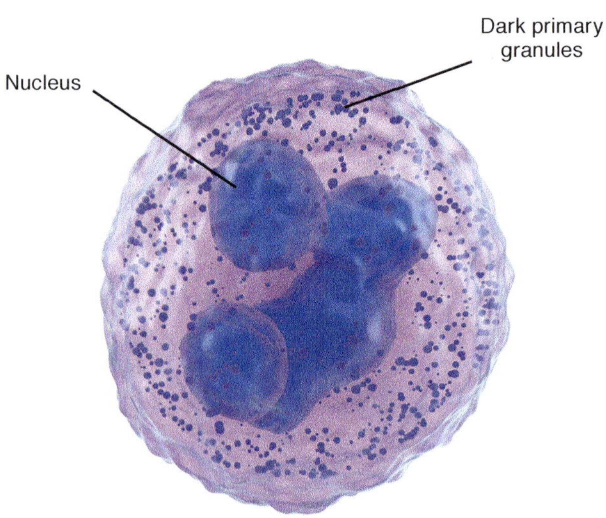

Figure 2.4 *Major structural features of a neutrophil polymorphonuclear granulocytes.* Note: *Irregular nucleus and lack of rough endoplasmic reticulum.*

The following factors must be overcome by neutrophils in order to engulf bacteria:

i. **Electrostatic repulsion** due to ionic cloud surrounding the cell as a result of a negative charge on the cell membranes attracting Na^+ cloud (zeta potential). This is overcome by opsonization (Ab or complement C3b coating of bacteria) (see Figure 2.5).
ii. **Nature of bacteria membrane**; for instance, neutrophil membrane is hydrophobic, making it capable of ingesting bacteria with hydrophobic coat, for example, Mycobacterium spp. more readily than carbohydrate-coated *Streptococcus pneumoniae.*

Engulfment of bacteria is facilitated by **chemotaxis**-directed movement under the influence of chemical substances, for example, **IL-8** (produced by macrophages, fibroblast, epithelial cells, and endothelial cells), **leukotrienes** (small lipid molecules), **bacterial peptides** containing unique amino acid—formylated methionine.

Neutrophils do not float in blood; they crawl on endothelial lining of blood vessels. Adherence is facilitated by **adhesion proteins—integrins** and **selectins,** secreted by the vessel wall.

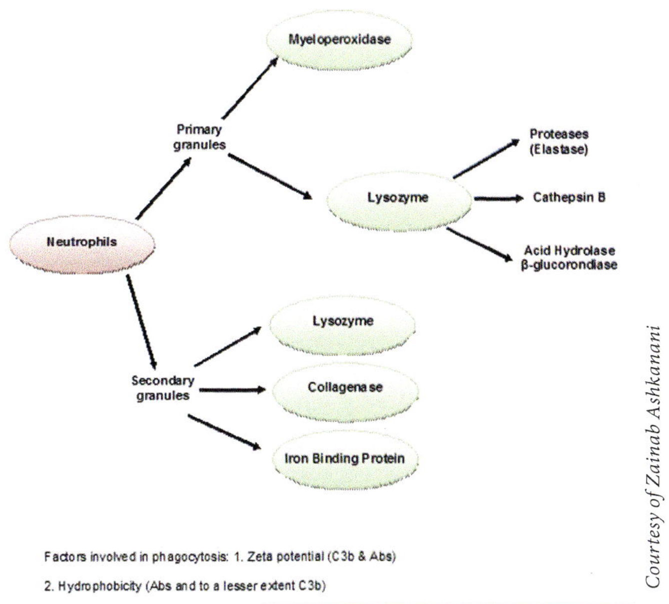

Figure 2.5 *Factors involved in phagocytosis: Zeta potential (C3b and Abs) and hydrophobicity.*

The neutrophils are the first responders to challenges among cells of the innate immune system. It is, therefore, not surprising that in diagnostic settings they are observed in large numbers in blood films as markers of an infection, especially of bacterial nature. They are released a lot from the bone marrow during infection because the pluripotent stem cells of the marrow are in such instance committed to neutrophil generation. They leave the bone marrow and pass through tissue into the blood stream, but they do not live long. The attack they mount against infecting agents is intensive, they virtually "fight and die", and so they are continuously produced during such infection episodes. The life span is between 24 and 48 hours. If they were being maintained in culture, they will survive for an average of 24–36 hours. They measure about 12 μm in diameter. A careful observation shows that there are two populations of granules: the fine electron dense ones, which are rich in bactericidal enzymes, such as myeloperoxidase and lysozymes, tissue degrading enzymes such as neutral proteases and elastases, acid hydrolases, glucuronidase, and cathepsin B. The secondary granules are coarse nonelectron dense, they are pale, and contain collagenase and an iron-binding protein, lactoferrin. They deprive bacteria of iron by virtue of their lactoferrin content, and because bacteria need iron for their propagation, their growth is impaired. Neutrophils have a lot of glycogen, which is a source of glucose for them, and they need glucose for energy generation; they generate ATP by autoglycolysis, by the Embden Meyerhof pathway.

The nucleus is lobulated, the extent of lobe formation is indicative of the age of the neutrophil. Neutrophils that have been pushed prematurely from the bone marrow into circulation, as occur in an acute bacterial infection, have fewer lobes compared to those found in a chronic infection. Neutrophil "surge" from the marrow is characterized by immature neutrophils in circulation and is indicative of a need due to infection. The less lobulated nucleus that characterizes this condition is designated as a "shift to the left." A shift to the right would be more mature ones that may indicate a normal situation or chronic infection. The fact that the neutrophil has organelles such as the Golgi apparatus indicates that it is capable of minimal biomolecular assembly.

In order for the neutrophil to efficiently engulf bacteria, it needs to overcome the electrostatic repulsion (zeta potential) previously mentioned. This repulsion arises from a potential generated by ionic cloud around cells. Cell membranes have a negative charge, so sodium ions (positive charge) form a cloud of ion around it that will attract chloride ions (negative charge). That cloud creates a potential that is named "zeta" potential. The Zeta potential must be overcome before neutrophils can reach the bacterium. This is usually done by opsonization. Opsonin is the name of those proteins that bind to receptors on microbes and then bind to receptors on neutrophils. Also, the cells of the innate immune system must overcome the problem involving the nature of the membrane of the bacterium. Some bacteria may have a hydrophobic membrane, making it easy for neutrophils to engulf them, for example, *Mycobacterium tuberculosis*, the causative agent of the disease tuberculosis. There are bacteria with a hydrophilic coating such as *S. pneumoniae*, which are more difficult for neutrophils to approach and engulf. This problem is overcome by opsonization because opsonization is independent of the relatedness of the membrane, but dependent on receptors (Figure 2.5). The mode of engulfment that is dependent on relatedness of membrane but is nonreceptor based leading to endocytosis exists and is not included in the example here.

The other aspect of engulfment of bacteria by neutrophils is that neutrophils must reach the location of bacterial invasion (see Figure 2.6). The way in which this is achieved is through chemotaxis: the sending of directional information by elaboration of cytokines, interleukin-8, and small lipids (leukotrienes, for instance), produced by other leucocytes at the proximity of invading bacteria. There are also bacterial peptides and formylated methionine which are released by bacteria that have infected the system.

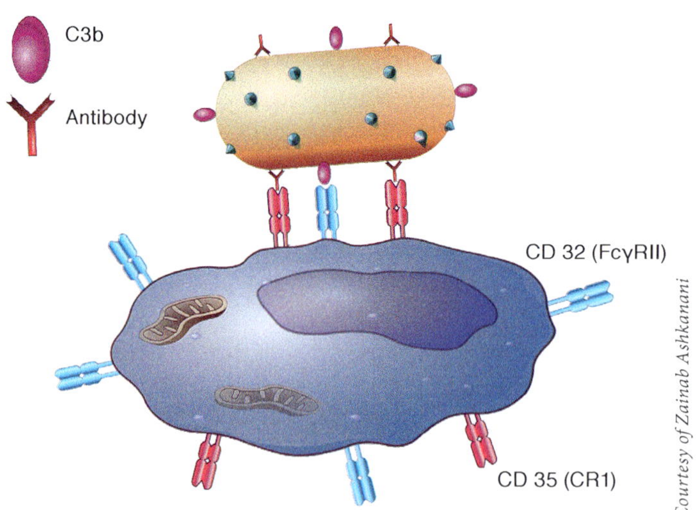

Figure 2.6 *The role of antibody receptors (CD32) and complement receptors (CD35) in the opsonization of bacteria for phagocytosis by neutrophils. Note that when antibody or complement-coated bacteria binds to these receptors, they stimulate phagocytosis.*

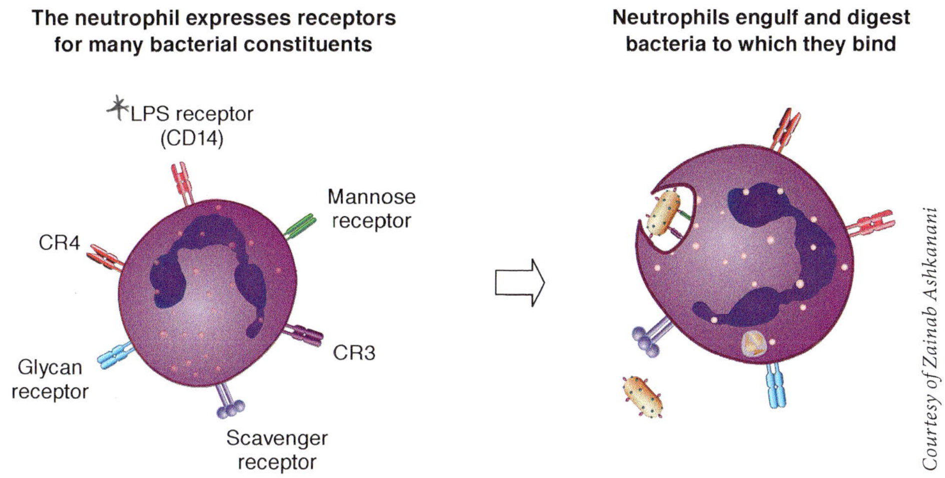

Figure 2.7 *Engulfment of bacteria by neutrophils.*

Figure 2.7 illustrates, neutrophil expression of receptors to many ligands of the bacterial cell including CD14 (LPS receptor), scavenger receptor (CD36), and mannose and glycan receptors, and CR3 and CR4. Once bound, the neutrophils engulf and digest the bacteria.

- Ingestion involves the **flow** of **pseudopod over** and **around** the **bacterium** with subsequent **engulfment**.
- The nature of bacterium affects the **ease** of **ingestion**. Neutrophil cytoplasm flows easily over bacterium with **hydrophobic lipid membrane**, for example, *Mycobacterium tuberculosis*, while for bacterium with **hydrophilic carbohydrate capsule** for example, *S. pneumoniae*, it is more difficult. **Abs** and **C3b** coating renders ***S. pneumoniae*** susceptible to engulfment.
- Destruction of organism involves (i) the release of **lethal oxidizing** agents which **oxidize bacterial lipids** and proteins, and (ii) the release of **lysosomal enzymes**.
- The release of **nitric oxide** is **not** very **efficient** in neutrophils. However, respiratory burst is very efficient (Figures 2.8 and 2.9).

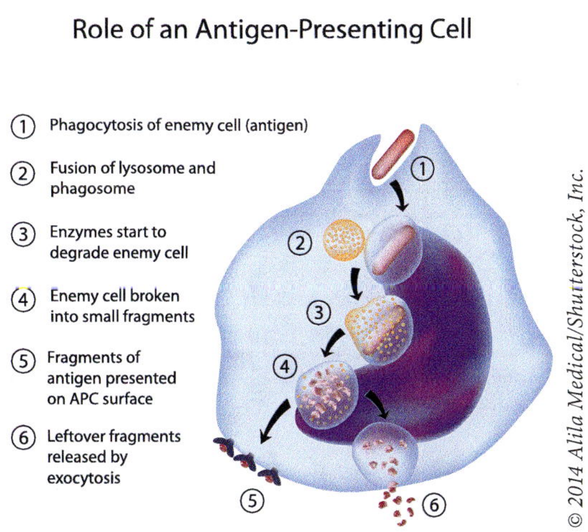

Figure 2.8 *Schematic representation of phagocytosis showing ingestion process and intracellular digestion.*

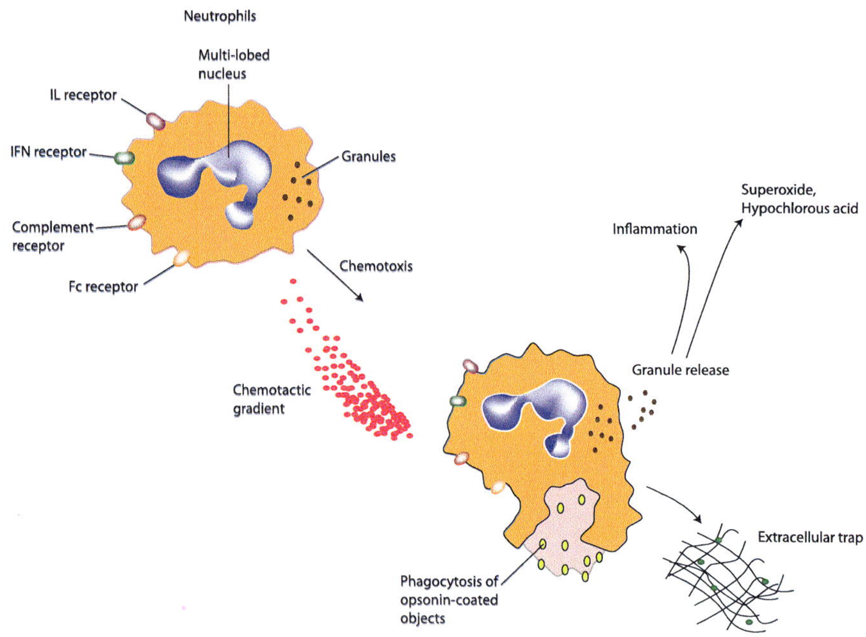

Figure 2.9 *The four basic steps in phagocytosis: chemostaxis, adherence, ingestion, and digestion.*

It is important to recognize how neutrophils move to the site of infection. They crawl on the endothelium by producing protuberances called "pseudopodia," as done also by amoebas. To facilitate the crawling amidst flowing blood, they need an adhesive surface which is provided by the production of adhesion proteins, integrin and selectin; so, infected surfaces release these proteins that will make it easier for neutrophils to crawl. It is when they crawl that they are able to pin bacteria against the wall of the vessel or the wall of the tissue and engulf them.

There are many other receptors that are at play during neutrophil interaction with bacteria, receptors such as lipopoly saccharides (LPS), the LPS receptors are named CD14 (clusters of differentiation 14). In addition, there are receptors to mannose binding proteins; these are capable of binding to proteins that bind mannose on bacterial surface. Bacterial surface is endowed with this particular hexose sugar, derived from mannitol oxidation. Also, there are receptors such as scavenger receptors that bind unwanted materials, usually these materials are modified, or have been changed from their normal configurations. The consequence of the binding of a typical receptor or collection of receptors to a bacterium is that the bacterium is internalized by the neutrophil, and it is then degraded.

The innate immune system, being nonspecific, will not only react to previous exposure but also react to new exposures. In the case of response to previous exposure, antibodies are mainly the opsonins at play with other factors (such as complement component) collaborating. In naïve animals, only nonspecific factors such as complement components (e.g., C3b) or mannose binding proteins are at play. The coordination of neutrophils to the site of infection before these ligands—receptor interactions depends on factors such as formylated methionine, leukotrienes, and interleukin-8.

The process of ingestion usually involves the flow of pseudopodia over and around the bacterium that is to be engulfed. The nature of the bacterium affects the ease of ingestion. Hydrophobicity makes it both easy and difficult. Antibodies and complement fragments make it easy to overcome such problems. Through release of lethal oxidizing agents, bacterial lipids and proteins are degraded.

Respiratory Burst Phenomenon

- Respiratory burst is the sequence of events starting with increased oxygen consumption and leading to the production of O_2^-, H_2O_2, and OCL^-.
- When foreign particles bind to neutrophils, oxygen consumption is increased 100-fold because a cell-membrane-bound enzyme NADPH oxidase is activated. This catalyzes the electron donation by NADPH, with oxygen acting as electron acceptor (Figure 2.10a and b).

NADPH Oxidase

$$NADPH + 2O_2 \longrightarrow NADP^+ + H^+ + 2.\ O_2^-$$

- $NADP^+$ generated goes to pentose phosphate pathway as electron acceptor. O_2^- is toxic to bacteria cell content.
- Two molecules of superoxide interact in superoxide dismutase (SOD) reaction to produce H_2O_2.

SOD

$$2.\ O_2^- + 2H^+ \longrightarrow H_2O_2 + O_2.$$

- H_2O_2 is toxic to bacteria and relatively stable.
- H_2O_2 may be further converted to bactericidal compound when it reacts with intracellular halide ions
- (Cl^-, Br^-, I^-, or CN^-) to produce hypohalides in myeloperoxidase reaction.

$$H_2O_2 + Cl^- \longrightarrow H_2O + OCl^-$$

- OCl^- kills bacteria by oxidation.

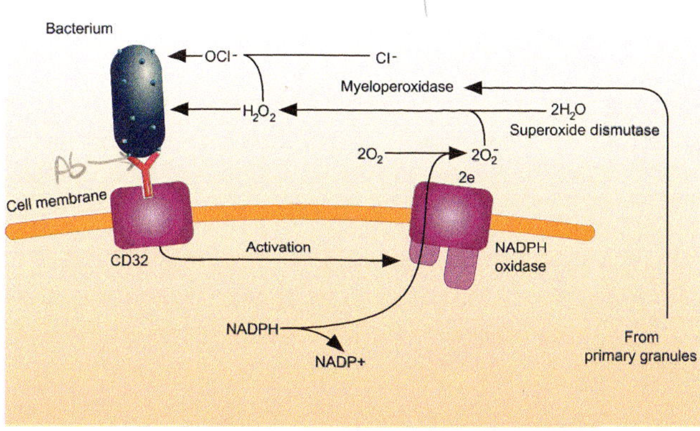

Figure 2.10 *Neutrophil respiratory burst. Bacteria binding to CD32 triggers activation of NADPH oxidase, with subsequent killing of bacteria by hydrogen peroxide and hypochloride ions.*

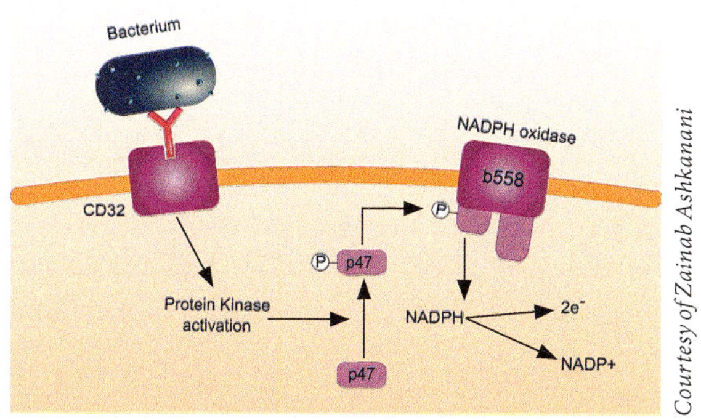

Figure 2.11 *Mechanism of activation of NADPH oxide. Binding of an antibody-coated particle to CD32 leads to activation of a protein kinase. This enzyme phosphorylates the p47 subunit of the oxide as thereby activating it.*

- Neutrophils are **short-lived**. They **die by apoptosis**. It usually involves macrophages recognition of an alteration in **dying neutrophil membrane lipids**. This **elicits** the release of **TNF** which binds to **TNF-R** on **neutrophils** and activates **FasL–receptor interaction**. This is death signal. It generates a **sequence** of events leading to mitochondrial oxidation and release of **cytochrome c**.
- Neutrophil lysis is usually **not permitted** because its **lysosomal** content would cause **tissue inflammation** and **damage**, so they are **engulfed** by **macrophages**.

Whenever an organism secures access to the animal's body and infects the systems, neutrophils drafted to the infection site begin to take up oxygen about 100 times more than they would have done ordinarily. This is described as respiratory burst. It is this respiratory burst that results in production of toxic radicals. Ordinarily, without infection, there is consumption of oxygen by neutrophils; the oxygen is exposed to changes in which NADPH oxidase transfers electrons from NADP, which is an electron carrier, to molecular oxygen. Whenever that happens, there is formation of superoxide. This is because in the outer orbital of oxygen there are two electrons in opposite spin which is meant to stabilize the orbital. Any factor that changes the pairing of electron in this outer orbital renders the orbital unstable and makes it very reactive. That kind of oxygen that is unstable is a radical and will always want to be stabilized. In its quest for stability, it attracts electrons from electron-rich center such as membrane proteins or lipids and cell deoxyribonucleic acid (DNA). It is on this basis that they are called free radicals and are toxic to cells including bacteria.

It is important to note that reactive oxygen species are generated naturally when consumed oxygen is reduced from molecular oxygen to water by the mitochondrial respiratory chain. The whole of this process usually requires that electrons are moved by biomolecules called reducing equivalents, so called because they are specialized in moving electrons and releasing them when required. Electron carriers finally become reducing equivalents, flavin, NAD (nicotinamide adenine dinucleotide), and so on. The electron carrier of special significance here is the $NADP^+$ (nicotinamide adenine dinucleotide phosphate), which is just the same NAD but has a phosphate group attached to it. Electron carriers vary according to cell type and depend on the nature of the reductive metabolic processes in which they are involved. In the case of NADPH, the acquiring of electron occurs in the popular pentose–phosphate pathway, also known as hexose monophosphate shunt. There is a divalent movement of electrons in electron transport chain. If it is tetravalent or divalent, it results in reduction of oxygen to water; if it is a trivalent or monovalent movement, which will happen depending on the extent of oxygen consumption, then there is the generation of radicals due to incomplete reduction. This occurrence is not dangerous in normal body function because of the endowment of the animal system with the capacity to detoxify such radicals. The way it does it is to quickly scavenge the radicals by using enzyme systems that it has developed over its evolutionary cycle; the major player is superoxide dismutase, which reduces oxygen radicals to hydrogen peroxide. The hydrogen peroxide so formed in the animal system is not as toxic as superoxide. That hydrogen peroxide can be broken down by more than one means. If it becomes organic peroxide, it is acted upon by glutathione peroxidase, but as inorganic peroxide, it is acted upon by catalase. So, the toxicity of superoxide is eliminated by converting it to the less toxic hydrogen peroxide that is finally broken down by peroxidases. This is a routine process in the animal system, so the generated superoxide during infection-induced respiratory burst does not endanger the animal system as such. The danger is further eliminated by the fact that neutrophils have a life span of about 36 hours. It is important to note that massive death of invading bacteria, death of neutrophils, and tissue destruction following the actions of free radicals such as superoxide, hydrogen peroxide, and hydroxyl radicals, and products of myeloperoxidase reaction, hypochlorite, which are generated result in pus formation and boils seen during infection.

It is worth noting that despite the fact that the central dogma of reactive oxygen species generation is its toxicity, there are emerging facts that because of the role of antioxidants in the attenuation of such radicals, instead of the concept of killing molecules, attenuated radicals are viewed as signaling molecules; molecules that can switch genes on and alter cell physiology in a favorable way. However, free radicals involved in signaling are not as reactive as those involved in killing. The hydroxyl radical is not likely to be involved in such signaling and it would appear that superoxide dismutase is an important switch in the signaling process.

Neutrophil membrane has receptors to complement, antibodies (CD32), lipopolysaccharides (LPS), and others. In the case of antibody, its Fc region is the ligand to the antibody receptor. This interaction generates signals which may have consequences such as the opening of channels through which calcium can flow rapidly, and such rapid influx of calcium will usually change the behavior of enzymes inside the cell. So, inactive enzymes become active. The activation of enzyme in this instance results in the production of an active kinase by phosphorylation, the activated kinase catalyzes the reaction in which the P47 fragment of NADPH oxidase is phosphorylated. The active enzyme catalyzes the removal of electrons from NADPH, carrier of reducing equivalents. The need to use reducing equivalents for electron transfer across membrane is because since electrons are charged particles (negatively charged) they will not transverse membrane, but when they are taken up by $NADP^+$, it provides proton that binds to the electron, so the charge is no more obvious, and that way it can be moved through the membrane border. It is the released electron that is supposed to reduce oxygen to water, but because of the burst in respiration, reduction is insufficient, and so there is formation of superoxide. This superoxide on its own can kill bacteria. However, the animal system will produce superoxide dismutase, an enzyme that will scavenge the superoxide resulting in the production of hydrogen peroxide as already explained. Hydrogen peroxide is bactericidal, but bacteria can also destroy hydrogen peroxide using catalase which is produced by some bacteria. So, the smart thing to do is to make what will really kill the bacteria once and for all. This is achieved through myeloperoxidase reaction, which results in the production of hypochlorite. Hypochlorite will kill bacteria more effectively. The electron carrier $NADP^+$ goes back into the hexose monophosphate shunt to become reequipped with electrons, so the cycle continues.

Neutrophils are short lived, they die by the process of apoptosis (apoptosis is programmed cell death; it is different from the kind of death in which the cell swells and bursts, which is described as necrosis). Apoptosis is a gradual cell death that is not messy; a very clean cell death. One of the events that happen is that a cell that is about to die by apoptosis usually has receptors for a biomolecule we call Fas proteins, and when receptors on the cell interact with Fas protein, they activate a group of enzymes that are proteases called caspases. In summation, the following events will always follow: caspases are activated; cell starts shrinking and they will "round up." The cytoplasm becomes denser and the intracellular materials appear tightly packed. The chromatin becomes condensed and it will appear as if it was compact patches, and they are usually condensed against the nuclear envelope. The nuclear envelope becomes discontinuous, and then the DNA is fragmented. Now, the membrane begins to show an irregular appearance as if it had protuberances, showing what is called "blebbing." Then, the cells break into small pieces. Those small pieces are what are commonly described as apoptotic bodies. So, one of the hallmarks of apoptosis is that the dying cell usually has the interior part of cell membrane flipping over to the exterior, and the phospholipids that are usually found in the interior part of the cell membrane are now seen on membrane surface, specifically phosphatidylserine. When that happens, scavenger cells like the macrophage are localized in such environment to either pick up those pieces of apoptotic bodies or pick up the cell directly. The system cannot afford to allow neutrophils to lyse into the environment because it is endowed with tissue degrading enzymes.

The Eosinophil

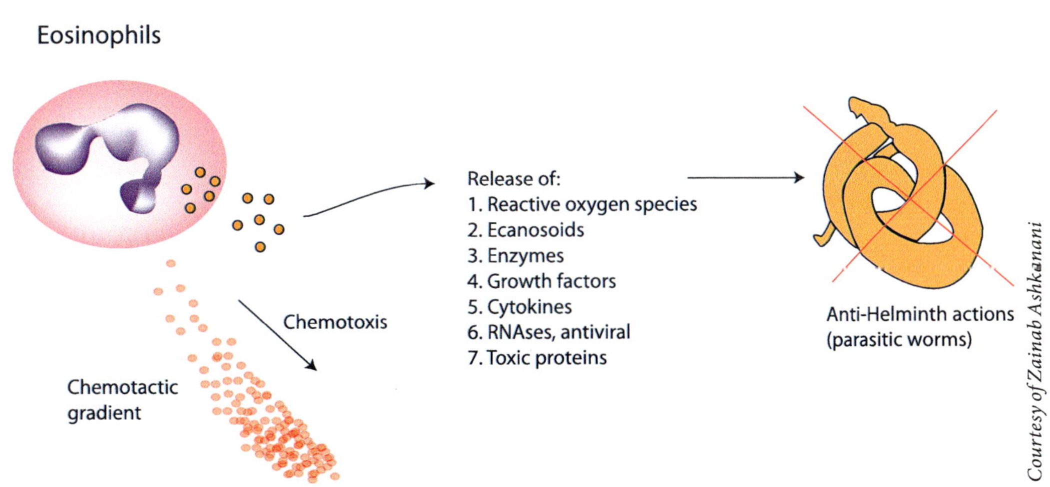

Figure 2.12 *An eosinophil. Note the characteristic pinkish granules containing an electron dense core.*

- Eosinophils leave the marrow **relatively immature**. They **mature** fully in the **spleen**. Their **half-life** is **30 min** after they are released into **circulation**. They migrate into **tissue**, where their **half-life** is **12 days**. In healthy humans, they constitute **2–5%** of leukocytes.
- They are phagocytic and their **granules** contain **acid phosphatase** and **peroxidase**. Eosinophil **peroxidase** are **efficient bactericidal**. They also contain **major basic protein (MBP)** which is **toxic** to **parasitic** worms (helminths).
- **Chemotactic** factors for eosinophils include **C5a, C567, histamine** and some metabolites of **arachidonic acid**.
- Eosinophils have **Ab** and **complement receptors**. Its **respiratory burst capability** may **exceed** that of **neutrophils**.
- Eosinophils are much more **suited** for **extracellular destruction** of **parasites** because they can **extrude** their **granules** into **surrounding** fluid.
- They **stick** to **parasites** and **extrude MBP**, and other **toxic proteins** to **destroy worm cuticle**.

EOSINOPHILIC GRANULE CONTENTS ARE AS FOLLOWS

- Acid phosphatase
- Arylsulfatase
- β-Glucuronidase
- Cathepsin
- Peroxidase
- Phospholipase

Eosinophil is another granulocyte, its granules stain pinkish (Figure 2.12). They are called "eosinophils" because they take up the eosin component of stain. Their levels are elevated in worm infection and allergic reactions. They leave the marrow a little bit immature and finally get matured in the spleen. Their half-life is 12 days when they are in the blood (in transit), so as soon as they are released from the marrow they pass through the spleen, and then go into the tissues; that is why there are of such low population in the blood. You never see more than 10% eosinophils in blood. They are 2–5% of circulating leukocytes. They are very phagocytic and are rich in acid phosphatases and peroxidases. Peroxidases, as previously said, are enzymes which hydrolyze organic peroxide, while acid phosphatases catalyze the removal of phosphate groups in acid medium. If they were alkaline phosphatases, it would be in alkaline medium. These cells can kill bacteria efficiently, but they are also endowed with the major basic protein (MBP). It is this biomolecule that is extruded from the cell (pushed out of the cell) when a patient is burdened with worms. In the case of intestinal worms, these cells are pushed into the tissue in the proximity of the worm, they extrude the major basic protein that coats the worm and helps to fragment it, thus killing it. It is because of such need that their population increases up to 10% in worm infections, or allergies. The role of eosinophils in allergic response will be further addressed when the topic about some soluble substances is treated later. The factors that attract eosinophils to the site where they are active, be they for bactericidal action or for parasitic killing, are factors such as complement factor C5a, which is a complement fragment. When the complement that we call C5 is fragmented into a small molecule C5a and a larger molecule C5b, C5b goes into the complement cascade; C5a remains in circulation and begins to act as an opsonin when it primes foreign agents by coating them. Eosinophil has a receptor for C5a on its membrane. Apart from the role of C5a as an opsonin, it also acts as a chemoattractant. An important chemoattractant for eosinophil is the molecule histamine. When eosinophil actually binds to antibodies especially IgE, for which it has a receptor, it begins to produce agents that can react against histamine; these are called antihistamines. In this way, histamine-induced allergic reaction is annulled by antihistamine reaction elicited by eosinophil. Biomolecules such as metabolites of arachidonic acid can also attract eosinophils to the site of need. Arachidonic acid is a C20 unsaturate (unsaturated fatty acids), which can be very reactive. It goes into the cycle of production of leukotrienes by the lipoxygenase pathway. Eosinophils are capable of undergoing respiratory burst in a way that is superior to what neutrophils do, they produce more radicals. They are more suited for destruction of extracellular bacteria and parasites, by extruding their organelles that contain MBP, which as previously described binds to parasite and shreds them.

The granules of eosinophil also contain aryl sulfatase, an enzyme that catalyzes the removal of phosphate and phenol groups from phenol sulfates, a complex that constitutes the tissue of lower organisms like parasites. Another biomolecule of interest is beta-glucuronidase which catalyzes the removal of glucuronides from proteins. Also present is cathepsin, a protease, which catalyzes the cleavage of proteins into its peptides and amino acids. As in neutrophils, there are peroxidases and phospholipases which convert phospholipids to fatty acids and fatty acid-related molecules, so the phosphate group is released; thus a cascade of actions that destroy bacteria and parasites can occur.

The Basophil

- Basophils are about **0.5%** of blood **leukocytes**. They are **not normally** found in **extravascular** tissue. They may **infiltrate** under the **influence** of **lymphocytes**. They are **proinflammatory**. Their granules have **vasoactive amines** e.g. **histamines** and **serotonin**.

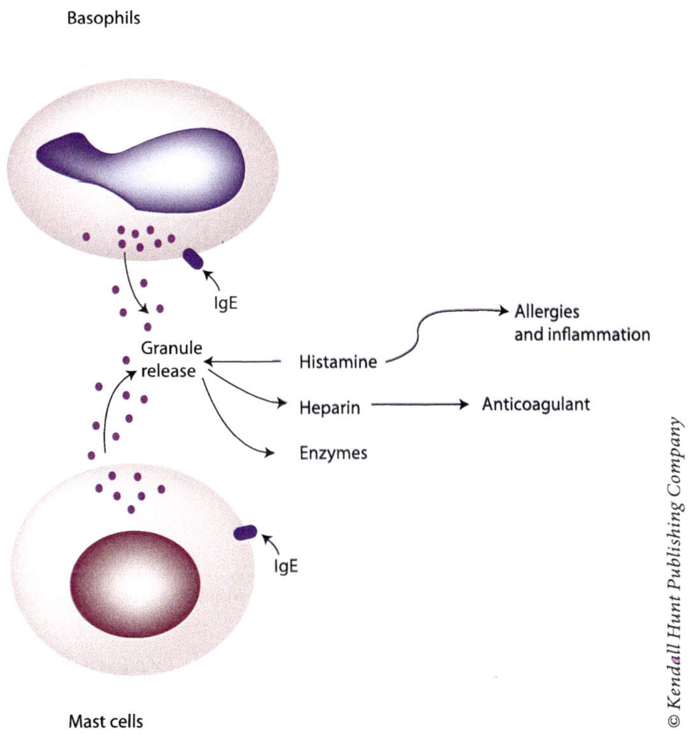

Figure 2.13 *A basophil.*

The basophils are so called because their granules react with basic component of dye such as hematoxylin (Figure 2.13). They are so few, in blood film they may be 0–0.5% of white cells population. They move into tissue under the influence of lymphocyte cytokines, depending on need. They produce amines that are "vasoactive," such as histamines and serotonin (5-hydroxytryptamine) which can dilate the blood vessels. Basophils like eosinophils also have receptors for IgE, but when they bind them, unlike eosinophils, they produce histamine, while eosinophils produce antihistamine.

The Macrophage

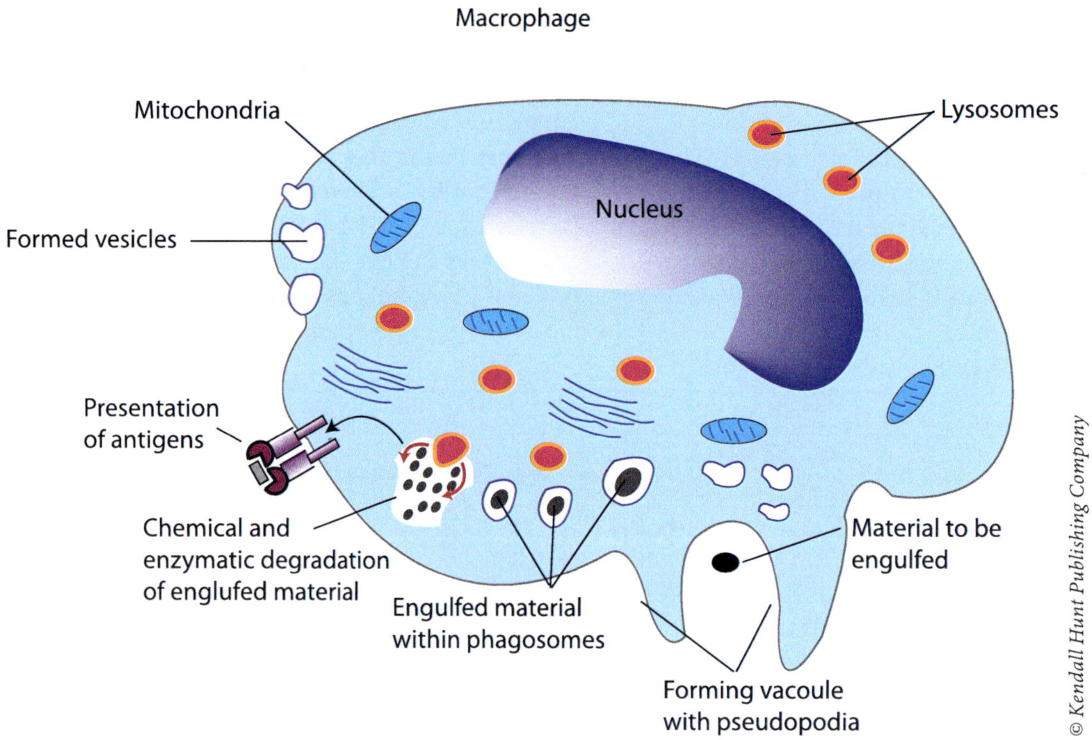

Figure 2.14 *Major structural features of a macrophage. Note the extensive Golgi apparatus and rough endoplasmic reticulum, indicating that this cell can synthesize and secrete proteins.*

- Macrophages are **widely distributed** in the body.
- They are **large**, about **14-20μm** in diameter with a single rounded nucleus.
- They are **avidly phagocytic**.
- They are **Ag Presenting** Cells.
- They secrete **proteins** that **amplify immune** response.
- They control **inflammation and healing**.
- They remove **dead, dying** and **damaged** tissues.
- They develop from **stem cell** through **monocytes** in blood and are taken to bone, liver, brain, connective tissue and other tissues.
- Their **cytoplasm** is **abundant**.
- Macrophages **stick to plate** in tissue culture.

Figures 2.14–2.21 illustrate various structural and functional aspects of macrophages.

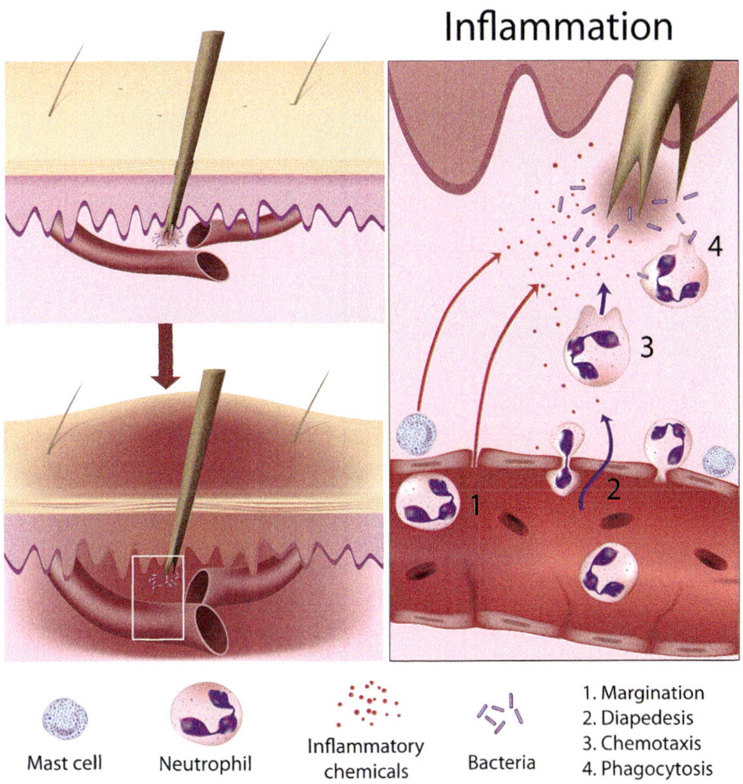

Figure 2.15 *Schematic of phagocytosis of infecting bacteria. It results in an inflammatory response including the release of cytokines, vasodilation, and increase vascular permeability.*

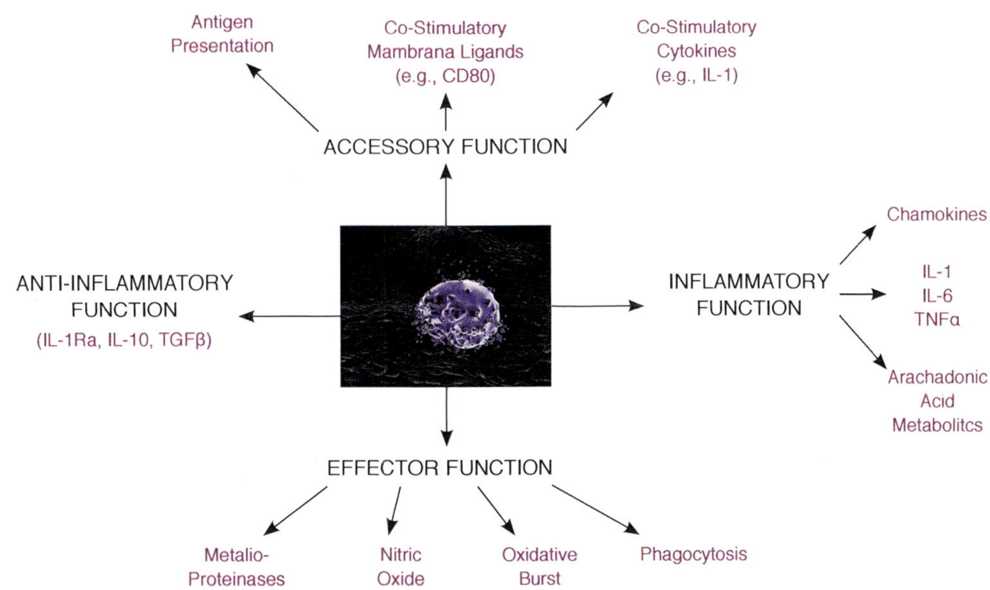

Figure 2.16 *Schematic of diverse functions of macrophages which are capable of many functional activities. Macrophages contribute both to the initiation of cell-mediated immune response and to the effector limb of those responses. During the course of the response, macrophages can display, at different times, both inflammatory and anti-inflammatory activities.*

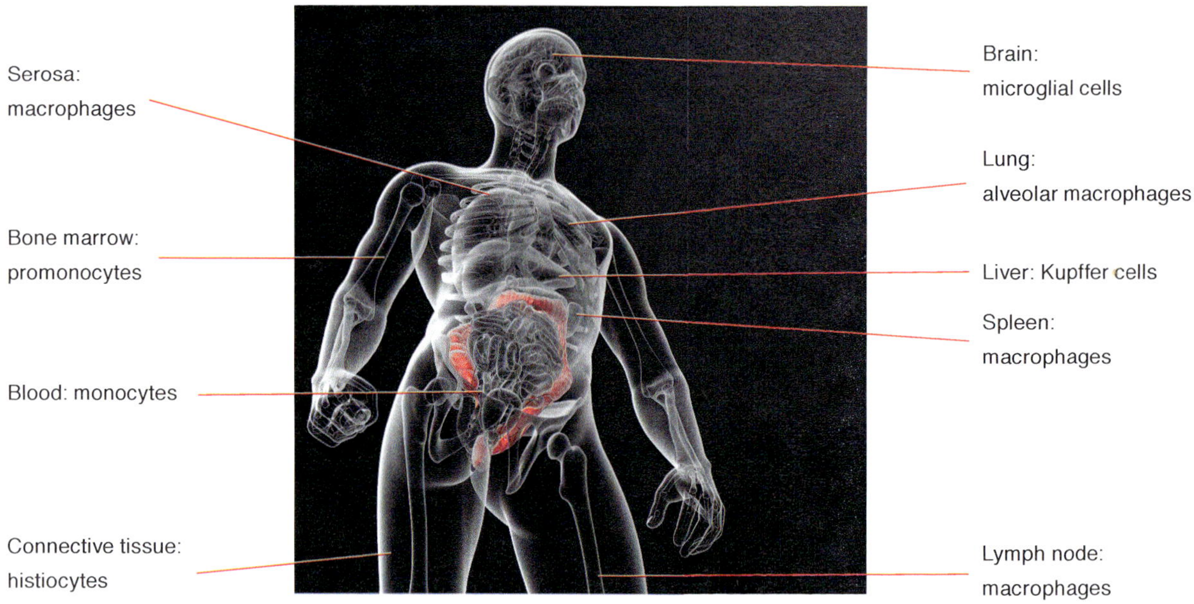

Figure 2.17 *Schematic of location of the mononuclear phagocytic system and its cells.*

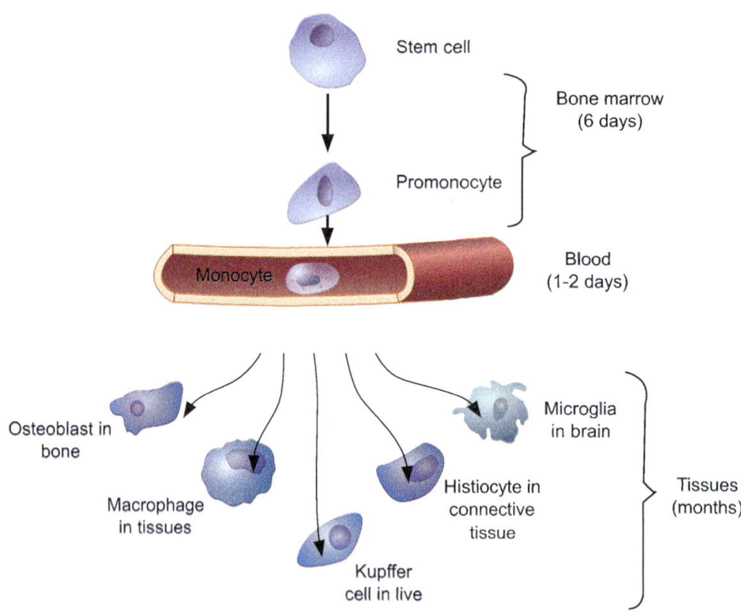

Figure 2.18 *Illustration depicting the progressive maturation of mononuclear phagocytic cells from a bone marrow stem cell through a monocyte stage in blood.*

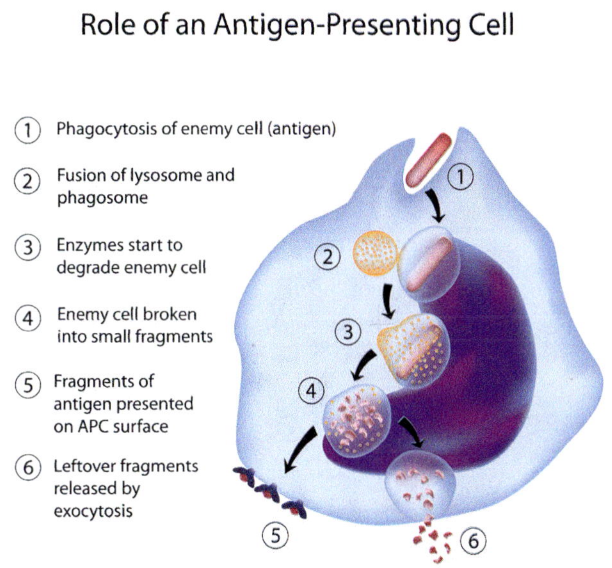

Figure 2.19 *Receptor-based phagocytosis of a bacterium by a macrophage. The bacterium binds to cell surface receptors and is engulfed into a vesicle called a phagosome within the cytoplasm of the macrophage. This degrades into a phagolysosome in which the bacterium is broken down.*

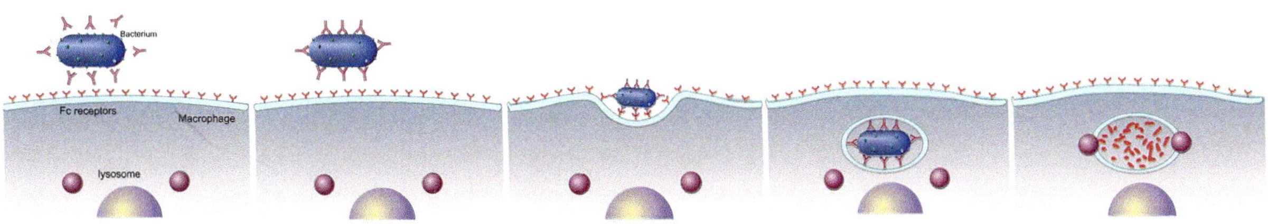

Figure 2.20 *Schematic showing breakdown of bacteria by a phagocyte. Fc receptors on phagocytes trigger the uptake and subsequent breakdown of Ab-coated bacteria.*

- Macrophages are **induced** to phagocytose invaders by stimuli including: **N-formylmethionyl peptides** from **bacteria, C5a, IFN-γ**, factors released by damaged cells or extracellular matrix (**collagen, elastin**, and **fibrinogen**).
- **Dying neutrophils** attract macrophages to site of microbial invasion.
- Macrophages destroy microbes by **oxidative** and **non-oxidative** processes. Oxidative processes involves the release of **ROS** ($\cdot O_2^-$, H_2O_2, OCl^-), **RNI** (NO, NO_2, NO_2^-, NO_3^-). **Non-oxidative** process involves **lysozymes** and **proteases**.
- Macrophages produce **NO** in the reaction of **inducible nitric oxide synthase** (iNOS). The enzyme **oxidizes** the **terminal nitrogen** atom of the guanidino group of **L-arginine** amino acid, leading to **the production** of **citrulline** and **nitric oxide**.

- **Nitric oxide** can react with $\cdot O_2^-$, to form $\cdot$**ONOO**$^-$, (peroxynitrite ion). This decays into highly toxic hydroxyl radical.
- $\cdot$**ONOO**$^-$ + H^+ = $\cdot$**OH**$^-$ + NO_2.
- Macrophages have **high protein synthesis capability**; they produce **IL-1, 6** and **12**. They also produce **TNF**. Most products **activate lymphocytes**.

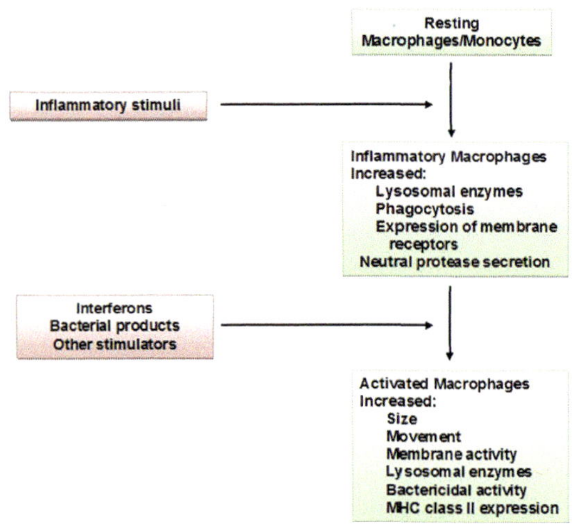

Courtesy of Zainab Ashkanani

Figure 2.21 *Activation of a macrophage.*

The macrophage is a giant cell. It is appreciably more complex, having more organelles such as Golgi apparatus, rough endoplasmic reticulum, mitochondria, and everything that it needs to be long-lived apart from its elaborately equipped nucleus. They are widely distributed in the body. This fact indicates that they must be very important! They are found generally in the brain, liver, lungs, peritoneum, and tissues. The blood macrophages are monocytes; they are usually large and heterogeneous, although they are all called macrophages. Their diameter is between 14 and 20 μm. The nucleus is usually one and rounded. They are avidly phagocytic and they come in at the later stage of the actions of innate immune response. They are scavenger cells; however, they also prepare the immune system for further action by production and elaboration of mediators. They behave as antigen-presenting cells. They engulf the organism, degrade it, and then select conserved peptides, unique peptides that will distinguish that organism from other organisms, even those that are closely related. The peptide is displayed on cell surface using the peptide carrying molecules called major histocompatibility complex. It is such peptide that is recognized by antigen recognizing cells (T cells) and result in acquired (specific) immune response. Other lymphocyte subpopulation cells recognize this display, memorize it and are able to produce heightened response in subsequent encounters. They are not the best antigen presenters because they are so avidly phagocytic, they sometimes destroy the conserved peptides themselves. A very important immune mediator produced by the macrophage is interleukin-1, which are proteins that activate other cell components of the immune system such as lymphocytes, and it activates them because the lymphocytes have receptors for IL-1, and the interaction results in the release of interleukin-2. The interleukin-2 so produced binds to receptors on lymphocytes causing the activation of the lymphocytes, clonal expansion of the activated lymphocytes, and the production of a population of memory cells. So, macrophages occupy a special place at the junction between innate immune response and acquired immune response.

Macrophages are induced to phagocytosis by N-formyl metionyl peptides from bacteria that are released by invading organisms. Thus, N-formylmethionyl peptides are chemoattractants. Interferon-γ is a cytokine produced by many cells, but mainly by leukocytes as a result of viral or bacterial infections; it is a macrophage activator. Also, factors that are released by damaged tissue, such as collagen, elastin, and fibrinogen are macrophage attractants. Dying neutrophils usually will attract the macrophages to the site of infection. Macrophage destroys microbes by oxidative and nonoxidative processes. It is oxidative if reactive oxygen species are produced, such as superoxide, hydrogen peroxide, and hypochlorite. Another oxidative process involves reactive nitrogen intermediates such as nitric oxide, dioxide, and trioxide of nitrogen, some of them carrying charges. The nonoxidative processes involve those enzymes that are proteolytic and destroy bacteria like proteases or other components of lysozyme, for instance, aryl sulfatases and others that can destroy organisms.

Something very special about macrophages is this capacity to produce nitric oxide (NO), in the reaction catalyzed by inducible nitric oxide synthase, iNOS, so called because infection will enhance the expression of the enzyme proteins and therefore accentuate the reaction. The enzyme oxidizes the terminal nitrogen atom of the amino acid L-arginine, the terminal group is called guanidine group, which is caused to release nitric oxide, and the remaining molecule is called citrulline.

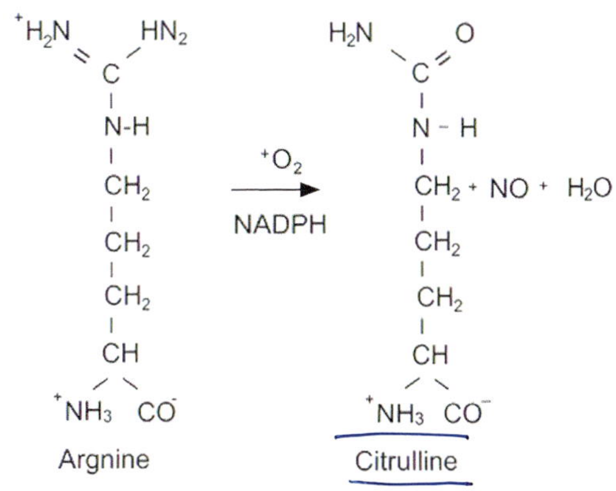

Courtesy of Zainab Ashkanani

Figure 2.22 *Production of bactericidal oxides of nitrogen, especially nitric oxide derived from the conversion of arginine to citrulline by nitric oxide synthase.*

Nitric oxide can kill bacteria through its decay products, those dioxides and trioxides of nitrogen and their decay products. Another decay product is formed when nitric oxide reacts with superoxide to produce peroxynitrite ion ($ONOO^-$). The formation of that ion is a process that supersedes any other reaction once you have nitric oxide and superoxide, even superoxide dismutase, which is a specific enzyme for superoxide, cannot withstand the speed of reaction between superoxide ion and nitric oxide. Peroxynitrite is highly toxic for two reasons: first, on its own it's very toxic, and second, its decay product, hydroxyl radical, is a great deleterious agent to membrane, as it destroys membranes. Macrophage as an immune mediator can produce agents that can draft other cells of the immune system to the site of challenge and activate them. Mediators commonly involved include interleukins- 1, 6, and 12, these are all called proinflammatory cytokines, and will also produce tumor necrosis factor.

One very important feature of macrophage is its wound healing capability. The biomolecular products of macrophage accelerate granulation process during wound healing.

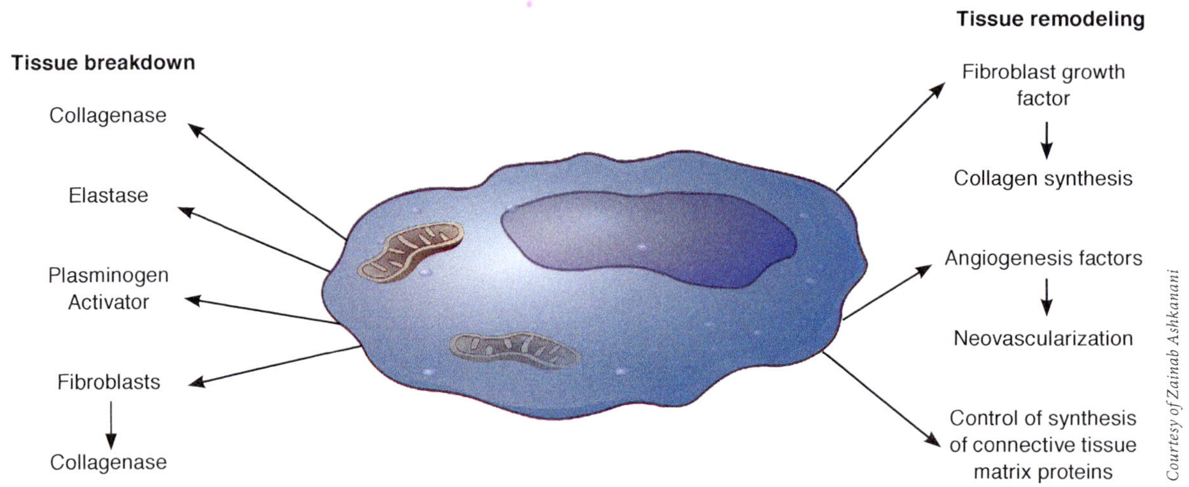

Figure 2.23 *Role of macrophage in wound healing. Macrophages are involved both in the breakdown and removal of damaged tissue and in the remodeling of newly healed tissues.*

The macrophage carries out wound healing by tissue breakdown and tissue remodeling. In tissue breakdown, it has to ensure that the dead cells and dysfunctional cells are removed and cleaned out before the process of remodeling starts. The biomolecules at play here are collagenase, a connective tissue degrading enzyme (the substrate is collagen), and elastase, also a connective tissue degrading enzyme (substrate is elastin). Plasminogen activator is a protein that activates a proenzyme that is called plasminogen. When plasminogen is activated, it becomes plasmin, which degrades fibrin and breaks down clots, thus it is a fibrinolytic enzyme. Having achieved that, it also induces the production of fibroblasts, which are responsible for remodeling of connective tissue through meshwork fibers and fiber formations. These have the role of connecting tissues together. To ensure that a neat arrangement is generated, fibroblast produces enzymes such as collagenase and elastase that can break down unwanted connective tissue in the repair process. It is this that gives the dark dot on healing tissue called granulation tissue. Now, once that is achieved, it can commence remodeling. During remodeling, fibroblast growth is enhanced and collagen is used to build up the new tissue. Angiogenesis factors responsible for the production of new blood vessels are elaborated, that is why there is neovascularization, because the new tissue that is forming must be nourished, and it is the angiogenesis factors that will provide the blood vessels that will supply the area. But if this process continues unabated, it results in an overgrowth. So, the controlling system is the regulation of the synthesis of connective tissue and matrix proteins (all those proteins that were responsible for bringing about meshwork formation and tissue relationship). The process must be terminated as soon as enough of connective tissue matrix is produced.

Macrophage also plays an important role in tumor destruction, thus contributing to how a normal functioning immune system will not allow any neoplasia, that is, formation of tumor cells. The macrophage contributes to tumor destruction by producing those proinflammatory proteins like interleukin-1 and other cytokines like interleukin-6 and interleukin-12; it also produces tumor necrosis factor, a protein that will attack tumor cells and destroy them.

An aspect of innate immune response that occurs if it were a viral challenge has the innate immune response centered on a group of cells that can kill cells that have been infected by viruses, the Natural Killer (NK) cells. NK cells: they are lymphocytes (but non-B cells and non-T cells), but they are considered part of the innate immune system.

They don't depend on the thymus; they are not like B cells that develop in the marrow, so they are unique. But they are innate and nonspecific. The element of specificity exhibited by NK cell is the capacity to recognize viral infected cells or tumor cells and kill them. That is why as said at this junction between innate immunity and adaptive immune response, you have a population of cells that will be performing a unique role.

SAMPLE QUESTIONS

INNATE IMMUNE SYSTEM

1. The predominant type of leukocyte in the blood is the
   a. monocyte
   b. eosinophil
   c. basophil
   d. neutrophil
   e. lymphocyte

2. The movement of neutrophils under the influence of external chemical gradients is called
   a. endocytosis
   b. chemotaxis
   c. phagocytosis
   d. chemolysis
   e. exotaxis

3. Which of the following is a potent chemotactic factor for neutrophils?
   a. C-reactive protein
   b. Interleukin-8
   c. Arachidonic acid
   d. Complement
   e. Immunoglobulin

4. For which one complement protein does the neutrophil contain a receptor important in phagocytosis?
   a. C1a
   b. C2a
   c. C3b
   d. C4a
   e. C5b

5. What is an opsonin?
   a. chemotactic factor
   b. type of granulocyte
   c. chemokine
   d. substance that enhances phagocytosis
   e. lysosomal enzyme

6. The key cell surface molecule that initiates the respiratory burst is
   a. hypohalide
   b. myeloperoxidase
   c. superoxide dismutase
   d. NADPH-oxidase
   e. singlet oxygen

7. When neutrophils die, they do so by a process called
   a. necrosis
   b. phagocytosis
   c. diapedesis
   d. endocytosis
   e. apoptosis

8. One function of eosinophil major basic protein is to
   a. destroy invading bacteria
   b. destroy helminth parasites
   c. cause acute inflammation
   d. cause asthma
   e. destroy normal tissue

9. Integrins are
   a. opsonins
   b. chemotactic factors
   c. cell surface adhesive proteins
   d. complement components
   e. antibody receptors

10. Bacteria are cleared from the bloodstream mainly by
   a. lung capillaries
   b. spleen and liver macrophages
   c. circulating neutrophils
   d. marginating neutrophils
   e. renal capillaries

Suggested Laboratory Practicals

- Case Studies designed to help students understand:

1. External and Internal Defenses
2. Cellular Defense Mechanisms
3. Phagocytosis Process
4. The role of Acute Phase Proteins

- Latex Agglutination Test for C-Reactive Proteins
- Demonstration of In vitro Phagocytosis
- White Blood Count and Differentials

CHAPTER 3

NATURE OF ANTIBODIES

An important fact about immune response is that for it to be efficient and effective, it must be accompanied by antibody production. This is because an effective response must also be accompanied by a lasting effect. In order for the response to be lasting, there must be a level of memory. The endowment of the immune cells with memory requires the process of antigen presentation which in part is accompanied by the making of antibodies. One of the advantages of such memory is that as soon as a familiar challenge occurs subsequently, there is rapid release of antibodies which act as opsonins and the innate immune system (professional phagocytes) combat the challenge easily. In the process of formation of antibodies, there is usually the need to activate B-cell system, and there is a population of B cells that will be clonally expanded to produce antibodies, while a small population develops into memory B cells. So, this process of antibody production is a pointer to the importance of memory cell formation. Therefore, a lasting immune response is usually accompanied by specific antibody production. Otherwise, if immune response terminates with the innate immune response, then a repeated cycle of an infection may occur with each challenge. The innate immune response to a challenge to which an antibody has been elaborated is usually faster because of the opsonin effect of antibodies.

ANTIBODY

- A type of **glycoprotein** molecule, also called **immunoglobulin** (Ig).
- Produced by **B lymphocytes**, they **bind antigens**, often with a high degree of **specificity** and **high affinity**.
- The basic **structural unit** of an antibody is composed of **two identical heavy chains** and **two identical light chains**.
- **Amino-terminal variable regions** of the **heavy** and **light** chains **form** the **antigen-binding sites**.
- The **carboxyl-terminal constant regions** of the **heavy chains functionally interact** with **other molecules** in the **immune system**.
- In any **individual**, there are **millions** of different **antibodies**, each with a **unique antigen-binding** site.
- **Secreted antibodies** perform various **effector functions**, including **neutralizing antigens**, **activating complement**, **promoting phagocytosis** and **destruction of microbes**.

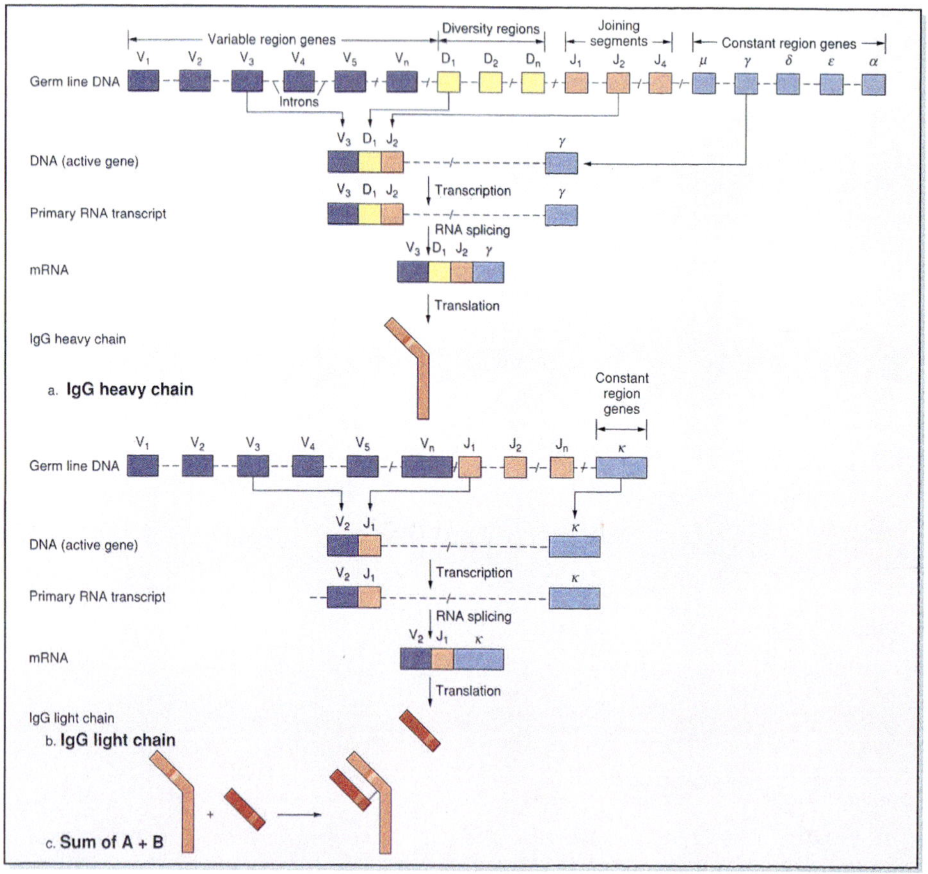

Figure 3.1 *Schematic representation of an antbody.*

NATURE OF ANTIBODIES

- **Found in** tears, respiratory tract, saliva, intestinal contents, urine, milk, and serum. Also on B cells as BCR.
- Demonstrate **electrophoretic mobility**. It is the subjection of charged particles to electrical potential at a standard pH (electrophoresis).
- Positive charge migrates to the cathode, Neutral charge remains stationary and negative charge migrates to the anode.
- Migration rate depends on the net charge.
- Serum can be fractionated into (from anode) Alb, α, β, γ-globulins, and fibrinogen.

The antibodies are complex biomolecules, having proteins and some carbohydrate contents, so they are glycoproteins. They are produced to a specific challenge which is presented as a specifically selected conserved peptide. There are many other molecules on the surface of each organism that can be described as conserved, so more than one type of conserved peptide will be presented for each organism; therefore, there are heterogeneous antibodies produced. This is beneficial because it gives room to a wide array of target for the antibodies to bind and more than one approach for killing the organism. The huge disadvantage is that in an instance where one is starting the study of antibodies using this complex source from this heterogeneous pool, it will be difficult to describe the antibodies and elucidate their structure. This was, however, a short-lived problem since the neoplasm of antibody-forming cells (B cells), called the myeloma cells resulted in the production of one clone of antibodies continuously. Thus, such monoclonal antibodies provided the opportunity for the elucidation of the antibody structure. The production of monoclonal antibodies shall be addressed later in this book.

STRUCTURE OF IMMUNOGLOBULIN

- IgG is the basic unit of immunoglobulin.
- It is a **monomer** linked by a disulfide bond.
- Each **heterodimer** has a **50–60 KDa**, called **heavy chain** linked by disulfide bond to a smaller chain **25 KDa** called **light chain**.
- In total, an **IgG** molecule consists of **four peptide chains**, **two heavy** and **two light chains**.

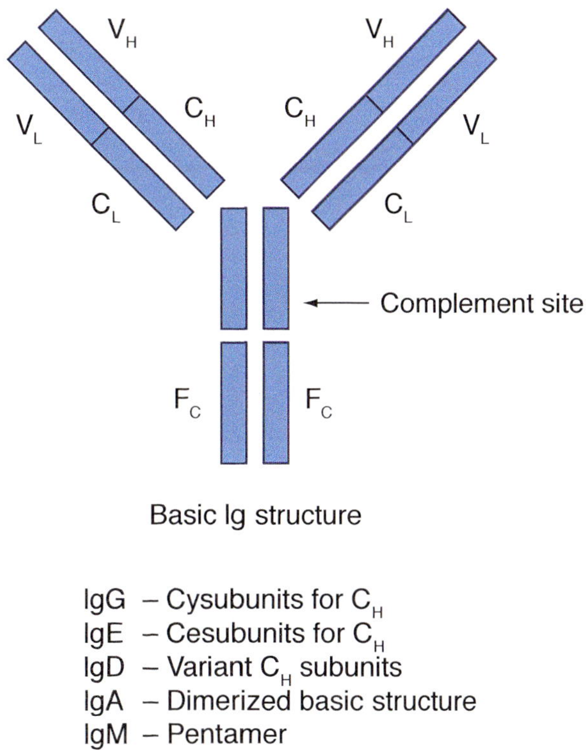

Figure 3.2 *A simple model of IgG molecule.*

The structure of immunoglobulin is, therefore, well elucidated using IgG as a model. It is important to note that IgG is a monomer, thus the generalized basic unit of immunoglobulin. It has two types of polypeptide chains: the heavy and light chains.

Antibodies are produced by B cells in response to specific antigenic stimulation and they react with the antigen specifically by binding to the site on the antigen that elicited their production. The antibody has two basic kinds of protein chain: heavy and light chains. Like every protein, the light and heavy chains have amino terminals and carboxyl terminals. Each of these chains also has an area that is variable, and an area that is constant. Areas of variability bring about heterogeneity of antibodies. The sequencing of the protein shows that the light chain has about half the amino acid as those in the heavy chain. The binding to a specific region (epitope) that has caused the production of the antibody usually occur on the antigen binding site on the antibody (Fab: fragment ab: antigen-binding site). On the constant region of the heavy chain, there are sites that can bind to complement, and subsequently bind to receptors on cells; these sites are located on the Fc region of the antibody. The reactive sites on the Fc region are not exposed for reaction on antibodies that are not bound to antigens. Conformational changes accompany antigen–antibody interactions resulting in the exposure of the reactive domains on the Fc region. The antibodies that serve as receptors on cells have a transmembrane region, which consists of more hydrophobic aminoacids, making it possible for them to associate with membranes. Apart from the capacity to act as an opsonin and bind complement, an antibody has other observable reactions when it interacts with an antigen. These include neutralization of the antigen, lysing of cells associated with antigen, and clumping of cells associated with the antigen.

The antibody has a hinge region which makes it flexible and able to rotate and the binding of each polypeptide linkage to the next is by disulfide bonds, which account for the flexibility of this molecule. The antibody has specialized protein clusters with defined functions, these areas are designated as "domains." Antibodies are found in tears, respiratory tract, body fluids, secretions, intestinal tract, urine, breast milk, and all openings to the exterior.

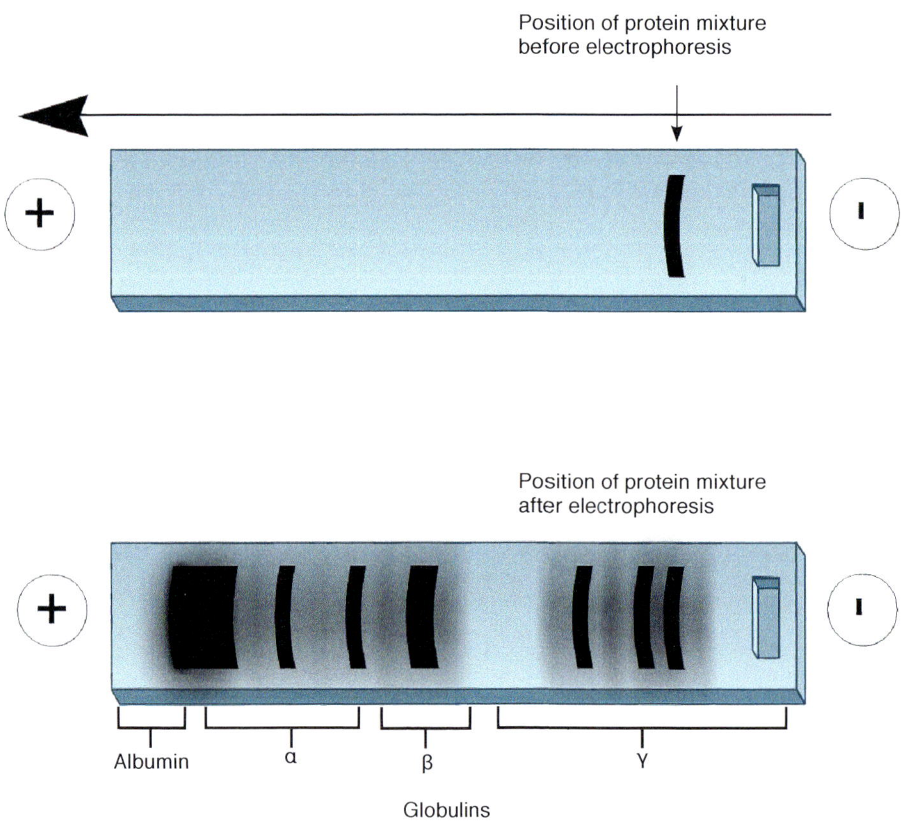

Courtesy of Zainab Ashkanani

Figure 3.3 *Electrophoresis of a serum sample on a strip of cellulose acetate. It can be resolved into about ten distinct bands in this way.*

They are studied in serum as proteins by exposure to an electric field (protein electrophoresis) as a basis for their classification. Usually, they are negatively charged, so they will migrate from the cathode to the anode. On such basis, they were found to be essentially globulins, specifically gamma globulins, although some of them are beta globulins.

The classification of antibodies is determined by the nature of the heavy chain, which is mainly how it moves in the electric field. If the heavy chain is an alpha chain, then it is an IgA; if it is gamma globulin, IgG; where it is an epsilon, it is IgE; a delta heavy chain is IgD; and mieu heavy chain is designated IgM. The antibodies produced during primary response are usually mainly IgM. In memory response, there is mostly IgG, which means it will be more in quantity at any time because it is likely that one has been exposed to an antigen in a repeated fashion.

ENZYME DIGESTION

- **Proteolytic enzyme (papain) splits IgG** into **three fragments**. **Two** of the **fragments (Fab) retain** the ability to **bind Ag**. The **third** fragment is non-**Ag binding (Fc)** but is **crystallizable**.
- Other proteolytic enzymes, such as **pepsin**, may leave **Fab fragments joined** together to **produce** the structure called **F(ab′)2**.

Proteolytic enzymes have physiological value in terms of antibody studies and use. The enzymes in common use are papain and pepsin. Antibodies can be raised and passively administered to individuals as passive vaccine, but the protection they provide rapidly wane within a short while because they are cleared by phagocytes. The problem immune globulins have is that the body clears them away since they are foreign. This occurs by virtue of the fact that antibodies would bind to scavenger cells like macrophages or monocytes with Fc receptor using their Fc-binding region. This scavenging accounts for the waning of passively administered antibodies. In order to reduce the clearance of the antibodies, advantage is taken of the ability of pepsin to cleave away the Fc region used for binding to phagocytes without compromising the antigen-binding capability. Another example of the use of enzymes is the reaction of antibodies with antigen, which can be enhanced and made more observable by hydrolysis using papain enzyme, and this makes room for enhanced binding and reduction of steric hindrances.

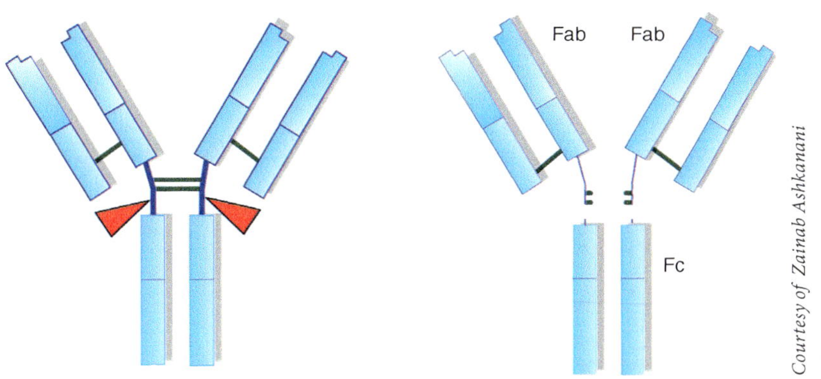

Figure 3.4 *Proteolytic cleavage by papain.*

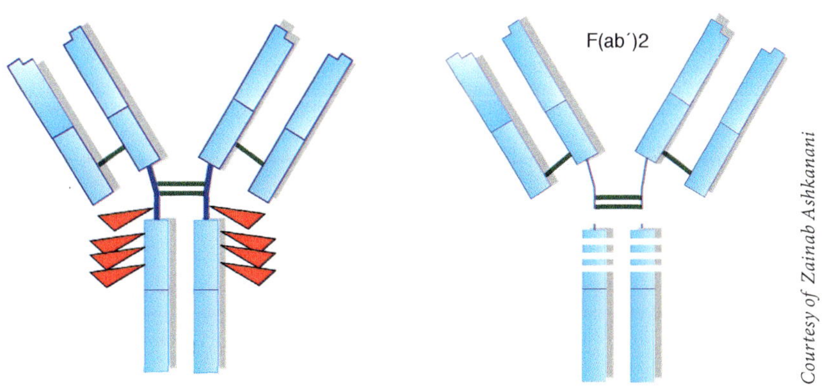

Figure 3.5 *Proteolytic cleavage by pepsin.*

IMMUNOGLOBULIN CLASSES

Figure 3.5 shows major immunoglobulin classes of humans, while Table 3.1 lists subclasses of human IgG.

IgG

- **Most abundant Ig.**
- Plays an important role in **Ab-mediated** defense mechanisms.
- It is **small in size** and can **escape** into **tissues** to **mount defense.**
- IgG can **opsonize**, **agglutinate**, and **precipitate** Ag.
- For **complement activation**, they are required in **large numbers**, and must **accumulate in correct configuration on Ag surface.**
- Each **heavy chain** of IgG has about **445** amino acids. In the center of the chain is an extended **flexible region** called the **hinge region.**
- The heavy chain has a variable **N-terminal** amino acid domain (V_H) and a constant **C-terminal** amino acid region (C_H) (Figure 3.6a and b).

IgM

- Next in abundance to IgG in mammalian serum. However, IgA has a higher concentration in human serum than IgM (see Figures 3.7–3.9).
- It is structurally a **polymer**, with **each unit** having **two Ag**-binding sites; therefore, a total of **ten binding** sites may be found.
- In **practice**, this may manifest as **five binding** sites because of **steric hindrance.**
- IgM **monomers** are **linked** by **disulfide bond** in a **circular fashion**. A small **cysteine-rich polypeptide** called the **J chain (15KDa)**, **coded** for by a **separate gene**, binds two of the units to **complete the circle.**
- **IgM** is the **major Ig** class of **primary response** with only a **little** produced during **secondary** response.
- It is more **efficient** in **complement activation**, **opsonization**, **viral neutralization**, and **agglutination.**
- As **receptors** on **B-cell** membrane, they exist as monomers.
- **Purification** of **myeloma proteins** make Abs **structural analysis** and **amino acid sequence** an **easy task.**
- Each light chain has about **214** amino acids.
- In the C-terminal domain **(constant C_L)** amino acid sequence is **identical**, while in the **N-terminal domain** **(variable V_L)** the sequence is **different** in each light chain.

TABLE 3.1 SUBCLASSES OF HUMAN IGG

POPERTIES AND BIOLOGICAL ACTIVITIES OF HUMAN SERUM IMMUNOGLOBULINS									
	IMMUNOGLOBULIN								
PROPERTY/ ACTIVITY	**IgG_1**	**IgG_2**	**IgG_3**	**IgG_4**	**IgA_1**	**IgA_2**	**IgM**	**IgE**	**IgD**
Molecular weight ($\times 10^{-3}$)	150	150	150	150	150 to 600	150 to 600	900	190	150
Heavy chain subunit	γ_1	γ_2	γ_3	γ_4	α_1	α_2	μ	ε	δ
Normal serum level (mg/ml)	9	3	1	0.5	3	0.5	1.5	0.003	0.03
Half-life (days)	23	23	8	23	6	6	5	2.5	3
Complement activation	+	+/–	++	–	–	–	+++	–	–
Crosses placenta	+	+/–	+	+	–	–	–	–	+
Found on B lymphocyte cell membrane	–	–	–	–	–	–	+	–	–
Binds to phagocyte Fc receptor	++	+/–	++	+	–	–	–	–	–
Mucosal transport	–	–	–	–	++	++	+	–	–
Induces mast-cell degeneration	–	–	–	–	–	–	–	+	–

Activity levels; + + + = very high; + + = high; + = moderate; + / – = weakly; – = none. IgG, IgE, and IgD exist as monomers; IgA can exist as a monomer, dimer, trimer, or tetramer. Membrane-bound IgM is a monomer but, secreted IgM is a pentamer.

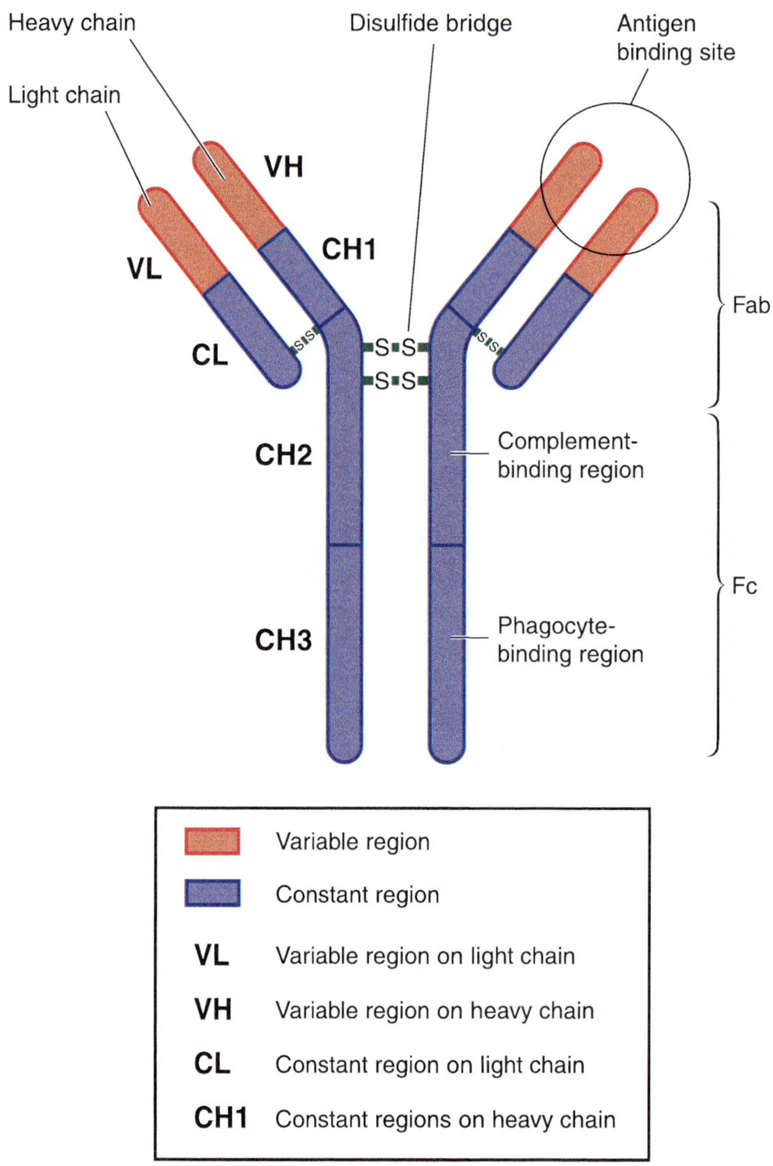

Figure 3.6 *Illustration showing IgG and locations of the variable and constant regions as well as the light and heavy chains.*

AMINO ACID SEQUENCE OF LIGHT AND HEAVY CHAINS

- **Antibodies** produced in response to antigenic challenges are usually **heterogeneous** because of **variation** in **antigenic determinant (epitopes)** on the challenger.
- **Sequence analysis** is usually **not possible** on this. However, in **plasma cell neoplasms**, only a **clone** of plasma cells results.
- Therefore, antibody elaboration is **absolutely homogeneous (monoclonal)**. As the tumor grows, the serum of the individual is dominated by monoclonal antibodies.
- The **tumor** of **plasma cell** is called **myeloma**; the antibodies elaborated are called **myeloma proteins**.

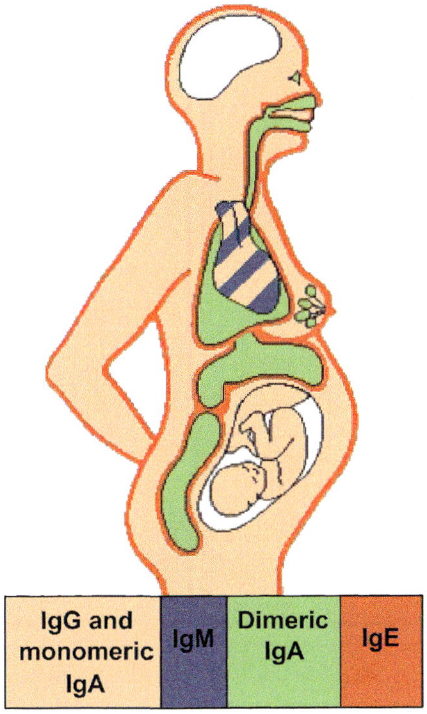

Courtesy of Zainab Ashkanani

Figure 3.7 *Distribution of immunoglobulin isotypes throughout the body.*

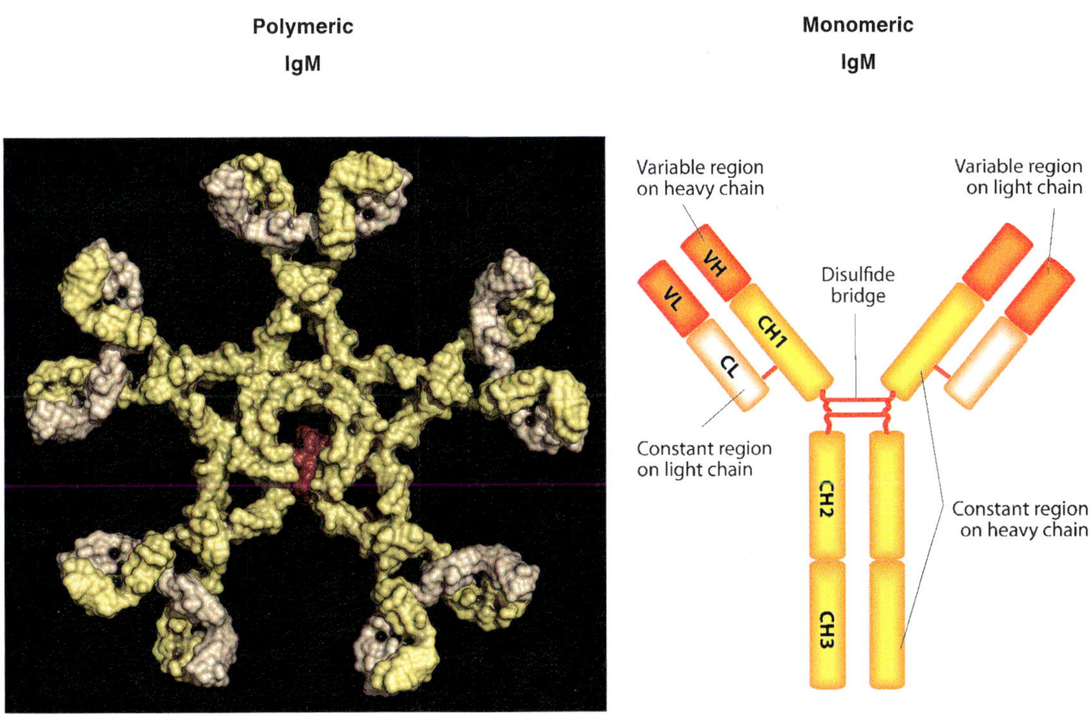

© 2014 molekuul.be/Shutterstock, Inc.

Courtesy of Zainab Ashkanani

Figure 3.8 *Structure of IgM.*

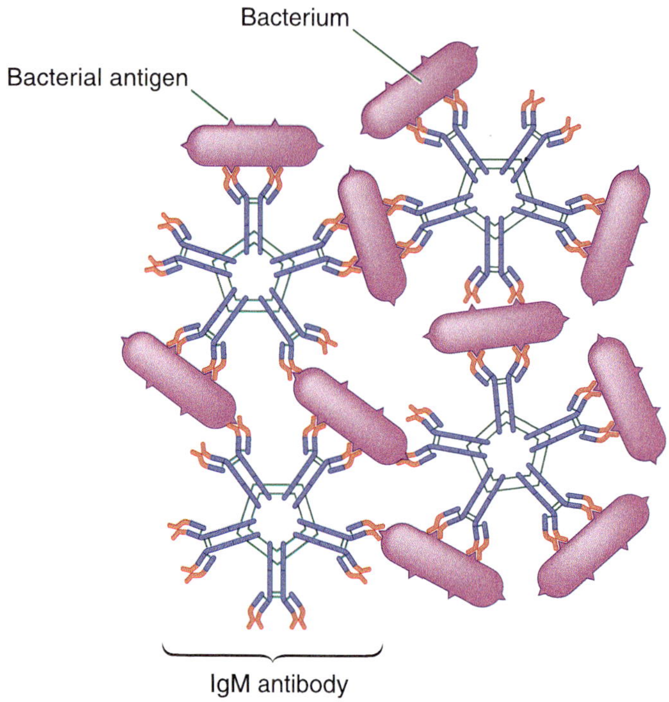

Figure 3.9 *Generation of a pentameric IgM from a monomeric IgM and J chain, so called to be described as a joining chain. Monomers are cross-linked by disulfide bonds to one another and to the J chain.*

IgA

- Occurs naturally as a **dimer**; the two monomers are joined by **J chain**.
- A **membrane bound** form of **IgA** acts as receptor **on B cells**. It **differs** from the **secreted form** in having a **hydrophobic membrane binding** sequence at its **C-terminus**.
- In humans, IgA is subclassified into **IgA1** and **IgA2** based on **differences** in **heavy chain** structure.
- An IgA2 **variant** that lacks disulfide bond is known, it is held together by **noncovalent** forces.
- IgA is **secreted** into **intestinal lumen** and **blood** and taken up by **intestinal epithelium** and **hepatocytes**.
- During **this period** they are **bound** to a **glycoprotein** of **71 KDa** known as secretory component to form a complex molecule called **secretory IgA** (sIgA).
- **sIgA** is a **form** that is **protected** from **hydrolysis** by **intestinal enzymes**, it is the form that **protects** the **body surfaces** from **invading microbes**.

IgD

- Has **no inter** chain disulfide bond between its heavy chains, so it is very **susceptible** to **hydrolysis**.
- IgD cannot be found in **serum** because during **blood clotting**, **proteases** generated **hydrolyze** them. But some are found in **plasma**.
- Like **IgE**, **IgD** is **thermolabile**. IgD is **primarily** a B-cell **antigen receptor**.

IgE Allergies

- Has extraordinarily **low concentration** in serum of **unparasitized individuals**, varying from **20–500** ng/ml; this is approximately **1/40,000** of the concentration of **IgG**.
- IgE does **not neutralize Ag**.
- It is important in **activating mast** cells and **basophils** during **allergies (type 1 hypersensitivity)** and activating **antiallergic** actions of **eosinophils** and **immunity** to **invading parasitic** worms.
- **The Fc region of IgE binds to Fc receptors of mast cells, basophils, and eosinophils with very high affinity. The receptor-binding site is the 12 N-terminal amino acids of the C_H3 domains.**

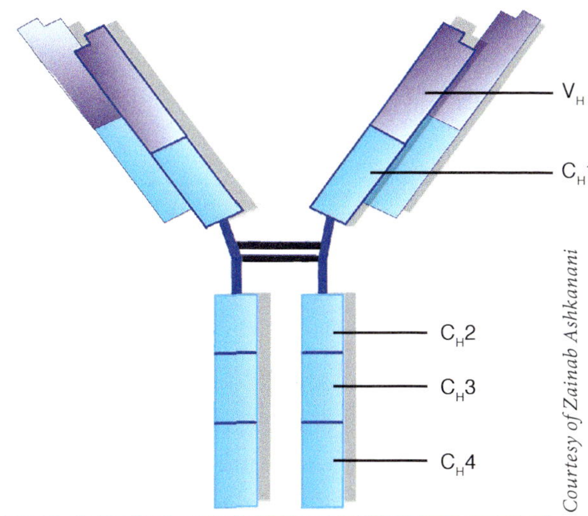

Figure 3.10 *Structure of IgE. Note the additional domain that permit the IgE to Fc receptors on mast cells.*

IgG. As the most abundant immunoglobulin in serum, IgG plays an important role in antibody-mediated defense mechanism (Figure 3.10). Since they are small in size and are the basic unit of antibodies, they can pass through tissue boundaries to mount defenses within intercellular spaces.

IgG can coat (opsonize) any invading challenge that they have been produced to react with. They can also cause agglutination, defined as the clumping of cells. If they are not on organized surfaces, they can cause precipitation, but if they are on an organized cell surface, they will cause clumping. They can also neutralize the effectiveness of an agent. IgG can activate complement, but for them to do it, they need to act at least in pairs; they must be able to accumulate in the right pattern (configuration) on the surface of the antigen in order for them to cause complement activation.

IgM. These are the preponderant antibodies of primary response. These antibodies are naturally occurring and are produced as blood group antibodies especially of the ABO blood group. They are next in abundance to IgG in serum in mammalian cells for obvious reasons, except in humans where sometimes IgA are more abundant than IgM. Immunoglobulin M is a polymer, usually a pentamer, that is, five IgG units. A typical IgG usually has two antigen binding sites; so, IgM will have ten. In real binding, it cannot utilize all ten binding sites because each adjacent binding site will create steric hindrance as one binding site impedes the action of adjacent sites; so, finally there are five active binding sites. When IgM exists as a cell surface receptor, they are not polymers but monomers. As a pentamer, individual units are joined together by disulfide bonds in cyclic arrangement that is concluded by a small piece of 15 kDa protein that is coded for separately; this is called the J chain. By virtue of their multiple binding sites, they are more efficient as complement activators. It is for the same reason that they are more effective at neutralization of viruses and cause agglutination more effectively. They are able to cluster on cells better. On B cells, where they are found as receptors, they are usually found as monomers.

There are subclasses of IgG due to variability of the heavy chain in the variable region, so you can have γ_1, γ_2, γ_3, and γ_4, giving rise to IgG_1, IgG_2, IgG_3, and IgG_4. There are no subclasses for IgM.

It is important to note that IgG has the greatest half-life in terms of days for the obvious fact that it is the antibody that remains for a long time, providing the required immunity after a primary response. IgA is found at virtually all portals of entry in the body, thereby serving as the first line of defense by preventing the entry of any specific antigen that it has been raised against. IgA is about twice IgG because apart from having different domains in the heavy chain region, it commonly exists as a dimer, with a J piece holding the two together, that is the way it is secreted to mount adequate defense at the portals of entry. IgE is usually very low in individuals that do not have allergies or parasites.

Antibodies are produced specifically in response to particular antigens, but because an antigen usually is on a point on an organized surface, you are likely to have many antigens on one surface. If a cell membrane was analyzed for protein distribution, the complex proteins covering the membrane will be a lot of different types; thus a lot of antibodies can be raised to one cell, and there is need for such response for effective and efficient protection because it makes the protection against a challenge multidimensional. The specific antigen on such organized surfaces is commonly described as "epitope," which are the antigenic determinants on the cell system challenging the host. On an organized cell surface, there are specific molecular arrangements that antigen presenting cells select as peptides to be presented on the molecule that has been fashioned to display it, the antigen presenting molecules (MHC). Having presented such biomolecule, the antibody produced will normally have a surface that can fit that arrangement; the epitope will always produce an antibody that has the binding sites that are specifically arranged to fit into it. The arrangement on the antibody that specifically binds the epitope will be called the paratope. It is not the whole of the paratope arrangement that determines this fitting during this interaction between epitope and paratope, it is a selection of small amino acids that we describe as complementarity-determining region.

It is important to note that the antibodies that are found in the neonate and the infant are predominantly antibodies that can be transferred from the maternal system into the fetus, and these are usually IgG. There is the conventional understanding that the capacity of IgG to transverse the placenta wall into the developing fetus is related to the size of IgG, but this assertion is not tenable because there are other small antibodies that do not transverse the placenta. Also, it is not all the IgG subclasses that will pass through the placenta, which is why the issue of size is not the point. A more plausible explanation for the IgG's capacity to cross the placenta is their endowment with a placenta transfer site which makes them meander through the placenta wall. At the point of delivery, the neonate has IgG as the main antibody in their circulation. The antibody levels wane, such that at 9 months postpartum, there is a total decline. However, at about this time, there is an increase in new IgM and IgG because of environmental antigens and the appearance of naturally occurring antibodies in the system. Also, the infant will begin to get exposed to infections which will elicit the production of IgM as the primary response antibody.

IgA. It occurs naturally as a dimer, you have seen that many times. The two monomers are held together by the J chain. A membrane-bound form of IgA normally acts as a receptor on B cells. The polypeptide that binds to membrane needs a hydrophobic amino acid sequence. The difference between the secreted and membrane-bound form is the C-terminal region. In humans, IgA is subclassified into IgA_1 and IgA_2 based on differences in the heavy chain structure. An IgA_2 variant that lacks disulfide bond is also known, it is held together by noncovalent forces. IgA are secreted in intestinal lumen and blood, and they are found in the endothelial lining and hepatocytes. The secreted IgA is held by a secretory component, which is a 31 kDa protein, such IgA is represented as sIgA. It is this piece that protects the IgA from hydrolysis by intestinal enzymes. This is different from the J piece which holds the antibody units together.

IgD. These are characterized with little or no interchain link, so they are easily degraded. They are not easily demonstrable in serum, because enzymes that are activated during blood clotting degrade most of the IgD. However, some of them can be found in plasma. They are thermolabile and can be found in association with B cells.

IgE. This immunoglobulin is of special importance in relation to an allergic response and is also in high levels in cases of helminthic infections. The concentration is low in individuals without these problems, making the level of IgE to IgG 1:40,000. It is important in activating mast cells and basophils during allergies (type 1 hypersensitivity) and it can also bind to eosinophils to release granular content (major basic protein), which can destroy the cuticle of parasites, especially worms, and kill them. The Fc region of IgE binds to Fc receptors of mast cells, basophils, and eosinophils with very high affinity.

The receptor-binding site is the 12 N-terminal amino acids of the CH_3 domain.

- In the variable region, there is a section of **hypervariability**, called the **frame work region** that binds to the **epitope** (Figures 3.11–3.14).
- It is the **amino acid sequence** in this **region** that **determines** the **shape** of the **antigen-binding site** (called **paratope**).
- This **region** is, therefore, **described** as **complementarity-determining region (CDR)**.
- Each **CDR** is **short**, consisting of **six–ten** amino acid sequences.

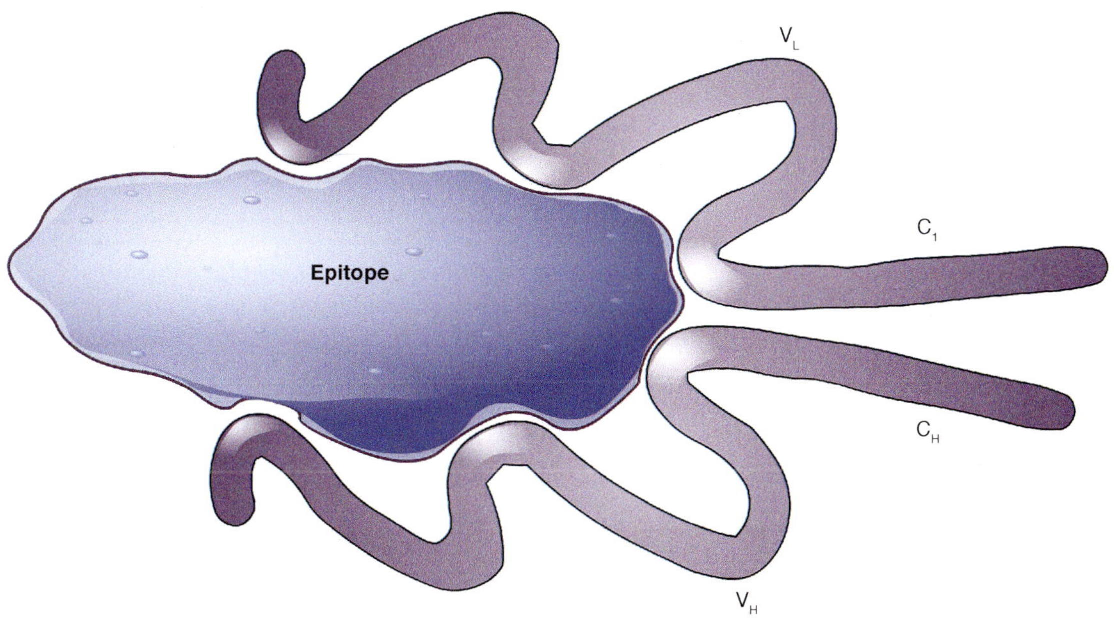

Figure 3.11 *A schematic diagram showing the way in which light and heavy chains are folded so that the three pairs of complementarity-determining regions in each chain form the walls of the antigen-binding groove.*

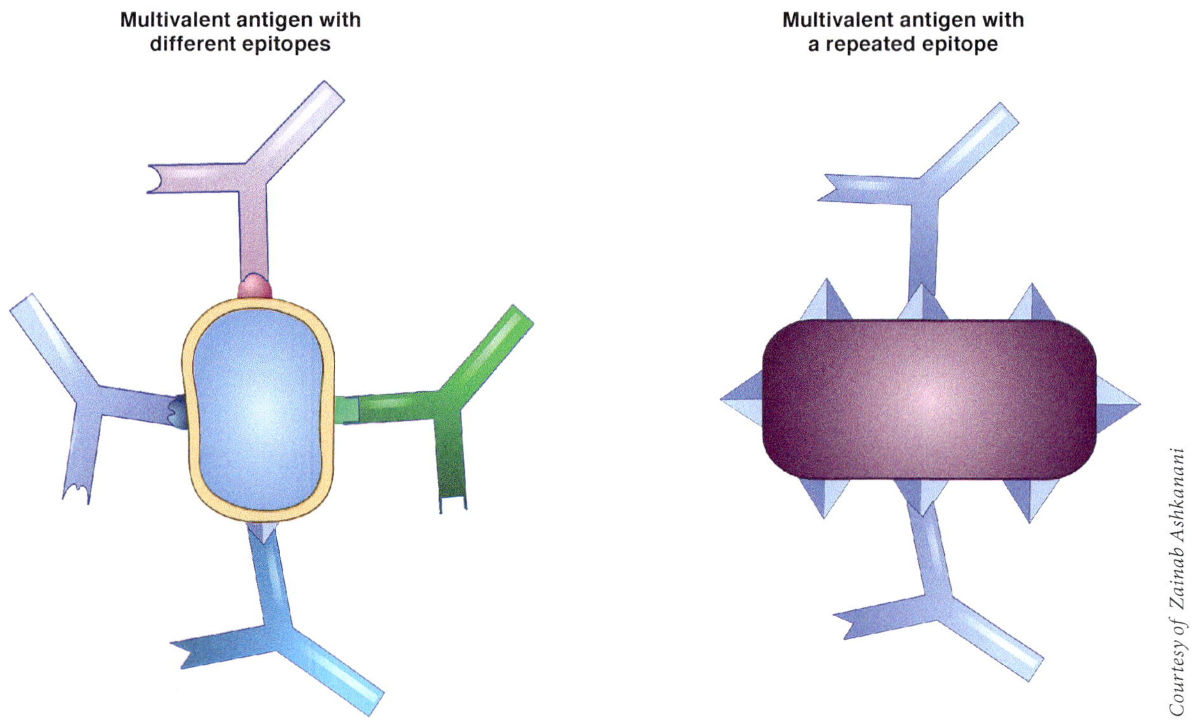

Figure 3.12 *Depiction of a multivalent antigen with either repeating epitopes or variable epitopes.*

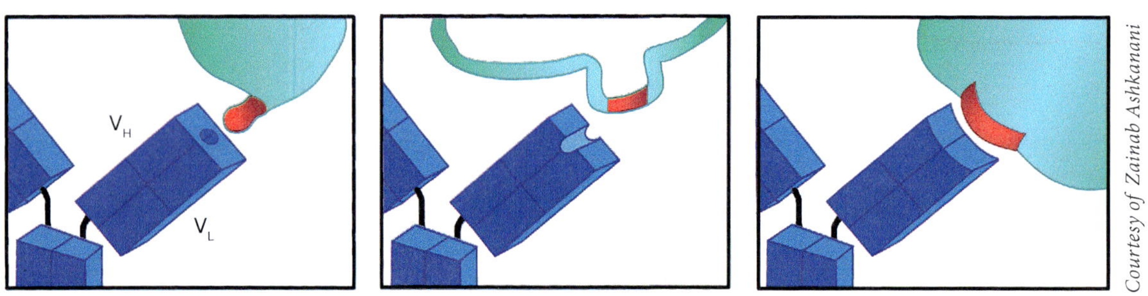

Figure 3.13 *Illustration of types of bonding done by epitopes to their complementary sites on antibodies, in pockets, in grooves, or extended surface areas.*

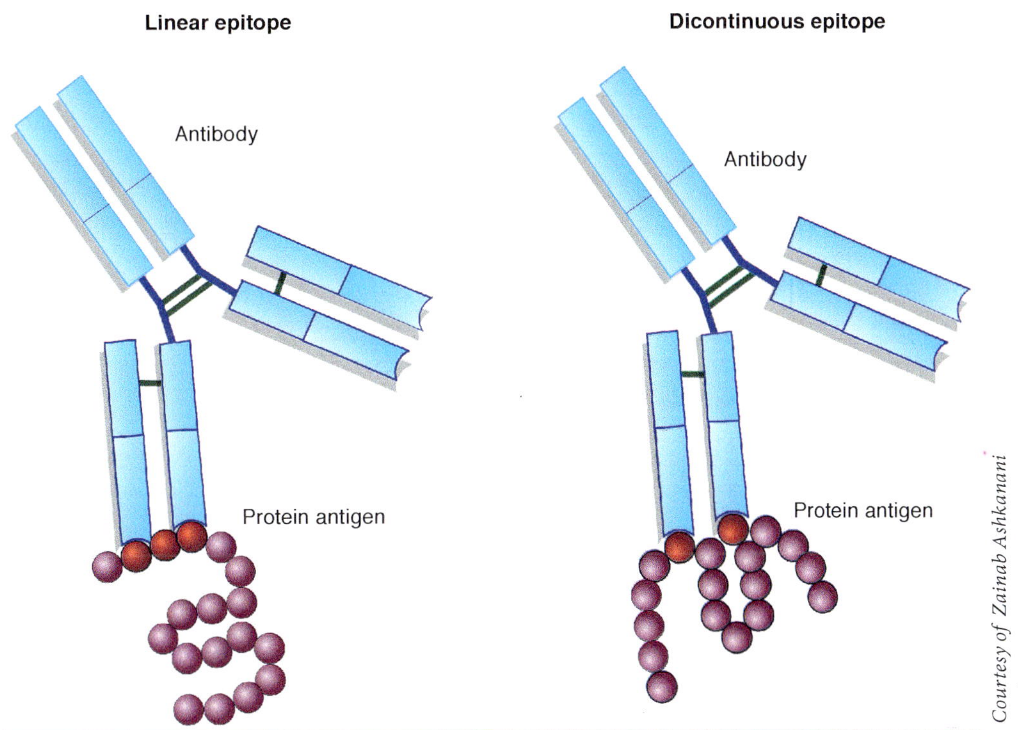

Figure 3.14 *Epitopes can be linear or discontinuous.*

- Ig **superfamily** is a general form of classification of **closely** related **proteins** with **related functions**.
- They are involved in **cellular interactions** and share **common ancestral origin**.

In the variable region of the antibody, there is the site that binds to the antigen, and there is a collection of amino acids responsible for this binding. This configuration constitutes the paratope. However, with this configuration are a small number of amino acids numbering six–ten that are patterned into a region described as the complementarity-determining region (CDR). The shaded areas are the points of complementarity and it is into this area that the epitope fits (Figure 3.14). Actually, the epitope is responsible for determining the arrangement on the paratope. Therefore, there are variations in the contour of the paratope because of varying epitope types.

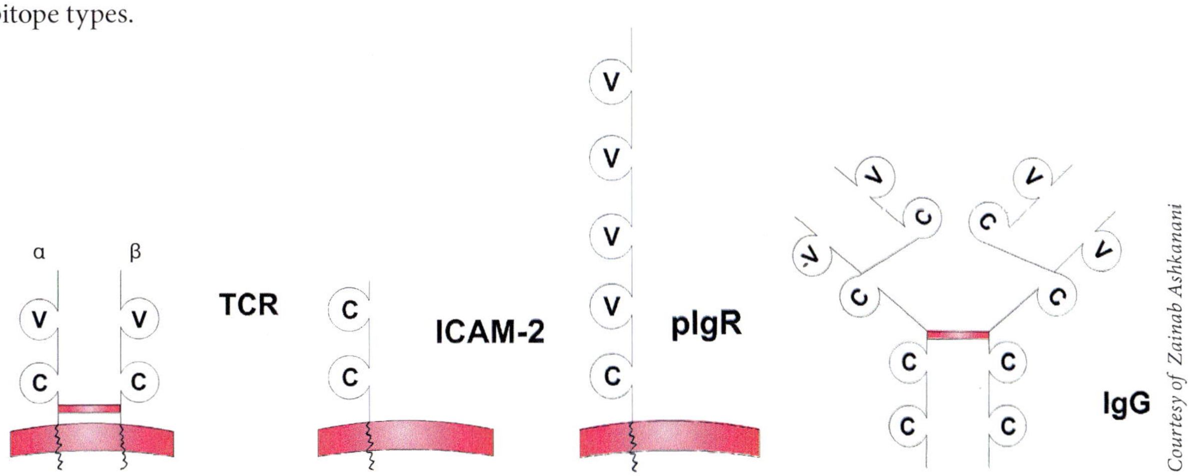

Figure 3.15 *The four major groups of immunoglobulin superfamily: (a) the antigen receptors, (b) the small receptors that contain one or two domains, (c) the large receptors that contain three or more domains, and (d) the immunoglobulins.*

Immunoglobulins are not necessarily free antibodies alone, some of them are bound to cell surfaces and are responsible for cell signals. All of these with diverse functions have been recognized as being of the same lineage, so we describe all of them as immunoglobulin superfamily. The concept of superfamily attests to the relatedness of antibodies and other immunoglobulins. There are categorizations of the immunoglobulin superfamily as illustrated above (Figure 3.15). Antigen receptors are typical examples of immunoglobulin superfamily members. The antigen receptors found on the T cell, for instance, the T-cell receptors, are members of the family. Major histocompatibility complex (classes 1 and 2) which are antigen presenting molecules are within the family. An important feature of the complex represented here is the configuration, the arrangement of the molecule on the membrane surface. It is important to note that it is a dimer with a pair of variable regions and a pair of constant regions; they have alpha and beta polypeptide moieties. The configuration is one of the structures that goes deeper into the cell and does not terminate at the transmembrane area, thus facilitating a more efficient signal transductional effect.

The example in the diagram with short signaling receptors and consistent protein pattern is not suitable for arrangement requiring variability.

T-cell receptors facilitate adaptive immune response and are able to respond to variable antigens; therefore, they have variable regions. The case is different for a bimolecular arrangement that binds constant ligands such as the binding of complement to complement receptors, the actions of adhesion molecules; the receptor arrangement has more constant regions. In some instances, the variable regions are more elaborate and the constant region is just one, illustrating the kind of need that the receptors fulfill. It is important to observe the depth of the receptor domain beyond the membrane into the cytosol, this reflects that signals generated can readily go deep into the cell. Whenever it is impossible to go deeper into the cell, the cell has a way of handing the signal. In the case of receptors like the LPS receptor, there is the assistive effect of the Toll-like receptor pathway, in which the pathway helps for deeper transduction.

In the case of antibodies (immunoglobulin), their relatedness to the superfamily is observable by the presence of variable and constant regions and domains.

IMMUNOGLOBULIN PEPTIDE CHAIN

- Each Ig molecule has light chains of one of the two types (**κ, kappa or λ, lambda**), regardless of their class or antigen binding ability.
- The ratio of κ to λ varies between species.
- In **humans**, about **65%** of Ig molecules have κ and **35%** λ chains. Mice and rats have **95%** κ chains, while cattle and horse have **98%** λ chains. Monkeys or the baboons have **50%** of each.
- Variation in heavy chains of Ig results in structural variants known as **subclasses**, which has effects on **structure** and biological activities.
- All normal persons possess all four subclasses (**IgG_1, IgG_2, IgG_3, and IgG_4**).
- **IgG_3** has the **shortest half-life**, the **lowest synthetic** and **highest catabolic rate**, and an **unusually** high number of **interchain disulfide bonds**.
- **IgG_4** is functionally **monovalent**, and will **not precipitate** or **agglutinate Ag**.
- **Autoantibodies** to **clotting factors** tend to belong to the **IgG4** and **autoantibodies** to **DNA** belong to **IgG1** and **IgG3** subclasses.

The diversity of the heavy chain of antibodies and the impact of this on the naming (as various classes) has been explained. The light chains, however, have some diversity of their peptides also; they are either kappa (κ) or lambda (λ).

Some Definitions

- **Idiotypes—heterogeneity** of Abs due to **varying epitopes**.
- **Allotypes—minor** sequence **variation** contributing to **structural** differences and **functions**.
- **Isotypes**—structural variation resulting in classification and subclassification.

ANTIGEN—ANTIBODY BINDING

- It involves the chemical groups on the surface of the **epitope** and the **complementarity**-determining regions on Ig molecules.
- The nature of bond operating is **noncovalent**, requiring close proximity of interacting molecules and **conformational fit** of **epitopes** to **CDRs**, likened to the specificity of a key to its lock.
- The **operating forces** are mainly **hydrophobic** and **hydrogen** bond.
- When half the Ig binding sites are occupied, the affinity constant is a reciprocal of the concentration of free epitopes. For example,

$$Ag + Ab = AgAb$$

- Defining strength of binding through mass action and affinity constant.
- **K = [AbAg]/[Ab][Ag]**, where [Ab] is the concentration of Ab-binding sites, [Ag] is the concentration of free epitopes, and [AbAg] is the concentration of immune complexes at equilibrium.
- So, if half the Ig binding sites are occupied, then K is a reciprocal of the concentration of free epitopes.

$$K = 1/[Ag]$$

- The average **affinity** of IgG–Abs **produced** during **Ag** stimulation increases as immune response progresses; in contrast, the average affinity of IgM remains unchanged.
- Thus, Abs that produce the greatest binding strength are found late during immune response.
- **Avidity** is the term **used** to **describe** the **strength** and **speed** of **binding**. Thus, a very avid Ag—Ab reaction occurs within a short time.

HIGH-AFFINITY ANTIBODIES

- Have the greatest binding strength.
- Are produced late in immune response.
- Are usually less specific.
- React with other closely related epitopes.
- Useful for viral and toxin neutralization.
- Useful for complement action and red blood cell lysis.
- High-**affinity antibodies** are **less specific** compared to **low-affinity antibodies** because high-affinity Abs **react not** only with their inducing **epitopes** but also with **closely related epitopes**.
- **High-affinity Abs** are more **useful** at **viral** and **toxin neutralization**, **complement activation**, and **red cell lysis**.

The easy way we measure antibodies is through antigen and antibody reactions. The reaction comes from the binding that is determined by the epitope and the paratope, more specifically the epitope and the complementarity-determining regions on the immunoglobulin molecule. The nature of the interacting bond is noncovalent and requires close proximity, so there must be adequate orientation of the antigen and antibody in a way that the fit can allow interactions. That is why in practice, it is important to have adequate dilutions in order to have optimum reactions. Appropriate dilution positions antigens and antibodies in an orientation that increases the tendency for interaction between the active surfaces. So, there is enhancement of the tendency for conformational fit of epitope to CDR. The operating forces during the interaction are mainly hydrophobic and hydrogen bonds.

The chemistry involved in the preceding explanation about the need to dilute samples for antigen/antibody interaction is the same as the laws guiding active masses. Whenever half the binding sites are occupied, the affinity constant, which is equivalent to the constant that is obtained in the law of mass action, applies. The affinity constant in this instance is the reciprocal of the concentration of free epitopes. It will also be the same as the concentration of free paratopes. According to the law of mass action in this instance, the reciprocal of either of the active masses varies as the constant. As the active masses increase, the constant decreases; therefore, for optimum constant, the active masses should be low, hence the need for dilution. In practice, there is need for a 2% dilution in the case of blood sample. So, if the law of mass action is applied, then the affinity constant is represented as follows: $K= [AbAg]/[Ab][Ag]$. Therefore, if half the immunoglobulin sites are occupied, then the constant of reaction is a reciprocal of the active masses of the interacting agents which are the epitope and the paratope. Thus $K = 1/[Ag]$.

If an animal were inoculated with an antigen, there is a primary response, followed by anamnestic response upon repeated inoculation. The IgG that is produced throughout the responses will continue to increase; therefore, it contributes more to immune protection than IgM does. Although IgM reacts more strongly, it doesn't offer better immune protection. It is important to note that affinity, which represents the attraction between binding sites, is different from avidity, which is the strength and time of reaction. An avid reaction produces observable strong reaction within a short time. The affinity of IgG produced during antigenic stimulation will increase as long as antigenic stimulation of the animal continues and is protracted. In contrast, the IgM level will wane. The antibody produced that has greater binding strength is usually found later in immune response, and these are IgG. Thus by implication, they have greater avidity but their affinity may be low, normal or high. The practical demonstration of avidity, therefore, involves allowing antigen and antibody interaction to occur and observing the time within which an observable antigen–antibody reaction manifests. So, avidity is defined as strength of reaction within a given time, whereas attraction of surfaces for each other within a given time, which may not be a strong reaction, is affinity. The practical application of this in immunology, apart from the use in optimizing antibodies for blood grouping, is in the optimization of vaccine for passive use.

Another important point is the fact that high-affinity antibodies, which are antibodies that have surfaces that are complementary to epitope, may be less specific compared to antibodies that have low affinity. It is for this reason that antibodies used as reagents are diluted to the point where they only react specifically with the antigen. However, for the purposes of vaccination, high-affinity antibodies are preferred because due to their nonspecificity, they will cross-react with epitopes in a broad fashion. This provides wider amplitude of immune protection. High-affinity antibodies are more useful for viral and toxin neutralization, complement activation, and red cell lysis, these are all processes that are related to immune protection. The essential characteristics of such antibodies are as follows: they have the greatest binding strength, are usually produced late during the immune response, and are less specific, so they react with other closely related epitopes as an extension of their lesser specificity.

BIOLOGICAL SIGNIFICANCE OF Ag—Ab INTERACTION

- **Opsonization** of invading microbes and **enhancement** of phagocytosis.
- **Immune complex formation, which** induces **signal transduction** that generates **complement cascade activation**, firm **binding** of invaders to **phagocytic cells**, initiation of **degranulation** of mast cells and bas ophils, and **most importantly** the further **production of Abs by B cells**.
- Blockage of **toxic sites** and prevention of **viral binding** to cells.
- Activation of **Antibody dependent cellular cytotoxicity, or ADCC**, which is carried out by **macrophages, neutrophils**, and some **lymphocyte** subpopulations. **Eosinophils** also **exhibit** such **effects** when Abs **coating helminthes bind to** their receptors.

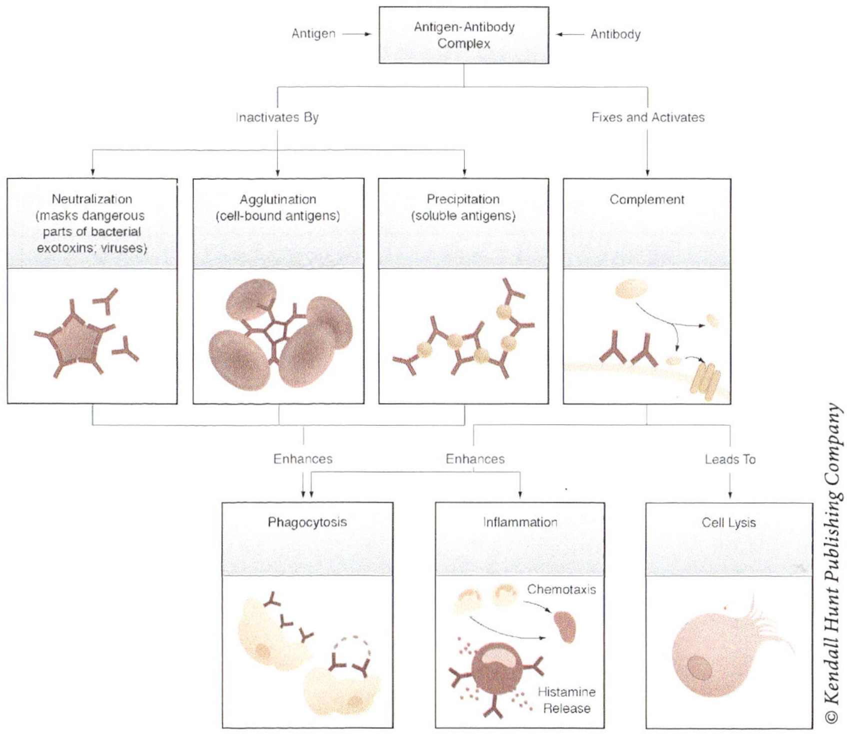

Figure 3.16 *Some of the biological consequences of the combination of antigen and antibody on the surface of the cell.*

The biological significance of the interaction between antigen and antibody (Figure 3.16) can be summarized as follows:

Opsonization. Antibody accounts for the opsonization of invading microbes and makes them easy to engulf.

Immune Complex Formation. If a free antigen that is not found on organized cell surface combines with its corresponding antibody, it forms an immune complex. If such a complex is deposited in joints, they can cause rheumatoid arthritis and other immune complex-mediated diseases. However, such complex can bind to professional phagocytes using the Fc region on the antibody and the complex would be engulfed. It is possible that the complex binds to complement and the complement then binds to a complement receptor on the phagocyte and the complex is engulfed. In other instances, if the complex arose from IgE binding to an allergen, then the IgE can bind to mast cells, resulting in degranulation and elaboration of histamine. If the IgE binds to eosinophils, then there is the production and release of antihistamine or histaminases.

Antibody (IgE) produced in response to the presence of helminthes can bind to eosinophil and cause the extrusion of granules in the eosinophil. This then results in those granules binding to the cuticle of helminthes, which finally elaborates the major basic protein resulting in the cleavage of the cuticle.

Antigen—antibody complex results in neutralization: The binding of antibody to toxic sites renders the site incapable of expressing toxicity, which is neutralization. If such site is a viral ligand that could be used for attachment to host cell, then the virus will not be able to bind to the cell, and therefore it would not be able to be internalized anymore, thus rendering the virus ineffective.

Antibody-Dependent Cellular Cytotoxicity (ADCC). This is the destruction of the cell that is mediated by antibody binding to antigen on those cells. In this situation, the cells that are invaded by viruses or have become neoplastic have markers on their surfaces that antibodies are produced against, the binding between those markers and the antibodies make it possible for destruction to occur to the cells. This mechanism facilitates the NK cells and cytotoxic T-cell killing capability. It is also useful for macrophage, neutrophil, and eosinophil immune actions.

SAMPLE QUESTIONS

NATURE OF ANTIBODIES

1. How many constant domains does the heavy chain of IgE contain?
   a. two
   b. three
   c. four
   d. five
   e. six

2. The antigen-combining site of an antibody molecule determines its
   a. isotype
   b. anti-idiotype
   c. allotype
   d. hypertype
   e. idiotype

3. Which class of immunoglobulin activates complement upon binding with antigen?
   a. IgM
   b. IgA
   c. IgD
   d. IgE
   e. all of the above

4. Serum IgM molecules usually have
   a. 10 light chains
   b. 10 heavy chains
   c. a pentameric structure
   d. a J chain
   e. all of the above

5. Molecules in the immunoglobulin superfamily share
   a. antigen-binding sites
   b. domains
   c. variable regions
   d. amino groups
   e. proline residues

6. The major forces linking antigen to antibody are
   a. hydrogen bonds
   b. coulombic bonds
   c. covalent links
   d. hydrophobic bonds
   e. ionic bonds

7. Immunoglobulin binding to receptors on effector cells (e.g., phagocytes, mast cells) is due to which portion of the immunoglobulin molecule?
   a. Fab
   b. Fc
   c. Fd
   d. light chain
   e. V region

8. The hinge region of an immunoglobulin is flexible because it contains a large amount of which amino acid?
   a. serine
   b. cysteine
   c. threonine
   d. tyrosine
   e. proline

9. The complementarity-determining regions of immunoglobulins
   a. activate complement
   b. bind to cells
   c. mediate opsonization
   d. bind to antigen
   e. make the molecule flexible

10. The strength of binding between an antigen and its antibody is called
   a. avidity
   b. valency
   c. hydrophobicity
   d. electrophoretic mobility
   e. affinity

Suggested Laboratory Practicals

- Case Studies on the following:
  1. Antibody Structure
  2. Antibody Classes
- Cleavage of Antibody by Pepsin and Papain
- Serum Protein Electrophoresis
- ABO Blood Grouping
- Demonstration of Bence-Jones Proteins in Urine and Serum

CHAPTER 4

THE LYMPHOID TISSUE

- Lymphocytes are derived from pluripotent hematopoietic stem cells. These cells appear already in the yolk sac of a developing embryo. They are later identifiable in the fetal liver. The bone marrow commences blood cell formation later in gestational life and continues after birth.
- The bone marrow has a total weight of 1300–1500 g in adult life, thus representing the largest tissue of the body.
- Bone marrow is the center of antigen-independent lymphopoiesis. Immature lymphocytes are released from the bone marrow and they travel to other primary lymphoid organs where further maturation takes place.
- One subset goes to the thymus and develops into T cells. In humans, it is accepted that B-cell maturation takes place within the bone marrow.
- The thymus is a small, flat, and bilobed organ found in the thorax or chest cavity below the thyroid gland and overlying the heart. In humans, it weighs about 22 g at birth, reaches about 35 g at puberty, and then gradually atrophies. Although the thymus diminishes in size, it is still able to produce T cells throughout a person's life span.
- Surface Ags are acquired as lymphocytes travel from cortex to medulla.

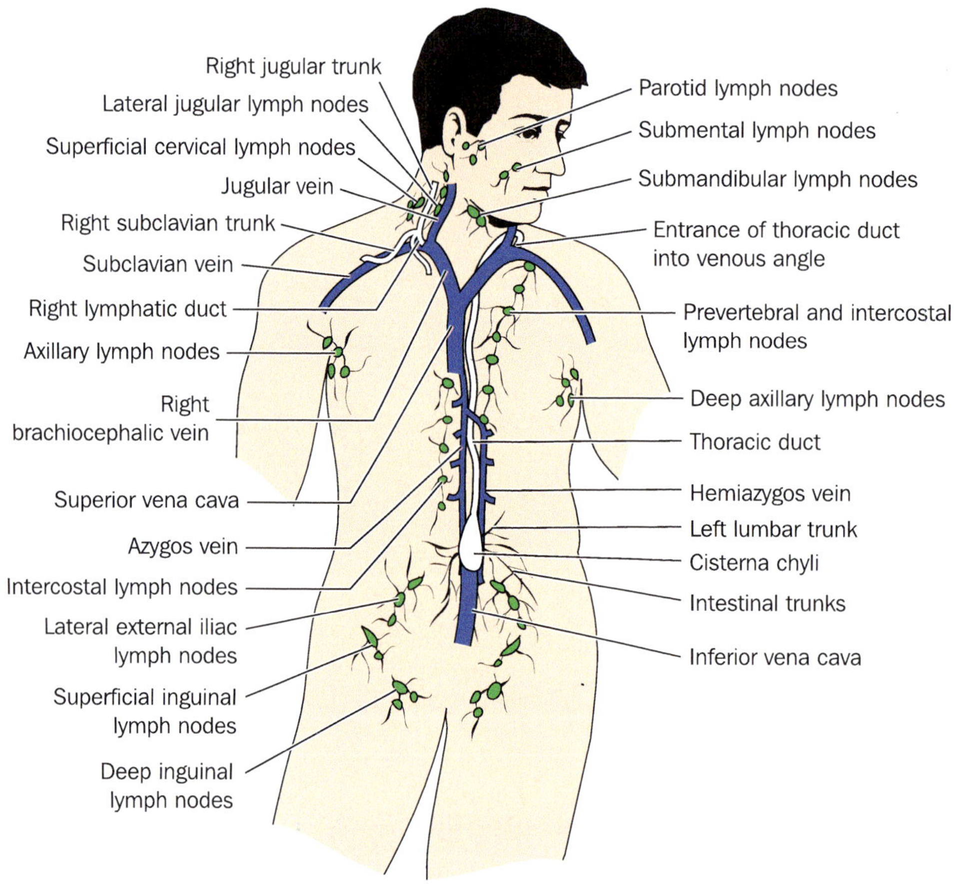

Figure 4.1 *Sites of lymphoid tissue within the human body indicating sites of maturation. For instance, B cells complete their maturation in the bone marrow whereas T cells migrate to the thymus to complete their maturation*

Lymphoid cells are a different group of cell population that originate from the hemocytoblast, the pluripotent stem cell in the bone marrow. These groups of cells are primitive and are capable of differentiating into any of the blood cell lines. The major subdivisions are the myeloid series, the lymphoid series, and the erythroid series. The erythroid series is of less importance in terms of immune protection, while the myeloid series has already been treated under the innate immune response. The lymphoid series is important in relation to lymphocytes and is mainly associated with acquired immune response. They are relatively long-lived and in this sense can be compared with macrophages. The lymphocytes can be subgrouped into two populations according to where they acquire their commitment as follows: B cells (those that become committed in the marrow before they are released into circulation) and the T cells (those that leave the marrow still immature and have to journey to the thymus to be committed. The B cell was originally named because they were first described in the cloaca of birds, which was found to be the repository of the bird's immune system. The population of cells involved in immune defenses in the cloaca area was concentrated in the Bursa of Fabricus. In circumstances in which these population of cells were cleared away in birds, as in Infectious Bursal Disease (Gumboro viral infection), the birds became immunodeficient. These cells, described as the Bursa cell

(B- cells), do not have an equivalent area of localization in humans, but the populations of lymphocytes that are sufficiently committed in the bone marrow appear to be equivalent of Bursa cells. There is a speculation that the bursa in the developed animal may be related to the Peyer's patches of the intestine. The name B cells was, therefore, retained and these cells may also be called bone marrow-dependent lymphocytes or B cells. The population of lymphocytes that must migrate to the thymus in order to be committed to their function, thus thymus-dependent (T cells), rapidly transverse the blood when released as immature lymphocytes from the bone marrow. The process of migration through the thymus enables them to develop into the group of cells that are capable of recognizing antigens expressed by challenges to the animal host; they are also capable of carrying memory of previous recognition. All their populations can produce soluble substances that regulate the immune system (immune mediators). The population of cells of this lineage is already present at the very early stages of gestation. In the yolk sac of the developing embryo, cells of lymphocyte lineage are already present; however, midway through pregnancy, it is the liver that is their site of presence. At the 7th month of pregnancy, the bone marrow becomes the site of formation of these cells and this situation persists for the rest of life. At the later stages of life, the bone marrow of the long bones no longer participates actively in their formation because it is replaced by fatty marrow; so the bone marrow that remains relevant throughout life is the marrow of membranous bones such as the scapular bones, the ribs, and that is why when there is a disorder afflicting these cells, the stress on the membranous bones manifest as aches and pain. When the disease becomes serious, the body reverts to the primitive way of producing the cells and so the spleen and the liver begin to participate in the formation of these cells. This is often accompanied by the enlargement of organs such as the liver and spleen.

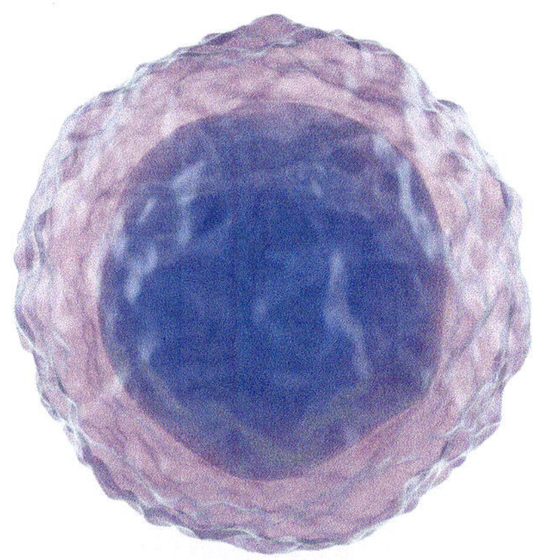

Figure 4.2 *Basic structure of a lymphocyte.*

There are two major populations of lymphocytes in peripheral circulation, the large and the small lymphocytes. However, functionally, these two are not known to be different. Generally, the nucleus is large with a tiny rim of cytoplasm (Figure 4.2).

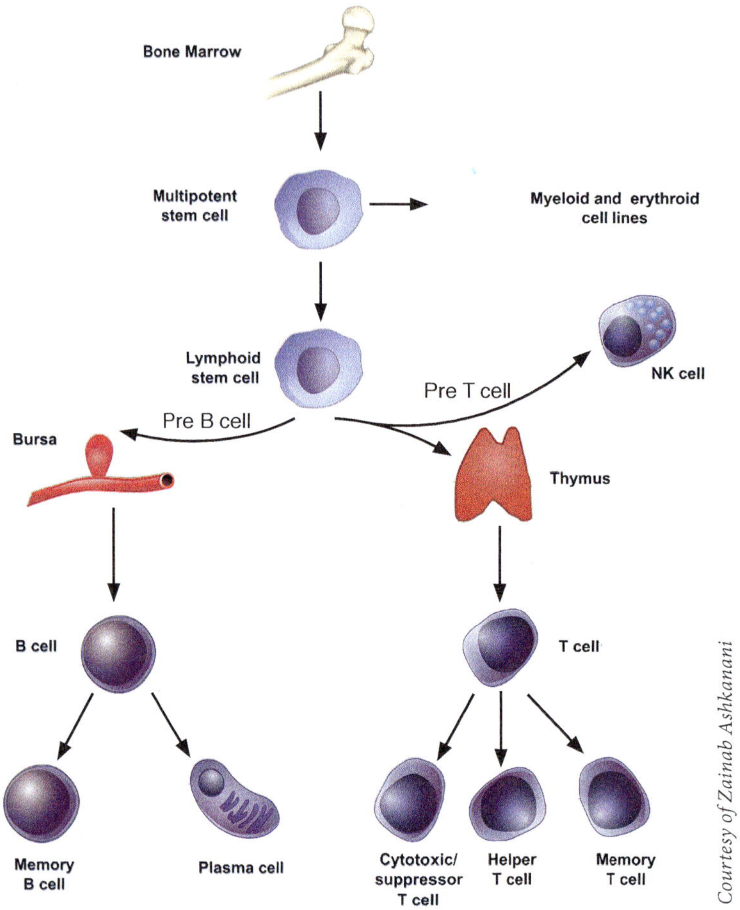

Figure 4.3 *The origin and development of B, T, and NK lymphocytes. The bursa is, of course, present only in birds. In mammals, its function is served by Peyer's patches or the bone marrow.*

The first group of cells that develop from the multipotent stem cell into the lymphoid series is the lymphoid stem cell; they can become B cells, T cells, or NK cells (Figure 4.3). They emerge from the marrow as pre-B, and pre-T cells. The B cells can be challenged to become antibody producing cells, the plasma cells, or cells that carry memory of previous challenge and therefore, with slight secondary challenge, they quickly begin to produce antibodies again.

The pre-T cells go to the thymus, they are not fully differentiated when they leave the bone marrow. In the thymus, they become fully differentiated and the ones that cannot become committed undergo apoptosis. The details as to how they selectively become specialized in function are reserved for the topic on tolerance. The T cells can become cytotoxic T cells, these are those subpopulation of T cells that kill other cells. They achieve this function through their secretions, through the markers that are on their surface and on the cell surface of the target cell. Some subpopulation may be suppressor in function (suppressor T cell), which regulate immune function. An important subset of T cells is the helper T cell, so called because they help the immune system to realize its function through their secretions of immune mediators (Figure 4.4).

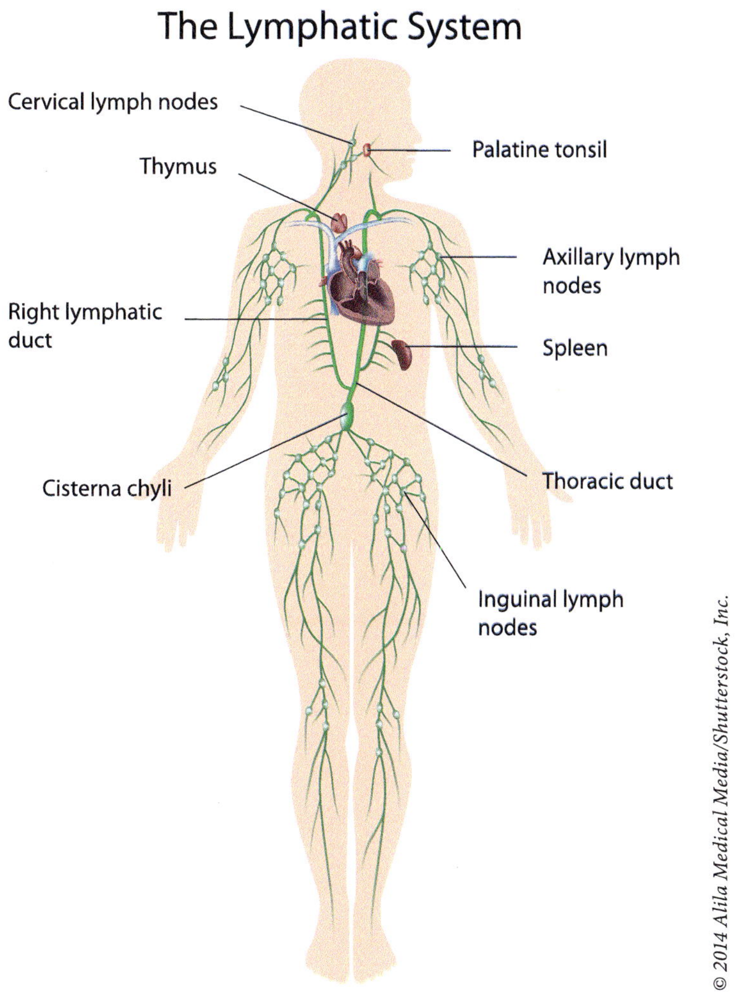

Figure 4.4 *Sites of lymphoreticular tissue. Primary organs include bone marrow and the thymus. Secondary organs are distributed throughout the body and include the spleen, lymph nodes, and MALT.*

The bone marrow is the largest tissue in the body, with a total weight of about 1300–1500 g in a normal adult. It is the site of antigen-independent lymphopoiesis (the development of lymphoid cells). The lymphocytes that are destined to become T cells go to the thymus for further development. The thymus is a small, flat, and bilobed organ, found in the thorax or chest cavity below the thyroid gland. It is located in the area anterior to the heart, posterior to the sternum. In humans, it gradually atrophies, a process described as thymic involution. Despite such atrophy or involution, the thymus continues to be a source of T-cell full development throughout an individual's life span.

The T cells, while developing in the thymus, acquire surface antigens (from the immunoglobulin superfamily, especially type I), as they travel from the cortex to the medulla. The subject of the acquisition of surface antigens and development of tolerance shall be addressed under the topic of tolerance.

T and B cells actually spend most of their life span in solid tissue, they only transverse the blood on their way to the tissues. The lymphoid tissues in which they spend most of their time are described as secondary lymphoid organs: the spleen and lymph nodes, tonsils, appendix, Peyer's patches in the intestine, and mucosal associated lymph tissues, also known as MALT. The primary lymphoid organs are the bone marrow and the thymus.

PRODUCTION OF LYMPHOCYTES

- Each individual lymphocyte, be it T cell or B cell, spends most of its life span in solid tissue, only traversing the circulatory system periodically to go from one secondary organ to the other.
- Lymphoid secondary organs include the spleen, lymph nodes, tonsils, appendix, Peyer's patches in the intestines, and other mucosal associated lymphoid tissue (MALT).
- Development of lymphocytes in the secondary tissue is strictly dependent on antigenic stimulation contrary to its development in the bone marrow. Most naive or resting lymphocytes die within a few days after leaving the primary lymphoid organs unless activated by Ags.
- When activated, they become long-lived memory cells and short-lived effector cells responsible for generation of immune responses.

The development of lymphocytes in the secondary lymphoid tissue usually depends on antigenic stimulation. This is distinct from what happens in the bone marrow, which is an antigen-independent stimulation. That is also why you cannot describe cells emanating from the marrow as really specific, because they have not been made so by a specific exposure to particular antigens. Most naïve or resting lymphocytes that emanate from the marrow, which are not stimulated and therefore have not gone through this process of antigen-dependent maturation, usually die within a few days after they have left the marrow or thymus. In contrast, when activated in the secondary lymphoid organ, they then become committed to specialized immune response, thus become long-lived, such as memory cells, or may become short-lived, but are able to produce immune mediators (cytokines), secretions that will have an effect on the immune system. The memory cells are capable of resuming the activity of protection upon subsequent stimulation down the road.

SPLEEN

- **Spleen** is the **largest secondary lymphoid organ**. It is located at the **upper left quadrant** of the **abdomen**, just below the **diaphragm**. It is surrounded by a thick **connective tissue** capsule. Its major function is to **filter** out **old** and **damaged cells** and **foreign Ags** from the body.
- The spleen consists of **two main** types of **tissues**—the **red** and **white** pulp (Figures 4.5 and 4.6).
- The **red** pulp makes up **more** than half the total **volume**; it plays a role in the destruction of **old red cells**. The **white pulp** contains **lymphoid** sheath (PALS).
- This sheath contains small and large lymphocytes, macrophages, plasma cells, and granulocytes.
- T cells are found close to the central arterioles, while B cells are located in the organization known as the primary follicles. B cells found here are not yet stimulated by Ags.

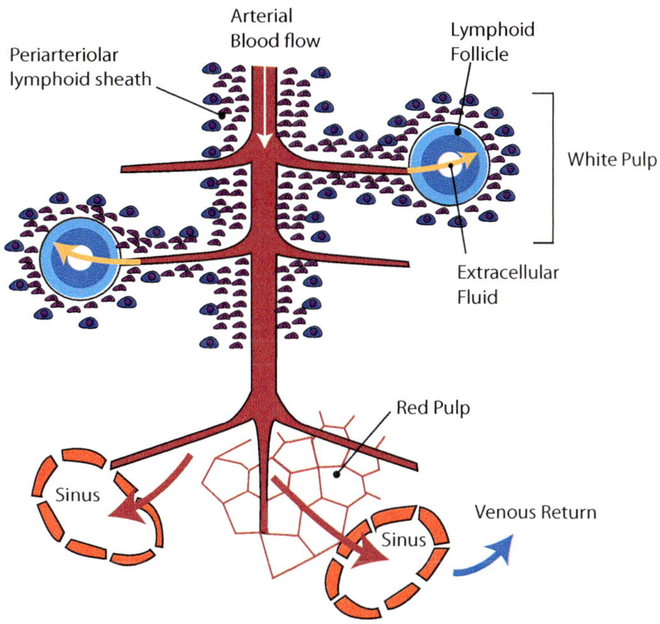

Figure 4.5 *Structure of spleen. The spleen has aggregates of lymphocytes similar to lymph nodes. Spleen weighs about 150 g and contains two distinct areas—red pulp and white pulp. Red pulp is formed when old and damaged red blood cells are removed from the circulation. White pulp is secondary lymphoid tissue.*

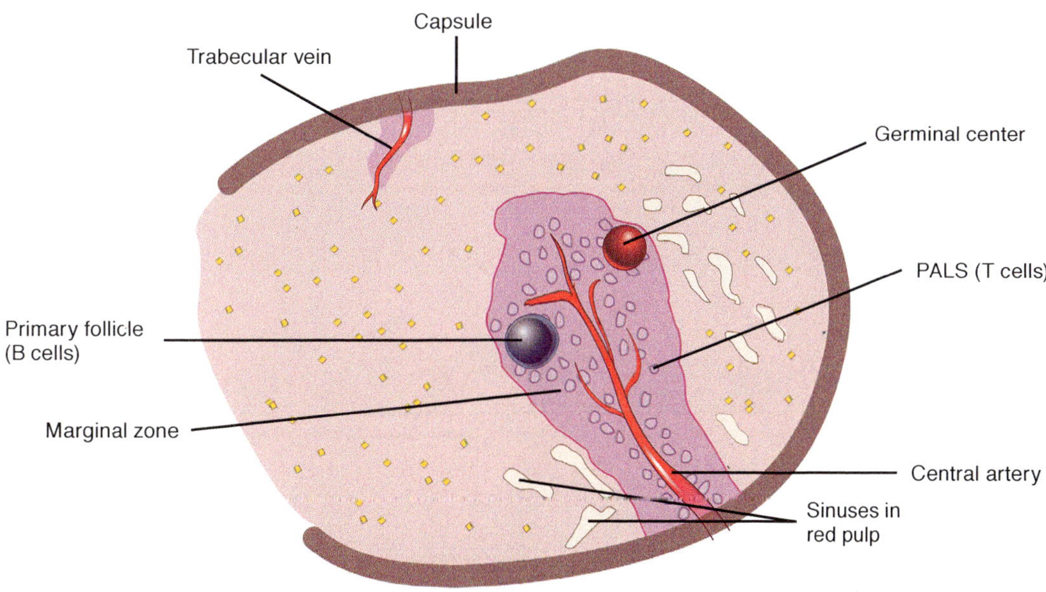

Figure 4.6 *Cross section of the spleen showing organization of the lymphoid tissue. T cells surround arterioles in the PAL. B cells are just beyond in follicles. When stimulated by an antigen, the B cells form germinal center. All of the lymphoid tissue is referred to as white pulp.*

LYMPH NODES

They are located along the lymphatic ducts (central collecting point for lymph fluid from adjacent tissues). Lymph nodes are especially numerous near joints and where arms and legs are joined to the body. Nodes range in size from 1 mm to about 25 mm in diameter. The tissue is organized into an outer cortex and an inner medulla. The subcapsular sinus (underneath the outer capsule) is lined by macrophages. Here, phagocytosis and Ag processing take place.

In primary follicles of the cortex are matured resting B cells, a small number of T cells, and specialized cells called follicular dendritic cells (responsible for Ag presentation and regulation of memory B cell activity).

- The secondary follicles consist of Ag-stimulated proliferating B cells. The interior of the secondary follicle is known as the germinal center because it is here that blast transformation of B cells takes place. Thus, plasma cells which actively secrete Abs and memory cells which transform into plasma cells are present.
- T cells are mainly located in the paracortex, the region adjoining the medulla. Here, T cells are in close proximity with Ag-presenting cells called interdigitating cells.
- The **medulla** is less **populated** but contains **some T cells** (in addition to B cells), **macrophages**, and small **plasma cells**.
- **MALT** is located in the **gastrointestinal**, **respiratory**, and **urogenital** tracts.
- The **tonsil**, **located** at the opening to the **oral** and **pharyngeal cavities**, is **endowed** with **macrophages** and **lymphocytes**. Its function is to **respond** to **pathogens entering** the **respiratory** and **alimentary** tracts.

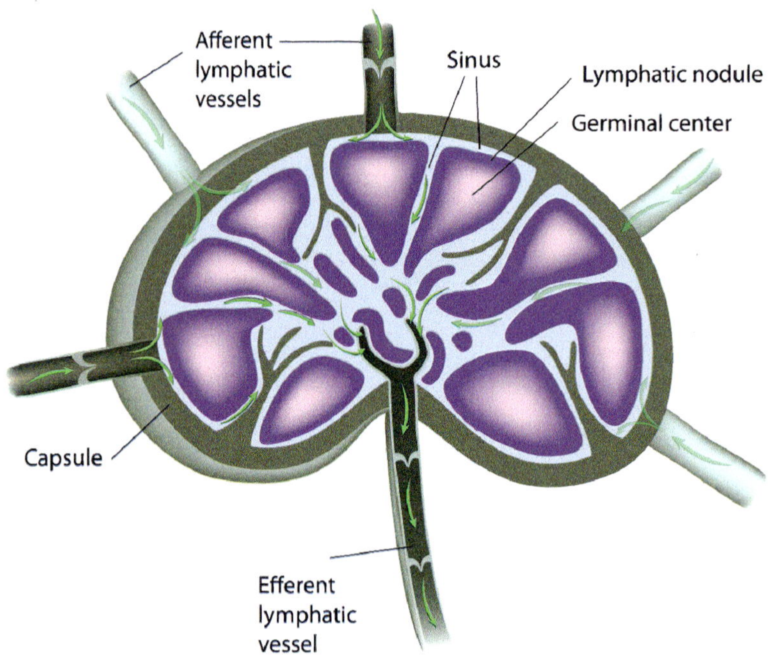

Figure 4.7 *Structure of a lymph node. A lymph node is surrounded by a tough outer capsule. Right underneath is the subcapsular sinus, where lymph drains from afferent lymphatic vessels. The outer cortex contains collections of B cells in primary follicles. When stimulated by antigen, secondary follicles are formed. T cells are found in the paracortical area. Fluid drains slowly through sinusoid to the medullary region and out of the efferent lymphatic vessel to the thoracic duct.*

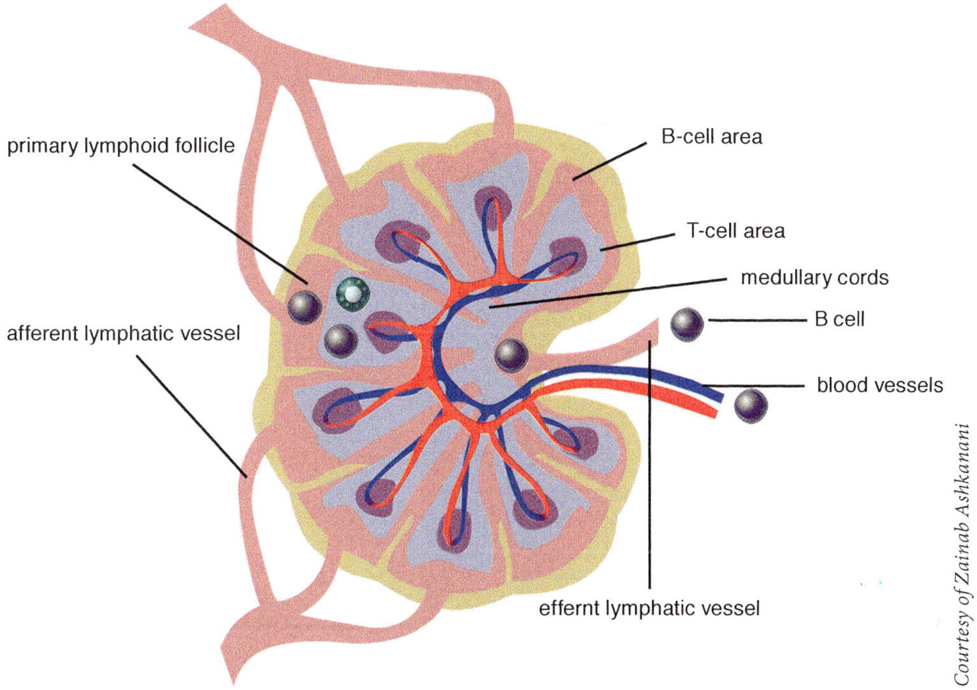

Figure 4.8 *B-cell circulation route in secondary lymphoid tissue: the lymph node. B cells are transported to the lymph node via the blood stream and enter the cortex through highly specialized high endothelial venules (HEV). If their specific antigen is not encountered in the cortex, the B cells will migrate out through efferent lymphatic vessel to eventually join the blood in the neck.*

Upon an immune challenge, the lymphatics draining that area transmit the infection and then the lymph nodes become swollen, because the cells are responding to the infection. Lymph nodes are especially numerous near the joints and where the arms and legs are joined to the body. They range in size from 1 mm to 25 mm, depending on which ones are being considered and whether they have been challenged or not (Figures 4.7 and 4.8). The lymph nodes are organized into the cortex, which is the external part, and the medulla, the internal part. The subcapsular sinus, which is the area beneath the thick covering called the capsule, is lined usually by macrophages. Here, phagocytosis and antigen processing and presentation take place.

The primary follicles of the lymph node have in their cortex, matured resting B cells, and sometimes a small number of T cells. Just as in the case of the spleen, the B cells have not been challenged, while in the secondary follicular centers, they have been challenged. The secondary follicles consist of antigen-stimulated, proliferating B cells. The interior of the secondary follicle is the germinal center. It is here that blast transformation of B cells takes place, so called because when cells begin to divide they assume a more primitive appearance, so that they can commence division. Plasma cells, derived from B cells, which actively secrete antibodies, and memory cells that develop into plasma cells are all found in the germinal center. Apart from the B and T cells, the primary follicles have a small number of special cells called follicular dendritic cells which are also responsible for antigen presentation, and they regulate memory B cells in addition.

The T cells are mainly located in the paracortex, which is the area of the cortex adjoining the medulla. It is here that T cells are in close proximity with those cells that will present antigens to them, the interdigitating cells. The medulla, which is after the cortex, is usually less populated but contains some T cells, B cells, macrophages, and plasma cells.

MUCOSAL-ASSOCIATED LYMPHOID TISSUES (MALT)

These are another group of secondary lymphoid tissue; they are located in the mucous lining such as gastrointestinal tract, the respiratory tract, and the urogenital tract.

THE TONSIL

It is located at the point where the mouth and the pharynx join; it is endowed with macrophages and lymphocytes. Its function is to respond to pathogens entering the respiratory tract and the alimentary canal.

THE LYMPHOCYTE

- Lymphocytes constitute 20–30% of circulating leukocytes, and they have a long life span. According to size, they are classified as small or large. Small lymphocytes are 8–10 μm, with a tiny rim of cytoplasm; they are either T or B lymphocytes. The large lymphocytes are about 16 μm and have more abundant cytoplasm with few granules.
- B lymphocytes constitute about 5–15% of circulating lymphocytes and they express surface immunoglobulin (sIg) which binds specifically to corresponding antigens.
- B lymphocytes have surface markers including immunoglobulin Fc receptor (CD16).
- B cells develop from committed lymphocytes. Already during early stages of fetal life, lymphopoiesis begins in fetal liver, and then later the bone marrow takes over and continues after birth. Maturation occurs in two stages: antigen independent and antigen dependent.

They constitute 20–30% of white blood cells and have a long life span. The recorded counts of lymphocytes are those transiting the blood on their way to the tissue from the bone marrow. The information obtained from such count is, however, quite useful because their increase in peripheral blood signifies an increase in release from the marrow, reflecting a positive stimulation of the marrow in response to infection, especially viral infection. As previously explained, they are either large (about 16 μm) or small (8–10 μm). Generally, they are either T or B lymphocytes, so there's nothing about that small size that determines the kind of lymphocyte.

The B lymphocytes usually are about 5–15% of the circulating leukocytes. They express surface immunoglobulins that bind specifically to their corresponding antigen, thus serving as receptors. Most of the surface immunoglobulins expressed are usually of the heavy chain μ, that is, IgM, but monomeric. However, there are a few IgGs; in that case, the heavy chain is γ, but in mucosal associated lymphoid tissue, the form of surface immunoglobulins are IgA, that is, the heavy chain constant region is α.

B lymphocytes have surface markers and also Fc receptors. These surface markers include CD16, complement receptors, CD11b, CD35, and MCH class II molecules. MHC molecules are antigen-presenting molecules. Other receptors include CD19, CD20, and CD21. B cells develop from committed lymphocytes already during the early stages of fetal life.

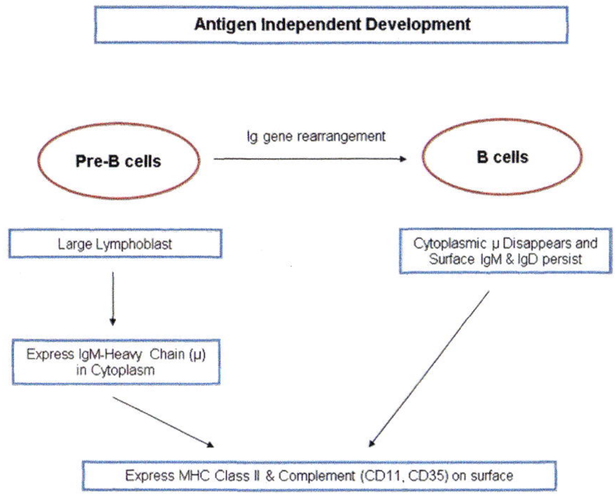

Courtesy of Zainab Ashkanani

Figure 4.9 *Schematic of antigen-independent development.*

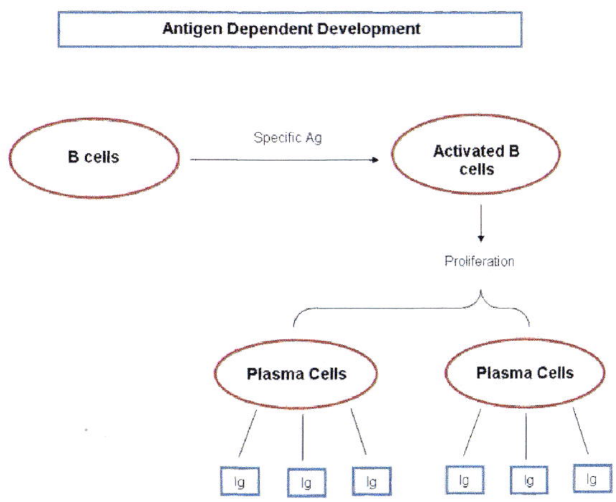

Courtesy of Zainab Ashkanani

Figure 4.10 *Schematic of antigen-dependent development.*

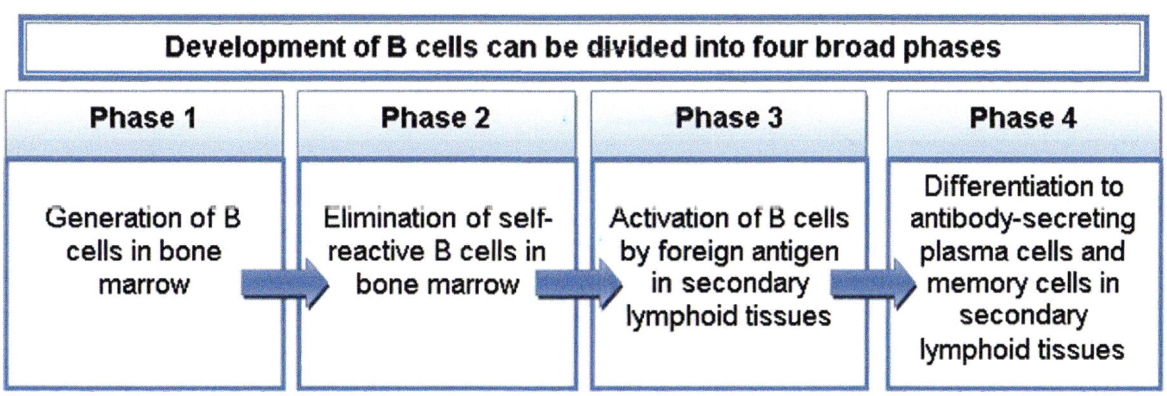

Courtesy of Zainab Ashkanani

Figure 4.11 *Four broad phases of the development of B cells.*

B cell maturation occurs in two stages: antigen independent, which is the continuous development in the marrow, but developed enough to have surface markers which are specialized that can be used to identify them. Then there is also the antigen dependent development (Figure 4.9–4.11). These B cells that migrate to the secondary lymphoid tissue become specific because of their encounter with antigen, this exposure changes course to antigen-mediated development.

In antigen-independent development, there is gene rearrangement in the lymphoblast resulting in the formation of matured B cells. The heavy chain μ can already be discerned in the cytoplasm (not on the surface) in antigen-independent development which is in the marrow. Also, they express MHC class II and complement receptors on their surface. At this stage at which they become fully matured B cells, their cytoplasmic μ disappears and surface IgM and IgD are now expressed.

When they encounter an antigen, especially a specific antigen, the antigen-dependent maturation sequence commences. The cells are activated, they begin to divide, and they become plasma cells which synthesize antibodies. Plasma cells do not have surface immunoglobulin expressed.

- Antigen-independent maturation begins when a stem cell destined to become B cell divides many times with immunoglobulin gene rearrangement and becomes a pre-B cell. Pre-B cell is a large lymphoblast expressing (1) IgM heavy chains in its cytoplasm (but not on its surface), (2) MHC class II, and (3) complement (CD11b, CD35) receptors on its surface. On full maturation, cytoplasmic μ heavy chains are no longer present but surface IgM and IgD are expressed.
- When B cells encounter a specific antigen, a sequence of development which may be described as antigen-dependent maturation commences.

  (i) Cell is activated, (ii) proliferation occurs, (iii) differentiation into plasma cells which synthesize and secrete specific immunoglobulins. Plasma cells do not express surface immunoglobulin.
- T lymphocytes constitute 80% of circulating lymphocytes; they have effector and regulatory functions. Effector functions include cytolysis of virally infected cells, tumor targeting, and lymphokine production. The regulatory function include increase or suppression of other lymphocytes and accessory cells.

Physiologically, about 20–30% of circulating leukocytes are lymphocytes. About 80% of them are T cells, thymus-dependent lymphocytes. They have functions that impact the immune system as follows: direct effect and regulatory effect on other cells of the immune system (by secretion of immune mediators). The effector functions include cytolysis, that is, the destruction of cells, such cells that have been virally infected carry markers on their surface that are recognizable by T cells, thus eliciting attack. Also, cells that are growing abnormally because of neoplastic changes will also be targeted for attack even if they are benign tumors. The effector function also results in cytokine secretion. The regulatory functions include increase or suppression of other lymphocytes and accessory cells (Figure 4.12).

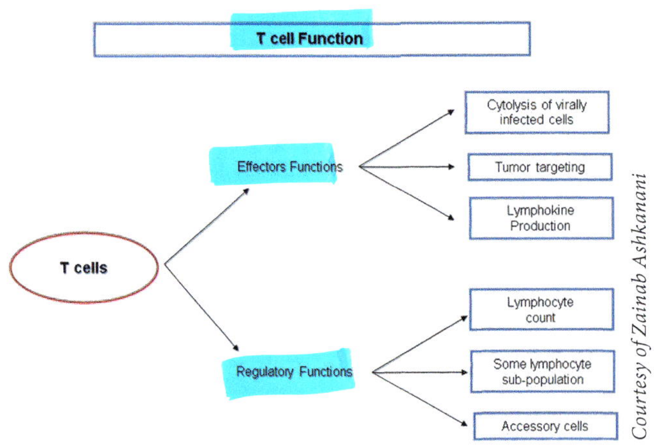

Figure 4.12 *Schematic showing T-cell function.*

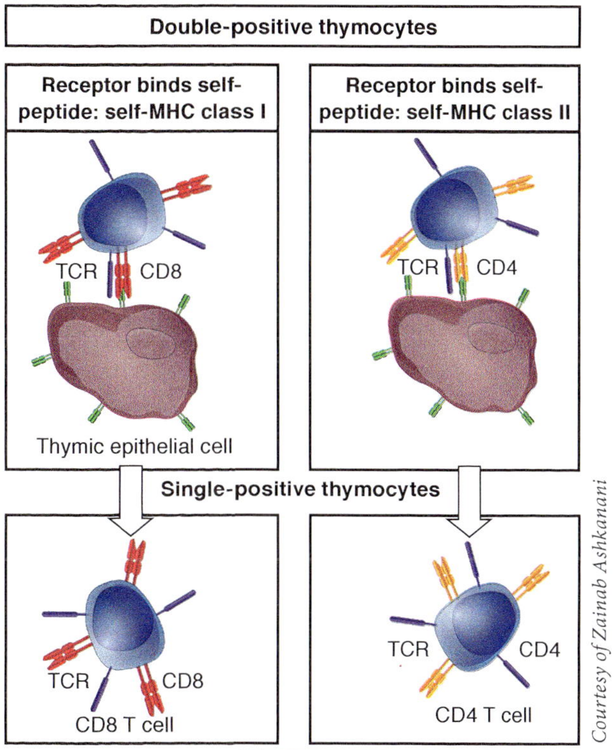

Figure 4.13 *Interaction of a double-positive T cell with a self-peptide–self-MCH complex. The interaction during positive selection determines if the T cell will become a CD4 or CD8 T cell.*

- T cells have the classical CD2 surface marker to which sheep red blood cells have a receptor (basis of classical erythrocyte rosetting). Also, all circulating T cells have CD3 which is associated with T cell antigen receptor complex.
- T cells have two important subsets expressing different CD markers and are functionally distinct: (i) helper T cells which express CD4 and (ii) suppressor T cells which express CD8.
- Pre-T cell maturation begins during fetal life in the liver, then in the bone marrow, and finally migrates to the thymus. Lymphocytes in the thymus are also called thymocytes. Pre-T cells contain terminal deoxynucleotidyl transferase (Tdt) in their nucleus, which serves as marker for primitive T cells.
- Initial maturation in the thymic cortex commences with the cell having CD2 and CD3 markers, subsequently there is coexistence of CD4 and CD8 cells along with CD2 and CD3. However, as they migrate into the thymic medulla, either CD4 or CD8 molecule is lost and at this point also, TdT is no longer produced (Figure 4.13).

T cells migrate as very primitive forms in the bone marrow to primary lymphoid tissue of the thymus and then migrate to the secondary lymphoid organs. The enzyme TdT usually plays an important role in DNA development. When they move from the marrow into the thymus, they become more mature and committed. At the point at which they enter the thymus, they are characterized by markers such as CD2 (responsible for rosetting of sheep erythrocytes), CD3 (antigen receptor complex), CD4, and CD8. They have lost the TdT. T cells have two important subsets expressing different CD markers, and of course, are functionally distinct. One set is the helper T cells that express the CD4, while the other ones are called suppressor T cells, because they are actually suppressing other aspects of the immune system in their functions. These express CD8 surface antigens. In the thymus, T cells are committed to become either CD4 T cells, which are helper T cells, so called because they help the immune system through their secretions and their action on challenges. It is important to note that these CD4 cells would have lost their CD8 marker. Or, on the other hand, they can be committed to become CD8 cells, and these have the general marker of the T cells, but not the CD4. The immature T cells that fail to get committed go through apoptosis. The initial maturation of T cells in the thymic cortex will commence with cells having CD2 and CD3 markers. All of these will coexist with CD4 and CD8, because they are not specialized yet. As they migrate into the medulla from the cortex, they become either CD4 or CD8 by losing the function of TdT enzyme, which is used up in the process of maturation. It is important to note that a cell type is CD 4 doesn't mean they are totally homogeneous.

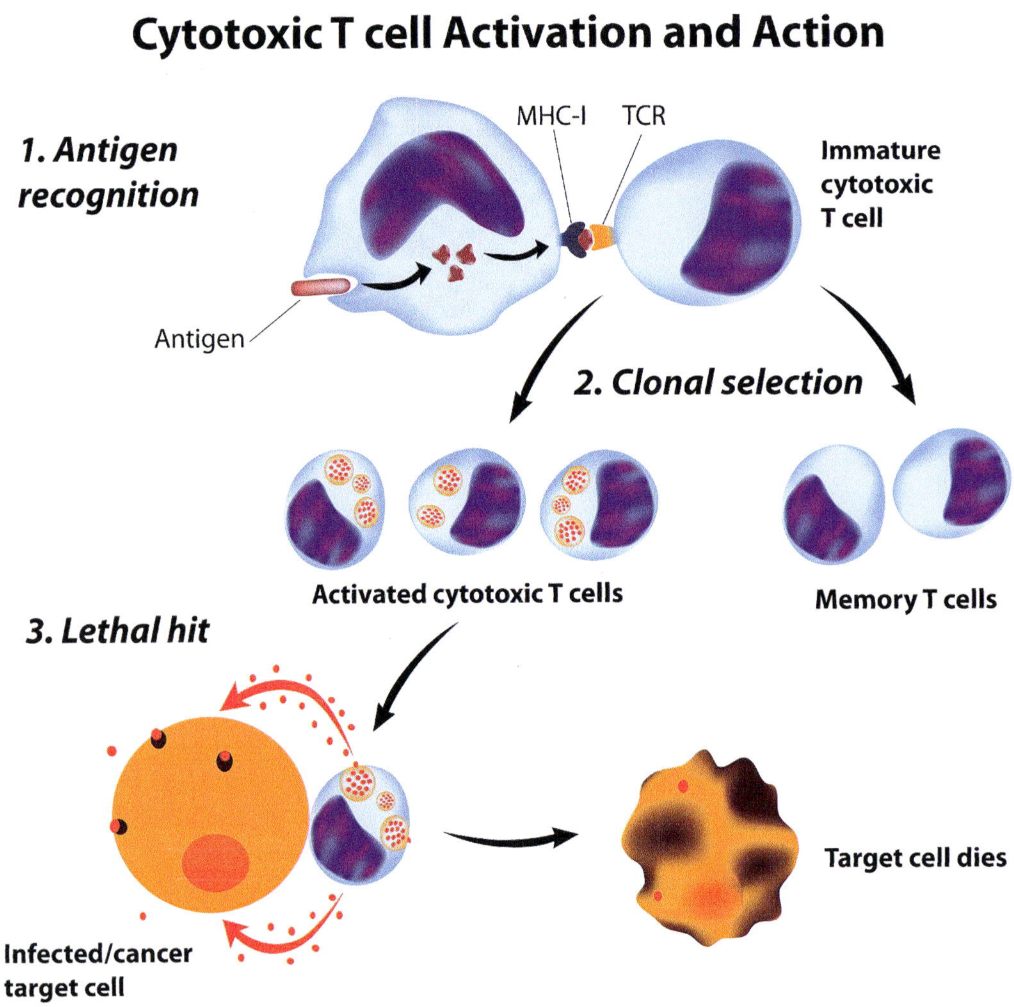

Figure 4.14 *Cytotoxic CD8 T cells selectively kill infected cells. Specific recognition of peptides–MCH complex on an infected cell by a cytotoxic CD8 T cell programs the infected cell to die. The T cell then detaches from its target cell and synthesizes a new set of lytic granules. Cytotoxic T-lymphocyte then seeks out and kills another target.*

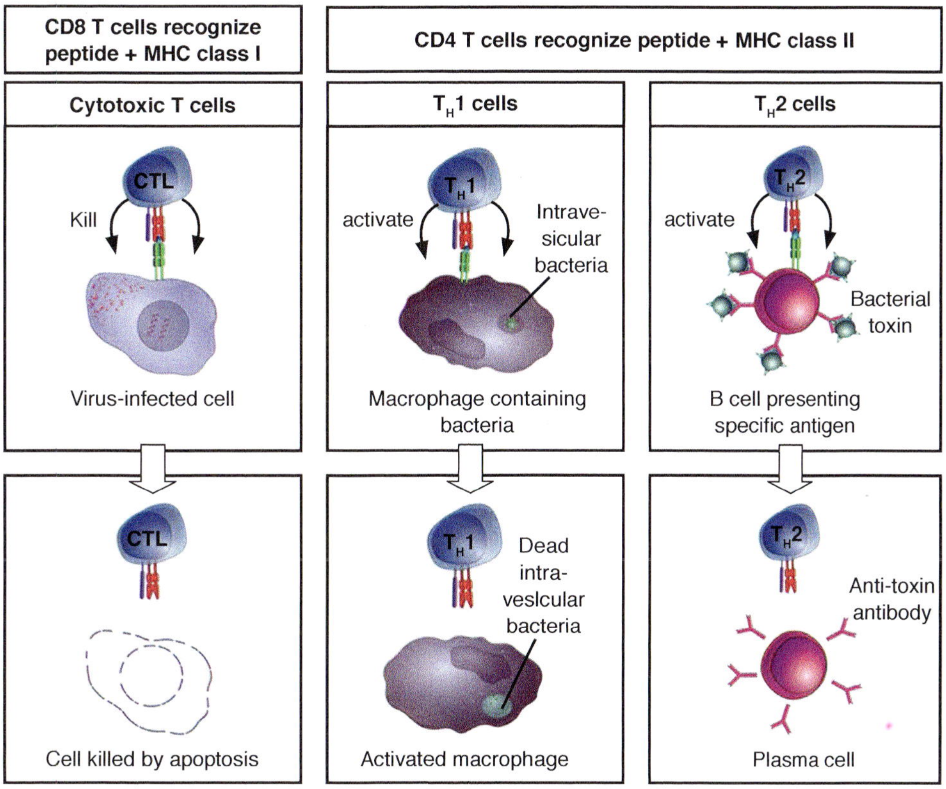

Courtesy of Zainab Ashkanani

Figure 4.15 *The three classes of T cells. These are specialized to deal with three types of pathogens. CD8 cells deal with viral infected cells, TH1 cells deal with bacterial peptides that have been phagocytosed and processed by macrophages, and TH2 cells activate B cells and control many aspects of the antibody response.*

The CD4 cells have subsets; some are heightened for cellular response such as the TH1 cells that usually activate macrophages and B cells, and production of opsonizing antibodies such as IgG_1. The TH2 cells are more heightened for humoral response, thus they activate B cells to make general antibodies (Figures 4.14 and 4.15).

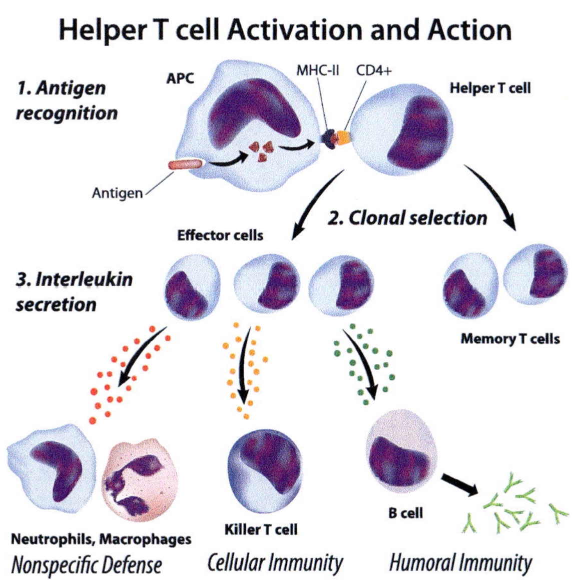

© 2014 Alila Medical Media /Shutterstock, Inc.

Figure 4.16 *Stages of the activation of helper T cells.*

The cytotoxic T cells have killing capability through receptor–ligand interactions.

The CD8 T cells recognize peptides that are presented. When cells present antigens, they use MCH molecules. The MCH class I specifically present molecules to CD8 cells, and it is usually related to viral infection, while the CD4 cells will recognize antigens presented with MHC class II. Therefore, an encounter with antigens and the various patterns to it is what the chart in Figure 4.16 is showing you. This aspect will be addressed under the topic of antigen presentation and the major histocompatibility complex.

There are numerous surface markers on T and B cells. Figure 4.17 below shows the profile of such markers.

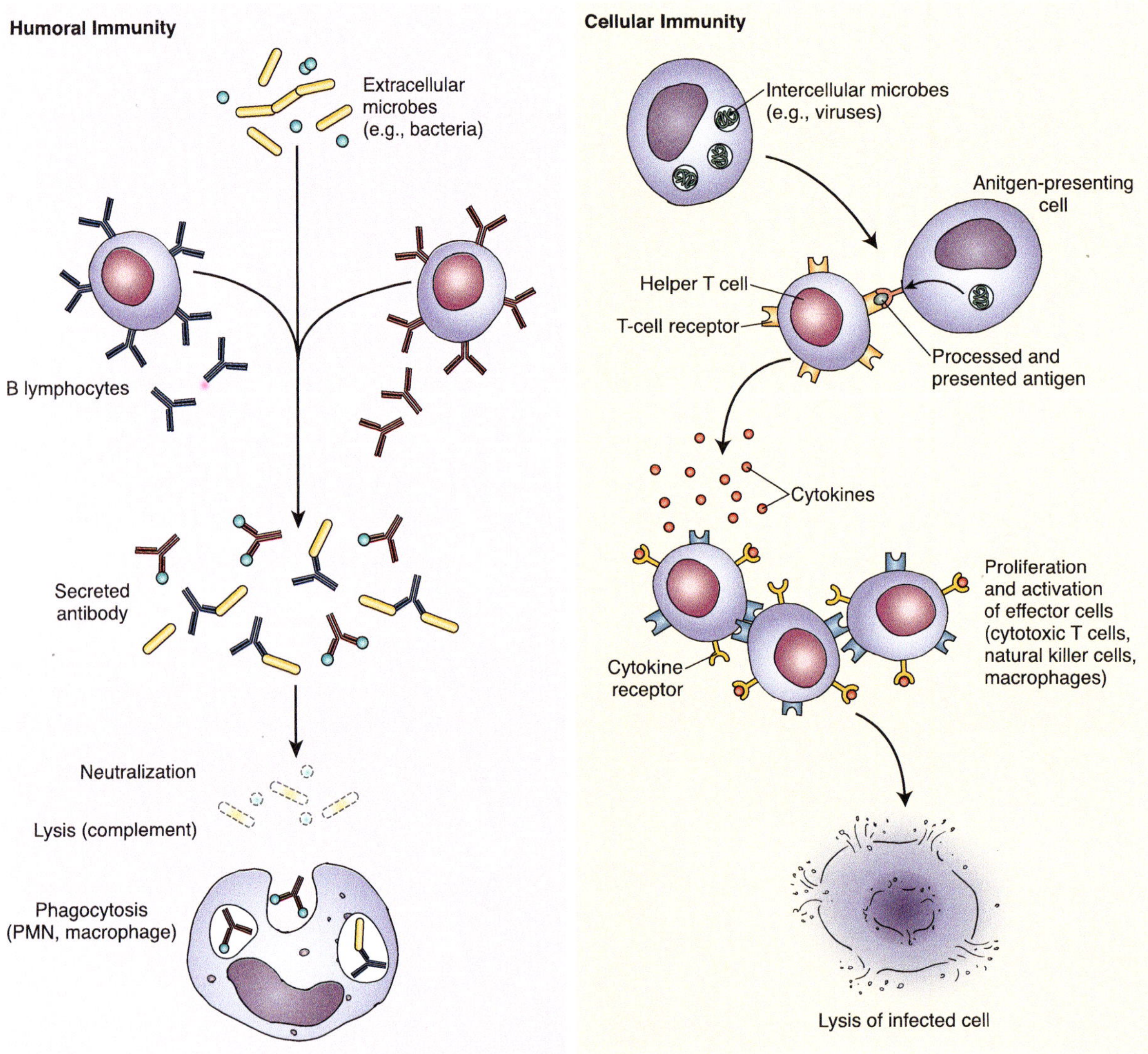

Figure 4.17 *Encounters with antigens result in naïve T cells becoming activated effector cells or long-lived memory T cells.*

SAMPLE QUESTIONS

THE LYMPHOID TISSUE

1. All of the organs below are part of the immune system *except* the
   a. thyroid
   b. thymus
   c. spleen
   d. Payer's patches

2. In which organ do T lymphocytes mature?
   a. marrow
   b. Thymus
   c. Lymph nodes
   d. Spleen

3. One characteristic cell surface molecule largely restricted to human thymocytes is
   a. CD4
   b. CD8
   c. TCR
   d. CD45
   e. Thy-1

Answer True or False to the following:

<u>Lymphocyte origins</u>

4. Lymphocytes are derived from pluripotent hematopoietic stem cells.
5. The bone marrow is the center of antigen-dependent lymphopoiesis.
6. Immature lymphocytes are released from the bone marrow and they travel to secondary lymphoid organs for continued maturation.
7. Lymphocytes that go into the thymus develop are T-cells.

<u>Lymphocyte production</u>

8. Each individual lymphocyte spends most of its life span in the circulatory system, only passing into solid tissue when it is needed there.
9. Secondary lymphoid organs include the spleen, lymph nodes, tonsils, appendix, Payer's patches in the intestines, and other mucosal associated lymphoid tissue.
10. Development of lymphocytes in secondary tissues is independent of antigenic stimulation.
11. Activated lymphocytes become long-lived memory cells and short-lived effector cells responsible for the generation of immune responses.

Spleen

12. The major function of the spleen is to filter out old and damaged cells and foreign antigens from the body.
13. The red pulp of the spleen makes up less than half the total volume, and it contains the lymphoid sheath.
14. The lymphoid sheath contains small and large lymphocytes, macrophages, plasma cells, and granulocytes.
15. B cells found in the spleen are found in the primary follicles, and they have not been stimulated by antigens yet.

Suggested Laboratory Practicals

- Case Studies on:
1. Primary Lymphoid Organs
2. Secondary Lymphoid Organs
- Laboratory Identification of Lymphocytes
- Cell Flow Cytometry
- Fluorescence Microscopy
- Enumeration of Viable and Nonviable Cells
- Use of CD2 as a T-cell Marker

CHAPTER 5

CELLULAR INTERACTIONS

WHY STUDY CELL–CELL INTERACTIONS IN IMMUNOLOGY?

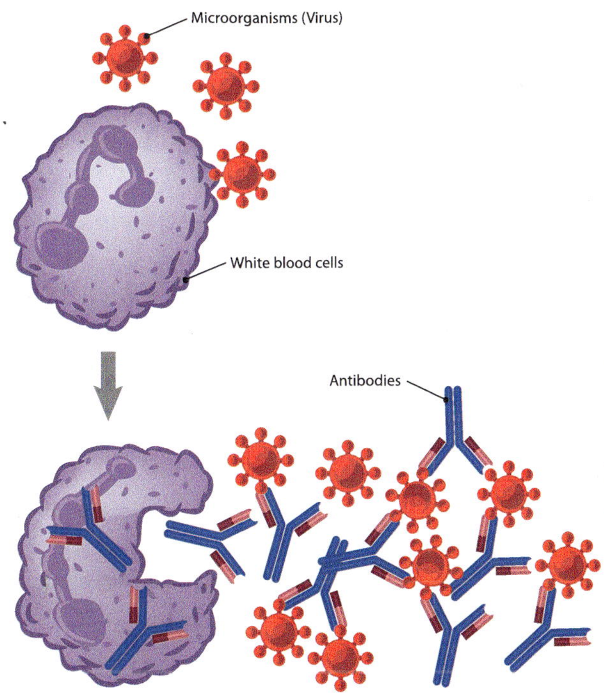

Figure 5.1 *Structure of an antibody and T-cell receptor. T-cell receptors are very similar to Fab fragments of antibodies, thus providing room for protein–protein interactions.*

In the sense of the immune system, a typical example of cellular interaction is the one involving a phagocyte to which an antibody binds after the antibody has reacted with an antigen on a bacterial cell surface (see Figure 5.1). The consequence of such interaction is the endocytosis of the bacterium, the digestion of the bacterium by lysosomal enzymes, the elaboration of immune mediators by the phagocyte, the selection of conserved peptide of the bacterium, and the presentation of the peptide by antigen-presenting molecules. This sequence of events usually initiates a new sequence of cellular interaction such as those that accompany antigen presentation by an antigen-presenting cell and recognition by an antigen-recognizing cell. Therefore, an understanding of the general mechanisms by which cells respond to changes in their external and internal environment is essential. The recognition process mentioned above results in the elaboration of cytokines that mediate further immune response. Thus, the surfaces of cells are lined with proteins that participate in the cell's functional processes. The orientation of the protein molecules and the functional groups that are exposed are useful in predicting and understanding the nature of reactions in which they are involved.

Cellular Interactions

- Nomenclature of cell surface proteins
- Dynamics of cell surface protein (endo and exocytosis)
- Membrane receptors and cell functions
- Adhesion Molecules

Some aspects of cellular interaction that a fair understanding of is needed include nature of the cell surface protein, the dynamics of cell surface protein, general types of receptors involved in cell signaling, and cell adhesion molecules.

CELLULAR INTERACTIONS

- Membranes have **fluid phospholipid** bilayer. **Attached** to or **embedded** within this phospholipid are **proteins** (cell surface proteins).
- Through these **proteins**, cells **communicate** with their **environment** (receiving and transmitting signals). These **signals** are **chemical** in nature in the case of the **immune system.**
- Reception and transmission of signals involve distinct steps which include
  - **ligand** and **surface** receptor interaction.
  - **transmission** of **information** on occupied receptor **to the interior** of cell.
  - **selective** turning **on** or **off** of **genes.**
  - Cell response: I° events—occur immediately after all receptors are occupied. 2° events—subsequent events.

The presence of proteins that affect cell functions make the presence of cells in close proximity a significant occurrence. The molecular facilitators of the enhanced close proximity of cells play a paramount role in effective interaction, efficient transduction, and transmission of signals.

A suitable example is the production of deliberate biomolecules like the adhesion molecules that can drive movement in a particular direction, just as in the case of neutrophils, which crawl on endothelial surface due to cell adhesion molecule elaboration, following the presence of bacterium, instead of floating in blood.

What are the steps involved in this process that is described as "signaling"? When a ligand adheres to a receptor, the outcome of such receptor–ligand interaction is the transmission of information about events at the cell surface to the deep interior of the cell without further movement as such from the cell surface. This kind of transmission of information without obvious movement is called signaling. Signals can be chemical or electrical. Most of the signals in immune response are chemical in nature (Figure 5.2).

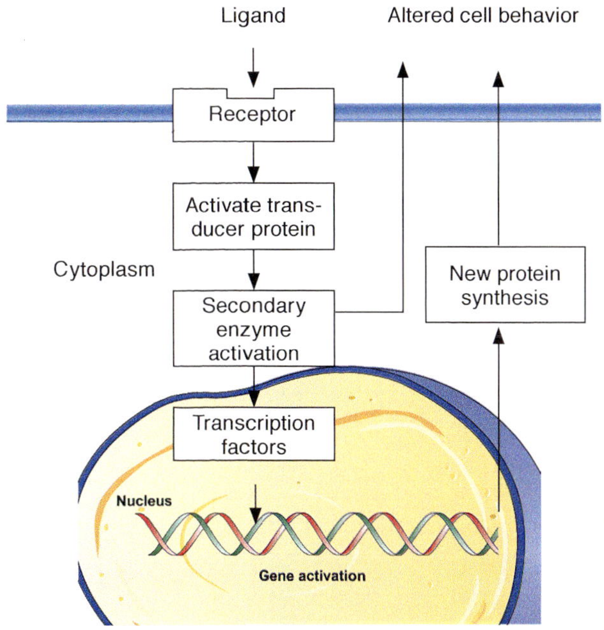

Courtesy of Zainab Ashkanani

Figure 5.2 *Basic features of the signal transduction pathways. Transductions are protein arrangements that bring about energy transformation.*

So, there is a ligand–receptor interaction and it starts in the cell exterior. This information is then transferred from the surface of the receptor where the ligand binds to, to deep within the cell, resulting in molecular events occurring deep inside the cell, events such as the switching on or off of genes. The overall effect is the change in cell behavior. Events can be early (immediate), intermediate, or late. Secondary response refers to subsequent events, such as intermediate and late events.

SURFACE PROTEINS

There are specialized biomolecules, mainly protein in nature, usually inserted in fluid phospholipid bilayer of membranes which allow cell–cell interactions. These proteins are specialized glycoproteins in nature.

CELL SURFACE PROTEINS

i. Loosely attached by hydrophobic bond and are easily removed.

ii. Integral membrane proteins.

- Cell surface proteins may be grouped according to their method of attachment to the membrane.
- Integral membrane proteins pass completely through the lipid bilayer once and are thus exposed to both the cytoplasm and extracellular environment.

TYPES OF INTEGRAL MEMBRANE PROTEINS

- Most are **type I** proteins in which the amino terminus is at the extracellular end and the carboxyl terminus is in the cytoplasm.
- **Type II** integral membrane proteins have a similar structure but their orientation is reversed.

- A **third type** is attached directly to the membrane lipid by a short phosphatidyl inositol linker chain.
- The **fourth** and **fifth type** of cell membrane protein pass through the cell membrane either four or seven times, exposing several sites to the cytoplasm and the extracellular fluid.

There are various cell surface proteins, some of them are usually loosely bound by hydrophobic bond, and can be easily removed; there are others that are integral membrane proteins, that is, they are deep proteins within the membrane, which are not easily removed. The integral membrane proteins which exhibit a level of permanence can be defined on the basis of their method of attachment to the membrane. Since proteins are not straight molecules as such but coiled, the nature of the functional group exposed to the cell exterior or interior plays an important role in their interactions and reveals information about the transductional processes in which it is involved. On the basis of the method of attachment to membrane, integral membrane protein can be classified into types I to V (Figures 5.3–5.7).

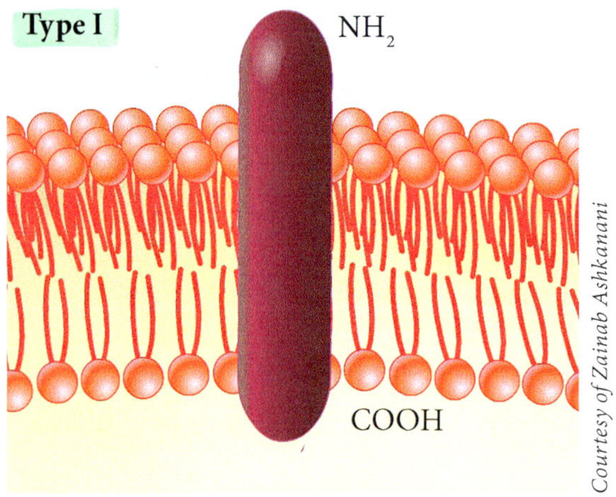

Figure 5.3 *Structure of integral membrane protein. Type I: Transmembrane proteins—single-pass polypeptides with their C-terminal in the cytosol, and the N-terminus outside. The domain that passes through the cell membrane is the hydrophobic sequence and this enables it to bind to membrane lipids. They are the most common form of surface proteins in leukocytes.*

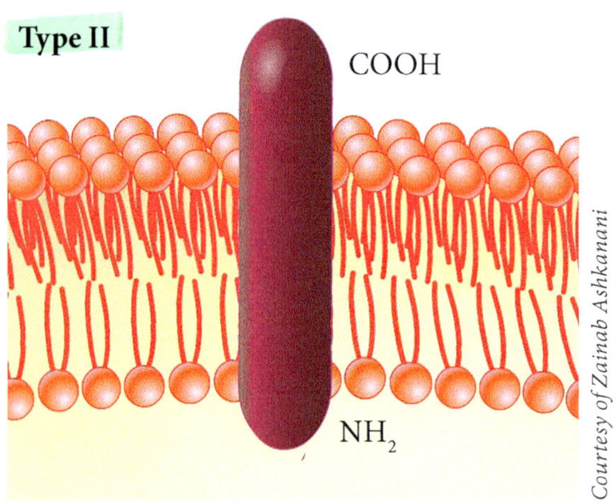

Figure 5.4 *Structure of integral membrane protein. Type II: They are also single-pass polypeptides but have opposite orientation to type I. The N-terminus is in the cytosol, while the C-terminus is extracellular.*

Most of them are types I or II. The type I has the amino terminus outside, with the carboxyl terminus facing the cytoplasm. Type II simply will have the same structure, but there is a reverse in the orientation of the functional group, the carboxyl terminus is on the outside, and the amino terminus is on the inside.

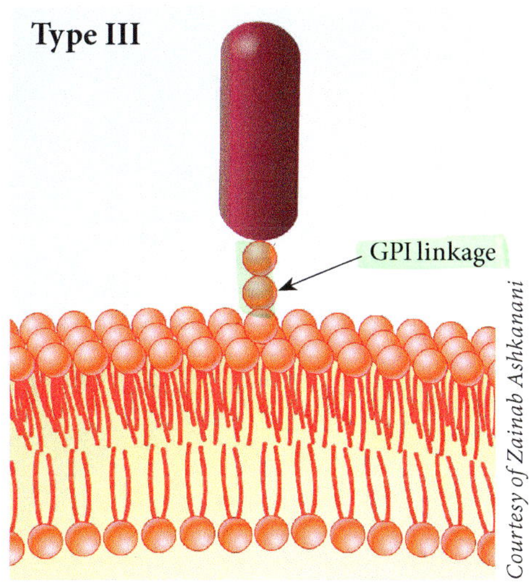

Figure 5.5 *Structure of integral membrane protein. Type III: They are covalently attached to cell membrane by glycosylphosphatidylinositol (GPI); for example, Ty-I molecules found in immature t cells.*

The third type is attached directly to the membrane lipid, usually there's a short piece of phospholipid, and the typical example is the one in which the phosphatidyl inositol serves as a linker chain. This linker chain appears to contribute to the amplification of a signal, a capability that is due to the attribute of phospholipids being a high-energy molecule.

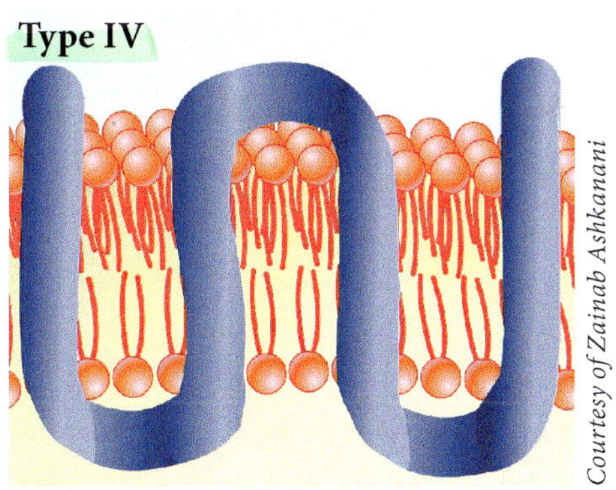

Figure 5.6 *Structure of integral membrane protein. Type IV: These are integral transmembrane proteins which pass through the membrane several times, specifically four times. They have hydrophobic and hydrophilic regions—the hydrophobic region is in association with membrane lipids, while the hydrophilic region is in association with aqueous tissue fluid. They are found not only on neutrophils but also on MØ and T cells.*

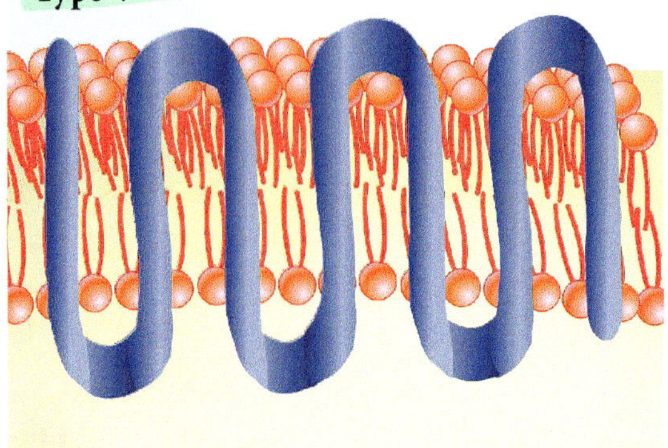

Figure 5.7 *Structure of integral membrane protein. Type V: Like type IV pass through membrane several times, usually up to seven times. They are common in macrophage and lymphocytes.*

The type IV and V transmembrane proteins are coiled either four or more times. This number of coils may be related to the extent to which they can interact with the appropriate ligand, because the exposed surfaces may be related to the tendency of interaction. There is a relationship between the distribution of protein type and what function the cell performs.

CELL SURFACE DYNAMICS

The proteins observed on cell surfaces are assembled in the cell interior and are coupled in intracellular structures such as endoplasmic reticulum and the Golgi apparatus. Also, there are components of the extracellular environment that are packaged within the cell before being spilled out, or components of the extracellular environment that are being internalized by the cell because of their enormous relevance to cell function. In this bidirectional movement, the process involves either the pinching off or invagination of biological particles on the membrane. If it is invagination that occurs, it leads to the formation of vacuoles. These vacuoles can be dismembered and their essential constituents are taken and assembled back into the cell. Endocytosis is the term used to describe the process of internalization of particles from outside. Those that are transported from the inside to fuse with the outer membrane and finally spill into the environment are said to have undergone exocytosis.

Newly formed complexes are sent to the exterior of the cell, they are exteriorized by the process of exocytosis, sometimes they will not be needed to be completely pushed out, and they need to be shifted to form an association with the interior part of the membrane, so it will fuse there. That is how a cell system becomes more and more complex.

CELL SURFACE RECEPTORS AND SIGNALING

In the interaction between cells, cells must be able to sense their surroundings and react accordingly. For example, neutrophils must detect the presence of bacteria and must be able to move purposefully toward the direction (by chemotaxis) where the challenge is present. Also, neutrophils become prepared for the actions needed for the killing of the bacteria before the intervention of other responses from other cells of the immune system. It is important to note that these events begin with interaction on the surface of the neutrophil. The conversion of these extracellular chemical events of receptor—ligand interactions to information that is transmitted deep into cell interior is called signal transduction.

CELL SURFACE RECEPTORS AND SIGNAL TRANSDUCTION

- In the **interaction** between **cells**, cells must be able to sense their surrounding and react accordingly.
- Membranes are endowed with receptors to which ligands bind; signals are generated and transmitted to the nucleus.
- The conversion of **extracellular signal** into series of **intracellular events** is called **transduction**.
- **There are four major types** of **mechanisms** by which **receptor signals** are **transduced**.
- Protein tyrosine kinases may be an **integral membrane protein** which is activated in the **cytoplasmic portion** of the molecule via ligand receptor interaction.
- Alternatively, the receptor protein to which the ligand binds may be **coupled to a separate cytoplasmic** protein tyrosine kinase.

There are four major types of mechanisms by which the receptor signals are transmitted.

Cell surface receptors are of four classes.

i. **Channel-linked receptors:** Receptors that use **transmitted ion gated channels** for rapid signaling as in nerve cells. Thus, the receptor itself is a channel, and **binding** to the agonist **opens** the **channel** and allows **ions to flow** through it. Channel-linked receptors are found in inflammatory and immune cells.

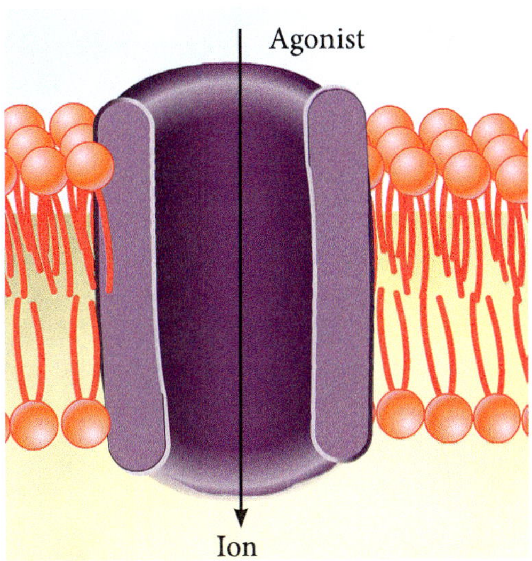

Figure 5.8 *A channel-linked receptor.*

The first example is the channel-linked receptors (Figure 5.8). It may also be described as ion-channel-linked receptors. These are receptors that use transmitted ion gated channels for rapid signaling. They are common in nerves, but recently have been described in macrophages. In this case, the receptor itself is constituted into a channel; it sits on a protein arrangement that constitutes what can be described as a channel. It is a protein arrangement that rapidly binds and release ions, thus allowing a continuous flow. In this arrangement, when the receptor binds the agonist, the "channel" opens and allows the ions to flow through it. Channel-linked receptors are found in inflammatory and immune cells.

ii. **Receptors with tyrosine-specific protein kinase cytoplasmic domain:** When a ligand binds to extracellular domain, a conformational change occurs that activates the intracellular kinase domain. Kinase activation triggers phosphorylation reaction which modifies protein function and structure, and initiates a series of changes in cellular activities. These receptors are common in cells of immune system.

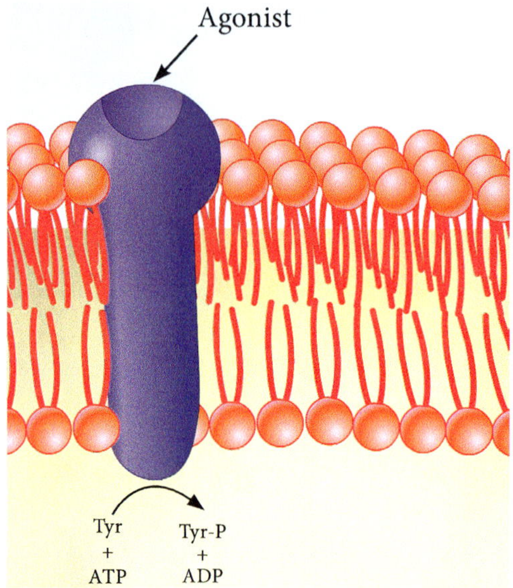

Courtesy of Zainab Ashkanani

Figure 5.9 *Receptor with tyrosine-specific protein kinase cytoplasmic domain.*

The second one is receptors with tyrosine-specific protein kinase cytoplasmic domain (Figure 5.9). When a ligand binds the extracellular domain of such receptor, a conformational change occurs that activates the intracellular kinase domain. Kinase activation triggers phosphorylation reaction which modifies protein function and structure and initiates a series of changes in cellular activities. Usually, the phosphorylating biomolecule is ATP.

iii. **Receptors associated with GTP-binding proteins (G-proteins):** G-proteins act as chemical switches. When inactive, the receptor, a protein complex, binds to GDP, when active it binds to GTP. When a ligand binds to the receptor having a G-protein complex, it rapidly loses its GDP and binds to GTP (thus energized). The activated G-protein can act on other substances, thus activating them. As control, the GTP is rapidly hydrolyzed by G-protein's GTPase component, thus turning off G-protein. These types of reactions take place in some cells of immune system.

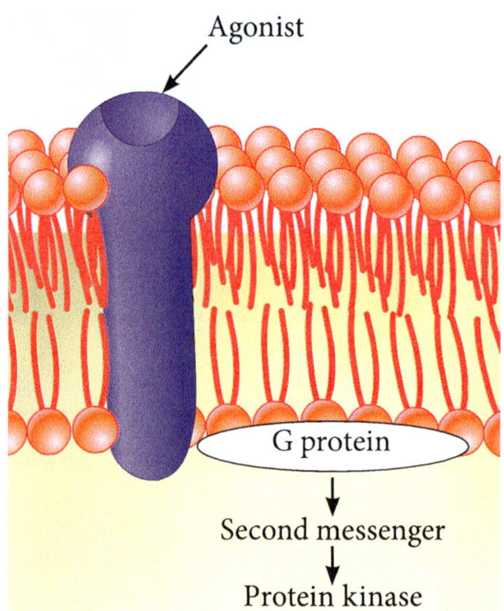

Courtesy of Zainab Ashkanani

Figure 5.10 *Receptor associated with G-proteins.*

The third example is the system that uses G-proteins which act as a chemical switch (Figure 5.10). When inactive, the receptor, a protein complex, is always bound to guanosine diphosphate, GDP, when active it binds to GTP. When a ligand binds to the receptor having G-protein complex, it rapidly loses its GDP and binds to GTP. The activated G-protein can act as a switch by initiating phosphorylation.

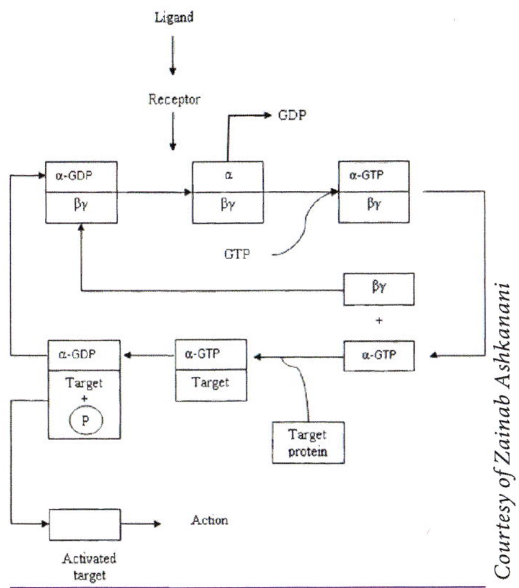

Figure 5.11 *Process by which a G-protein consisting of three units, α, β, and γ,* ***acts as a signal transduction****.*

The control of this system is the fact that as the process is switched on, there is activation of a phosphatase, guanosine triphosphatase (GTPase) which quickly quenches the G-protein energy by converting GTP to GDP. Cells of the immune system have this kind of receptor.

iv. **Receptors associated with sphingomyelin in cell membrane:** Such receptors activate sphingomyelinase, which splits off ceramide from sphingomyelin. Ceramide acts as the second messenger, that is, it initiates phosphorylation processes. This generates transcription factor, for example, NF–κB. Receptor for IL-1 and TNF-α employ this signaling method.

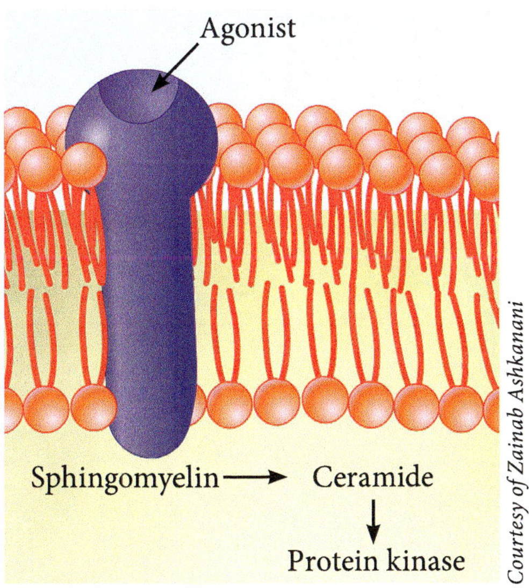

Figure 5.12 *Receptor associated with sphingomyelin in cell membrane.*

Then, the fourth example is of receptors that are associated with sphingomyelin (Figure 5.12). Sphingomyelin is a phospholipid. Usually, receptor–ligand interaction activates sphingomyelinase which splits off ceramide from sphingomyelin; ceramide is also a phospholipid which acts as a second messenger, so it initiates phosphorylation processes which generate transcription factors, for instance, nuclear factor KappaB. The receptors for IL-1 and TNF employ this signaling method.

CELL ADHESION MOLECULES

Adhesion molecules between cell and cell or cells to connective tissue is mediated by cell membrane proteins. There are four major cell adhesion molecule (CAM) families (Figure 5.13):

1. Immunoglobulin superfamily
2. Cadherin family
3. Integrin family
4. Selectin family

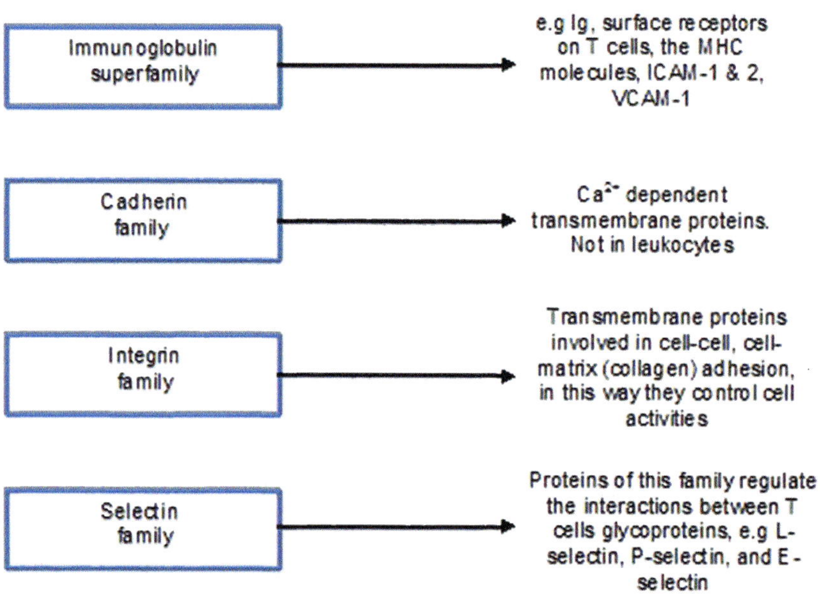

Courtesy of Zainab Ashkanani

Figure 5.13 *Four major cell adhesion molecule families.*

The cell adhesion molecules aid in cell movement in a deliberate pattern to facilitate their functions.

The immunoglobulin superfamily is a large group of cell surface and soluble proteins that are involved in recognition, binding, or adhesion process. They all possess domains known as immunoglobulin domain or fold. The members of the superfamily include antigen receptors, coreceptor, and coinflammatory molecules of the immune system. Also, molecules involved in antigen presentation to lymphocytes, cell adhesion molecules, certain cytokine receptors, and intracellular muscle proteins are members of this family.

Cadherin is a cell adhesion molecule named for "Ca^{2+}-dependent adhesion." They are transmembrane proteins. They play important roles in all cell adhesions, ensuring that cells within tissue are held together. The members of the family include: cadherins, proto-cadherins, desmoggleins, and desmocollins. They all share cadherin repeats, which are extracellular Ca^{2+}-binding domains. They are said to be absent in leukocytes.

Integrins are transmembrane proteins involved in cell–cell and cell–matrix interaction. They are receptors that mediate attachment between a cell and the tissues surrounding it. They play a role in signaling and they regulate cell shape, motility, and cell cycle. They do not only perform signaling involving extracellular sensing but also signal in an inside-out mode. This allows rapid and flexible responses to changes in the environment, for example, allowing blood coagulation by platelets to prevent intravascular leaks. Integrins work alongside other proteins such as cadherins, immunoglobulins, and selectin. They bind cell surface components to mediate cell–cell communications.

Selectins are proteins found on leukocytes. They recognize sialylated groups. They act as a homing receptor for leukocytes to enter secondary lymphoid tissues. Ligands present on endothelial cells bind to leukocytes expressing L-selectin, thus slowing leukocyte trafficking through the blood, thereby facilitating entry into secondary lymphoid organs. The receptor is commonly found on T-cell surfaces. Effector and memory T cells do not express L-selectin receptor, because they circulate in the peripheral circulation.

SAMPLE QUESTIONS

CELLULAR INTERACTION

Answer True or False to the following:

Channel-linked receptors

1. Receptors that use transmitted ion-gated channels transduce signals very slowly.
2. Channel-linked receptors are linked to another transmembrane protein, which is known as the channel.
3. When the agonist binds the receptor, the channel opens and allows ions to flow through it.
4. Channel-linked receptors are found only in inflammatory and immune cells.

Receptors with tyrosine kinase domain

5. When an agonist binds to the receptor, a conformational change activates the intracellular kinase domain.
6. Tyrosine kinase activity of receptor de-phosphorylates proteins inside the cell.
7. The actions of the kinase modify the function and structure of target proteins.
8. Tyrosine kinases can also act on serine and threonine residues of proteins.

G-protein-coupled receptors

9. G-proteins act as chemical switches.
10. Inactive G-protein complex binds GTP, but when activated, it binds GDP.
11. The activated G-protein is rapidly inactivated by the GTPase component of the protein.
12. The activated G-protein acts on other molecules which act as second messengers to transduce the signal deeper into the cell.

Sphingomyelin-associated receptors

13. When the sphingomyelin-associated receptor binds to its agonist, ceramide and phosphocholine are joined to form sphingomyelin.
14. Ceramide acts as a secondary messenger.
15. Sphingomyelin is a membrane phospholipid.
16. Another important phospholipid-associated signal transducing enzyme is Phospholipase C.

Suggested Laboratory Practicals

- Case Studies on:

1. Cell Structure
2. Cellular Compartmentation and Role of Macromolecules in Signal Transduction

- Experiments showing activation of Neutrophils and Lymphocytes
- Agglutination Reactions
- Rubella Testing
- Serial Dilution and Titrations

CHAPTER 6

ANTIGEN PRESENTATION AND MAJOR HISTOCOMPATIBILITY COMPLEX

ANTIGEN PRESENTATION AND MHC

- Antigen processing cells
- Major histocompatibility complex

The antigen-presenting cells are macrophages, dendritic cells, and B cells (Figure 6.1). These are professional antigen-presenting cells. In circumstances of need, such as during elaborate infections, any cell can be an antigen-presenting cell under the influence of interleukin-1.

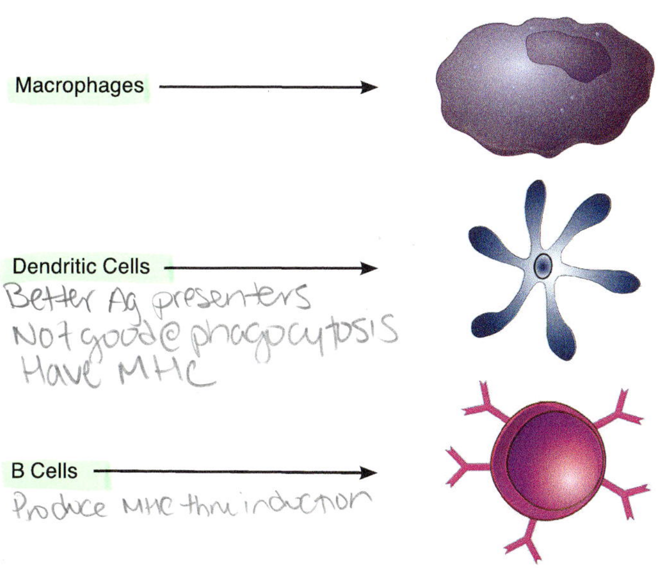

Courtesy of Zainab Ashkanani

Figure 6.1 *Antigen-presenting cells. All three cells secrete IL-1 and IL-12 in a varying relative proportion.*

The effective function of the antigen-presenting cells is moderated by immune mediators (the cytokines). Some of these mediators are elaborated by the antigen-presenting cells (Figure 6.2). Macrophage is not very effective at antigen presentation because it is endowed with the capacity to degrade phagocytosed microbes in a manner in which the conserved peptides are not delineable.

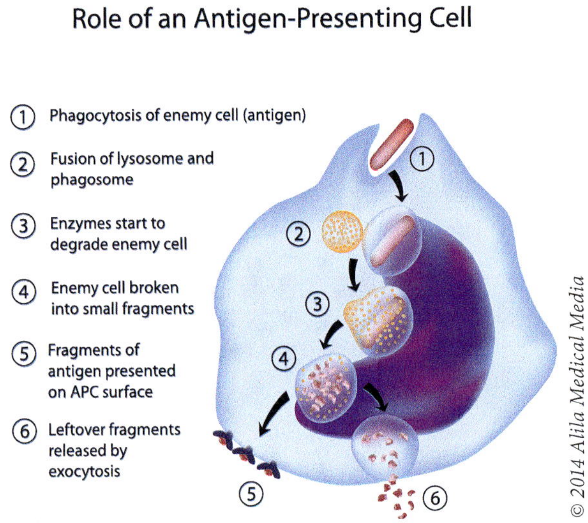

Figure 6.2 *Antigen processing and presentation. Antigen processing results in broken down peptides that can be presented via the MHC molecule.*

	Macrophages 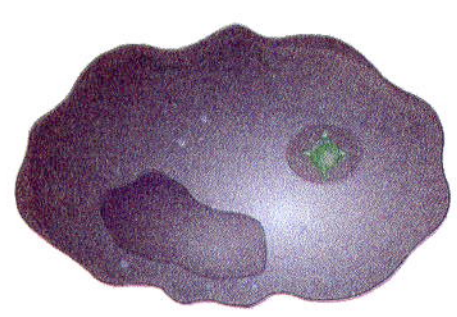	Dendritic cells 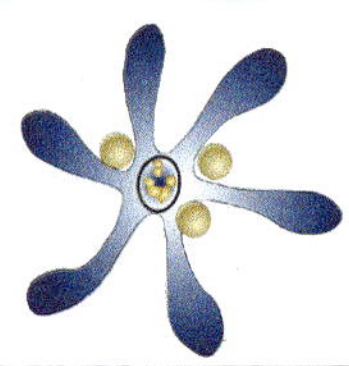	B cells 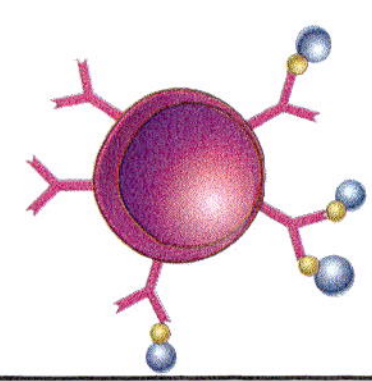
Antigen update	Phagocytosis +++	Phagocytosis by tissue dendritic cells +++ Viral infection ++++	Antigen-specific receptor (Ig) ++++
MHC expression	Inducible by bacteria and cytokines – to +++	Constitutive ++++	Constitutive increase on activation +++ to ++++
Co-stimulator delivery	Inducible – to +++	Constitutive in mature non-phagocytic lymphoid dendritic cells ++++	Inducible – to +++
Antigen presented	Particulate antigens Intracellular pathogens	Peptides Viral antigens (allergens?)	Soluble antigens Toxins Viruses
Location	Lymphoid tissue Connective tissue Body cavities	Lymphoid tissue Connective tissue Epithelia	Lymphoid tissue Peripheral blood

Courtesy of Zainab Ashkanani

Figure 6.3 *Activities of various types of professional antigen-presenting cells.*

MACROPHAGE

- Are important in presenting **Ags** that have **not** been **encountered previously**. This enables them to **engulf organisms** in the **absence** of Abs for **opsonization**.
- They are less important when there are **preexisting antibodies** because **B cells** and **dendritic** cells are capable of **handling** the situation.
- Ag presentation by macrophage is **ineffective** because most of the **Ag** endocytosed are **destroyed** by lysosomal proteases. Therefore, dendritic cells are better Ag presenters.

Macrophages can confront antigenic challenges by receptor and nonreceptor-based endocytosis; therefore, they are important for antigens that have not been encountered before. However, the endocytosed challenge is digested by lysosomal enzymes in a way that makes the presentation of antigen not as efficient as those that occur with dendritic cells. The presentation of antigen is the reserve of the antigen presenting molecules designated as major histocompatibility complex (MHC). These molecules are inducible. The presentation of antigens by MHC is followed by a recognition process carried out by antigen recognizing cells (Figure 6.3–6.5).

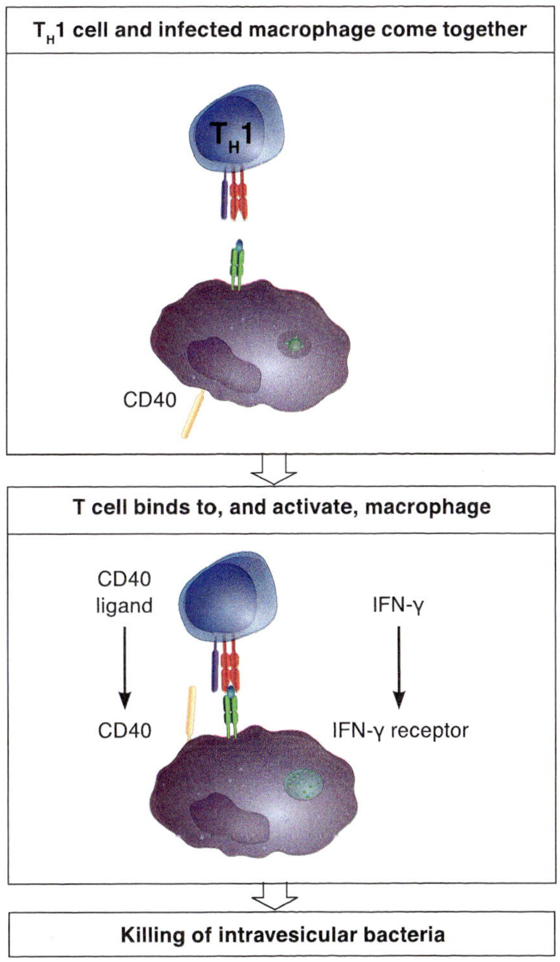

Courtesy of Zainab Ashkanani

Figure 6.4 *TH1 CD4 cells activate macrophage to become highly microbicidal.*

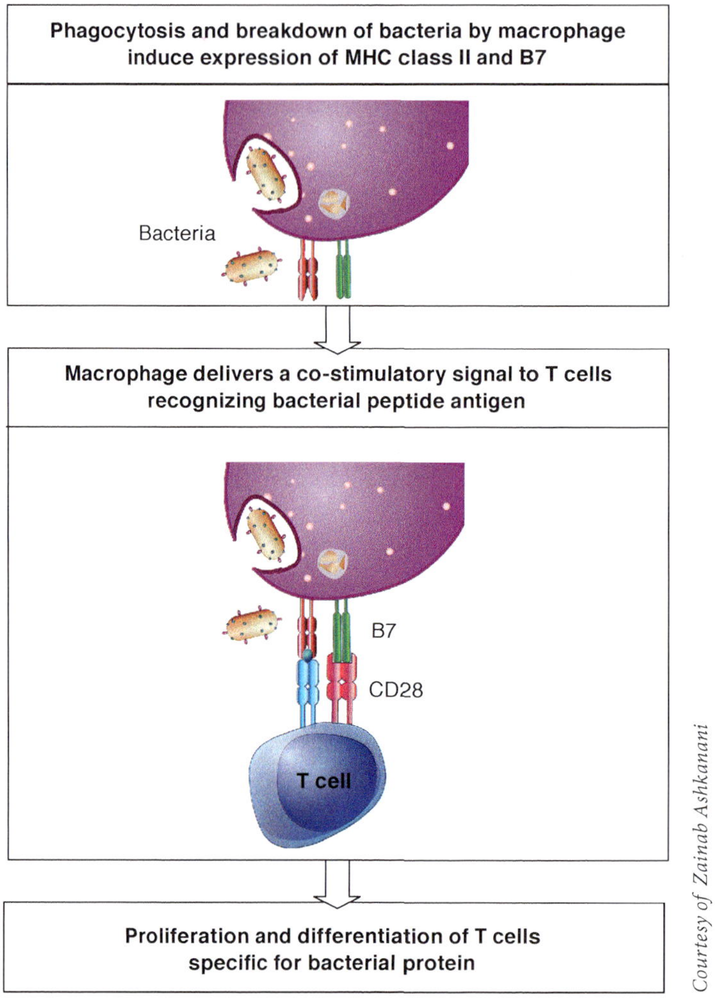

Figure 6.5 *Phagocytosis by macrophage. Microbial substances induce co-stimulatory activity in macrophages. Phagocytosis by macrophages and the subsequent breakdown by phagolysosomes induces the expression of MHC class II and B7 to promote adhesion to T cells to deliver peptide antigen.*

DENDRITIC CELLS

- They are located **throughout** the body but **more** in the lymphoid organs. They have long processes—called dendrites, have lobulated nuclei, and their cytoplasm is clear with characteristic granules called Birbeck granules.
- They have **Ab and complement receptors** but are poorly phagocytic. In the **skin**, they are described as Langerhans cells; here, they play an important role in skin allergies such as **delayed hypersensitivity** and **allergic contact dermatitis**.

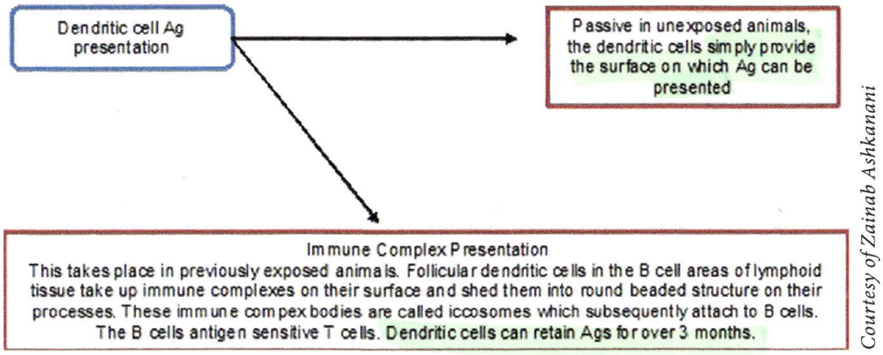

Figure 6.6 *Dendritc cell antigen presentation.*

Their strategic position in the secondary lymphoid organ compartments is indicative of a need for optimal interaction with challenges, in a manner that favor appropriate antigen presentation. It does not necessarily mean that they are not found elsewhere, but the lymph node is regarded as the site of maximal activation. The dendritic cells are not as efficient as macrophages in phagocytosis but as already mentioned, are better antigen presenters. Dendritic cells have the MHC constitutively; they are the most efficient of the professional antigen-presenting cells. They have antibody and complement receptors on their surface, but they are not efficient at phagocytosis. In the skin, they are the Langerhans cells; here, they play the important role of allergy, delayed hypersensitivity, and contact dermatitis. Dendritic cell antigen presentation is of two types: it can be passive, in unexposed animals, the dendritic cell simply provides its surface (because its surface area is very elaborate) on which the antigens can bind. In the other aspect, in a previously exposed animal that has elaborated antibodies, the antibodies interact with antigens to form immune complexes and they can be presented by dendritic cells (Figure 6.6). This second aspect of presentation of antigens occurs in the B-cell area of the lymphoid tissue, resulting in antigen presentation to B cells. The antigen-presenting complex is shed into round beads (thus, amplifying immune response), the beaded structures on the processes are called iccosomes and they attach themselves to B cells. The B cells ingest the antigen, and then present them to $CD4^+$ T cells (TH2 functional types heightened for antibody production). Dendritic cells can retain the antigen for over 3 months (Figure 6.7).

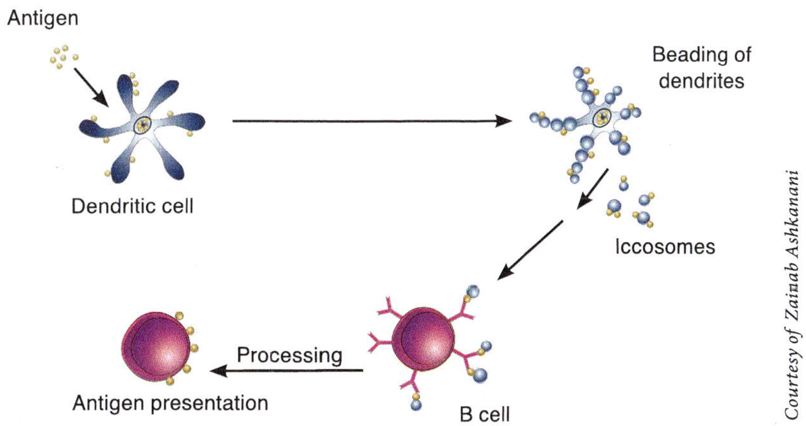

Figure 6.7 *Role of B cells in Ag processing. This depicts a suggested way in which iccosomes deliver antigen to B cells for processing.*

B CELLS

- They bind Ags by means of their Ag receptors. They then ingest, process, and present the Ag (conserved peptides) to T cells (memory T cells).
- Other cells such as endothelial cells, eosinophils, and keratinocytes can present Ag and even produce IL-1 under the influence of IFN.

The B cells are not phagocytic as such, but they have immunoglobulin receptors on their surfaces which are antigen specific. They are present late in immune response in this form, or in cases where there was previous exposure. In such case, they are primed, and this is expressed as specific antigen receptor on their surface. While macrophages elaborate cytokines that facilitate the production of MHC molecules, they are able to produce MHC molecules through induction. B cells have MHC molecules constitutively but it is increased upon activation. B cells present soluble antigens such as peptides and toxins. Whereas macrophages perform their function of antigen presentation in lymphoid tissue, connective tissues, and body cavities and dendritic cells carry out such functions in lymphoid tissue and connective tissue, the B cells perform this activity in lymphoid tissues and the peripheral blood. It is worth noting that the lymph nodes are the places where all the antigen-presenting cells are really distributed. The dendritic cells are found in the cortex, in close association with T cell. The macrophages are found all over, even in the medulla. The B cells are found in the follicles, the ones that are already primed, are in the germinal centers.

ANTIGEN-RECOGNIZING CELLS

These are T cells; there are two subpopulations, namely, $CD4^+$ and $CD8^+$ cells. For proper understanding of the antigen-presenting cells and their mode of action, there is need to know of the antigen-recognizing cells. The $CD4^+$ cells are the helper T cells and are of two functional types, TH1 and TH2 cells. In terms of antigen recognition, the $CD4^+$ cells of the TH1 types recognize antigens presented on macrophages by the antigen-presenting molecules of the MHC class II. The consequence of this recognition is the elaboration of cytokines that further activate the macrophage and facilitate phagocytosis, microbial degradation, the enhancing of

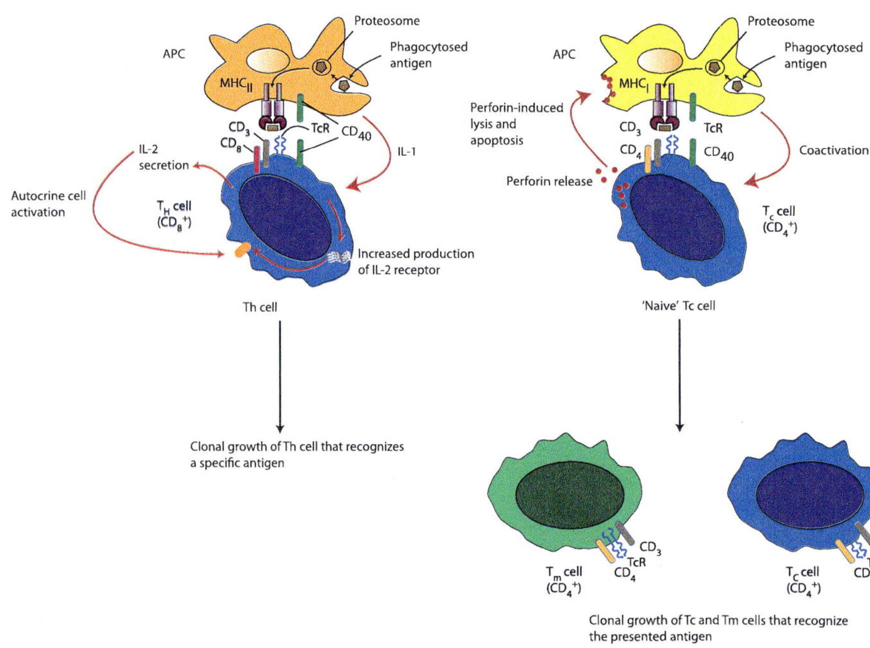

Figure 6.8 *Cytotoxic CD8 T cells recognize and kill virus-infected cells. CD8 T cells recognize virally derived peptides presented by MHC class I antigens at the surface of the cell.*

MHC class II molecule induction, and antigen presentation process. The cytokines that are the major players here are tumor necrosis factors superfamily member (CD40 ligands) and interferon-gamma. The TH2 cells recognize antigens presented by MHC class II molecules displayed on B cells. The consequence of such recognition is the elaboration of cytokines such as interleukin-2 which further activates B cells and leads to the clonal expansion of B cells and antibody production (see Figures 6.8–6.10).

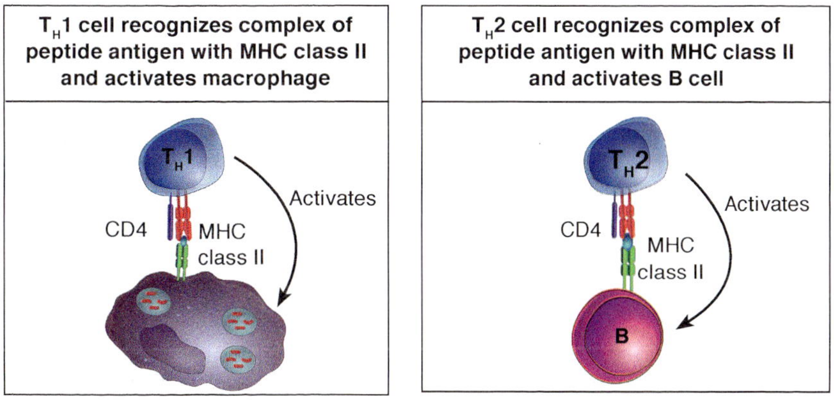

Courtesy of Zainab Ashkanani

Figure 6.9 *Helper function of CD4⁺ T cells. TH1 cells recognize antigen with MHC class II and activate macrophages and TH2 cells recognize MHC class II and activate B cells.*

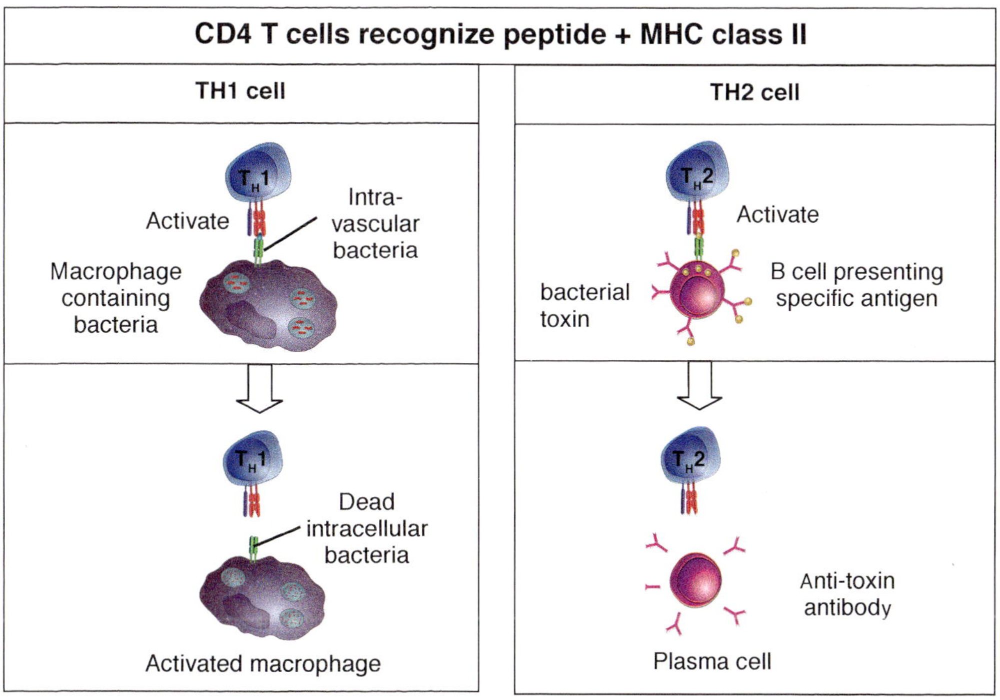

Courtesy of Zainab Ashkanani

Figure 6.10 *Recognition of antigens. Effector CD4 cells recognize antigens bound to MHC class II molecules. CD4 T cells also carry the coreceptor molecule, which binds to MHC class II molecules on the antigen-presenting cells and helps to stabilize T cell receptor–antigen binding. Effector CD4 T cells fall into two main categories: TH1 and TH2. TH1 cells are involved mainly in responding to antigens presented by macrophages, whereas TH2 cells respond to antigens presented by B cells, stimulating the differentiation of B cells to plasma cells and the production of antibodies.*

The $CD8^+$ cells are suppressor T cells and some functional populations are cytotoxic. In terms of antigen recognition, the $CD8^+$ cells recognize antigens presented on viral infected cells by the antigen-presenting molecules of the MHC class I type. The consequence of the event is the production of cytotoxins such as perforins and granzymes, which invariably will cause cell death and cytokines, such as Fas ligand (which will bind to Fas receptors on viral infected cell surface, thus inducing apoptosis), interferon-gamma, and tumor necrosis factors-alpha and beta (which impair viral protein synthesis, viral replication, and viral penetration into host cells). It is important to note that for proper antigen recognition involving MHC class I and $CD8^+$ cells, the costimulatory molecules B7 and CD28 are important players.

MAJOR HISTOCOMPATIBILITY CELLS

These are the major histocompatibility complex molecules. These antigen-presenting molecules are specialized receptor glycoproteins, inherited in a gene complex. It is the fact that it is genetically determined that is taken advantage of in typing tissues before such tissues are transplanted. It is noteworthy that their physiologic role is antigen presentation to antigen-recognizing cells, with the consequent elaboration of immune mediators that drive immune response in a specific acquired direction. All animals have the MHC genes, with great variation. In humans, it is located on the short arm of chromosome 6 and contains about 140 genes, spanning 3.6 megabase pairs. About half of these are known to have immune functions.

MAJOR HISTOCOMPATIBILITY COMPLEX

- These are **antigen presenting molecules**. They are **specialized receptor glycoproteins**, **inherited** in a **gene complex**. The absolute need to present antigen bound to MHC molecules is called **MHC restriction**.
- All animals have MHC gene in their genome. In humans, MHC is located in the short arm of chromosome 6. In mice it is found in chromosome 17.

There are three classes of genes that determine the MHC complex: the class I gene, the class II gene, and the class III gene (Figure 6.11).

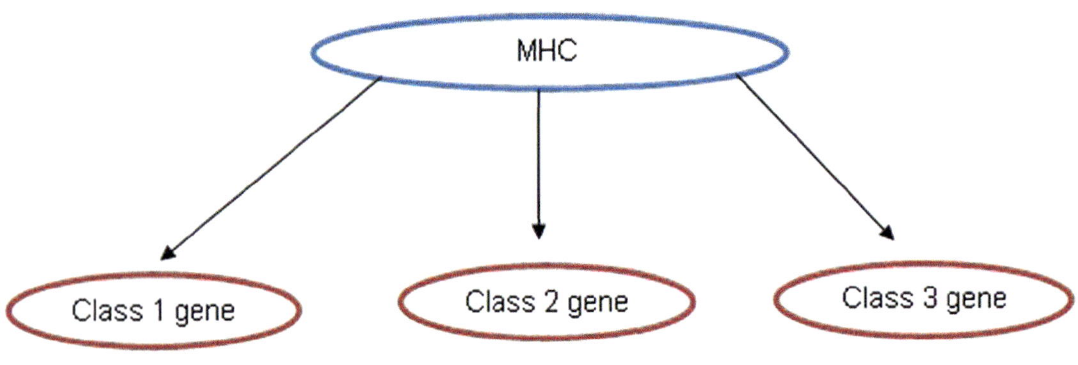

Courtesy of Zainab Ashkanani

Figure 6.11 *The classes of MHC genes.*

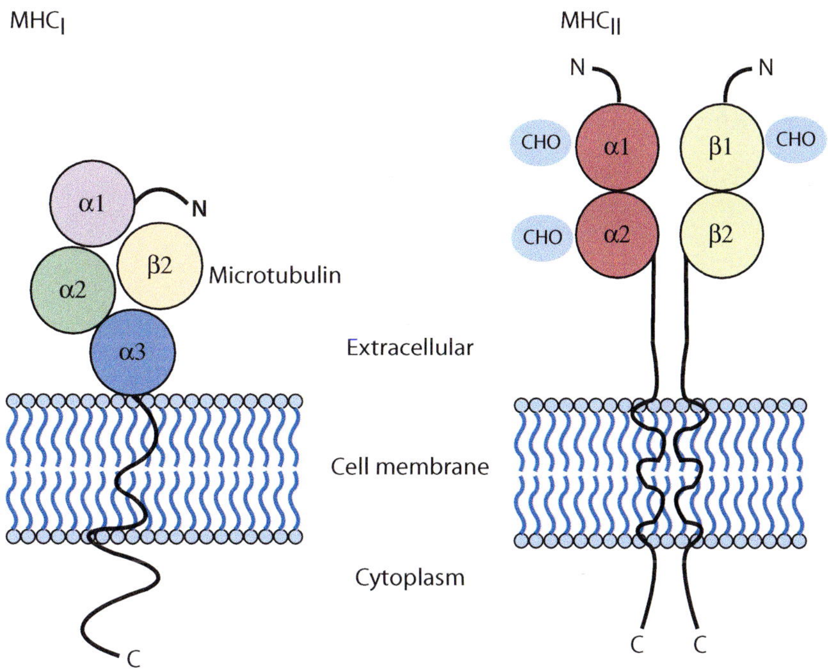

© Kendall Hunt Publishing Company

Figure 6.12 *Diagram of the two types of major histocompatibility complex proteins. MHC class I work with CD 8⁺ T cells and MHC class II work with CD4⁺ T cells.*

The class I gene codes for MHC class I molecule, they are found on all nucleated cell surfaces, including mouse RBCs. There are two types, depending on polymorphism, which mean structural differences in proteins that will result in functional differences. There is a subcategorization of the class I proteins, class Ia, which is more structurally diverse compared to the class Ib. The peptide binding proteins which class I genes encode present antigens to $CD8^+$ receptor borne notably on cytotoxic T cells and inhibitory receptors borne on natural killer cells. The class I genes also code for molecules aiding in antigen processing such as transport-associated protein (TAP) and tapasin. MHC class I receptors may be absent in rare inherited deficiencies.

Figure 6.12 shows major histocompatibility complex proteins and Figure 6.13 shows three major classes of genes found on mouse major histocompatibility complex.

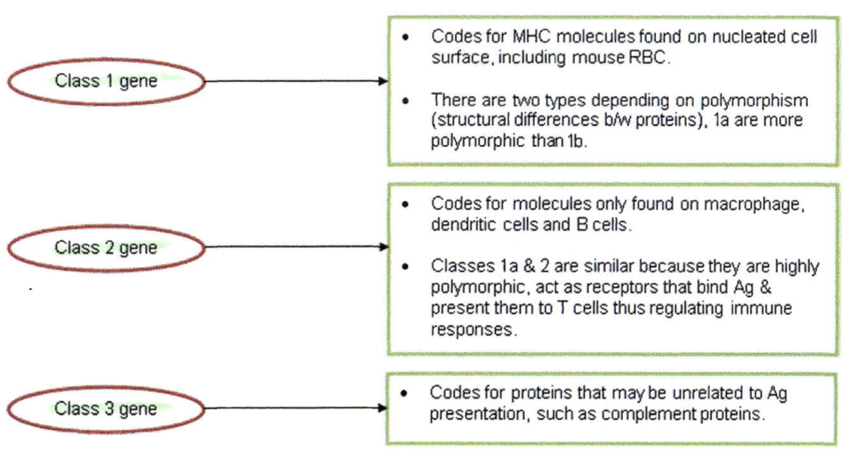

Courtesy of Zainab Ashkanani

Figure 6.13 *The functions of the major classes of genes.*

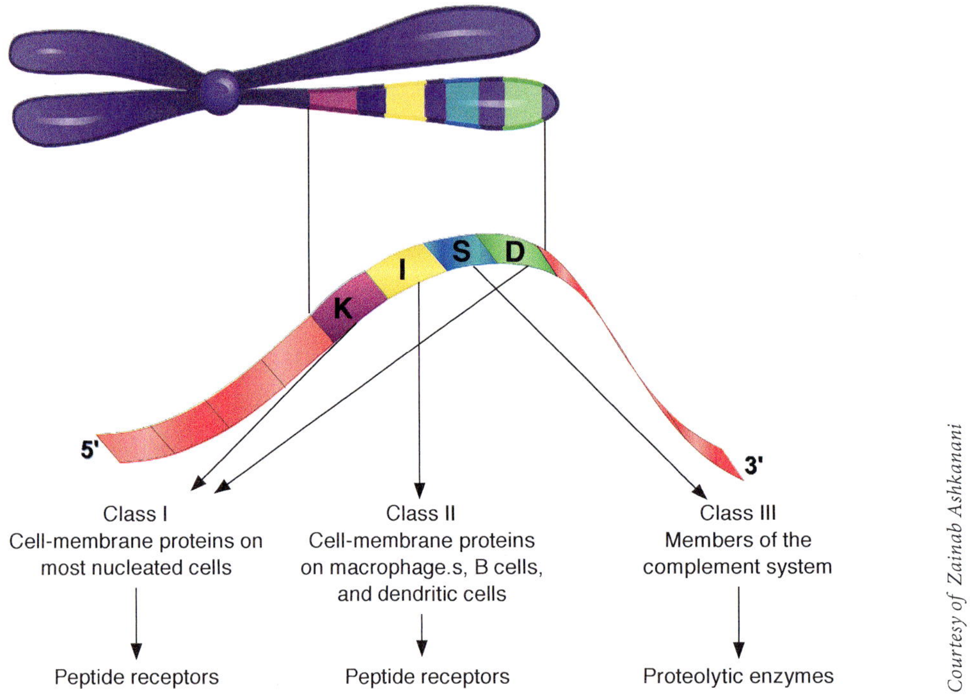

Figure 6.14 *The major classes of genes found in the mouse major histocompatibility complex and functions of their gene products.*

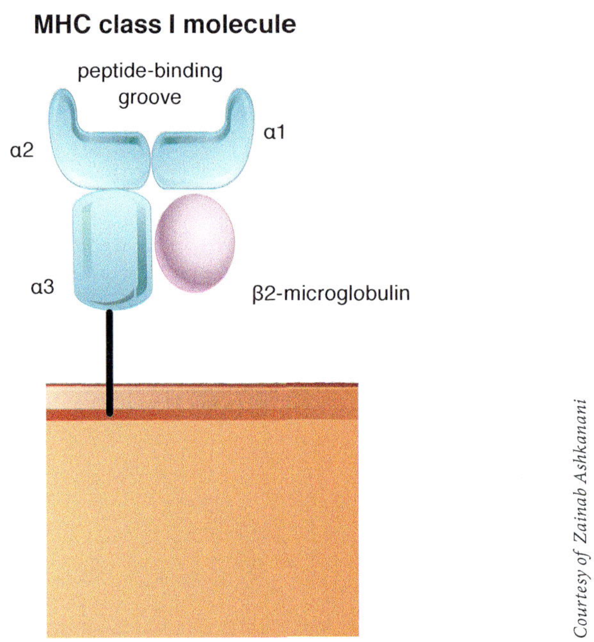

Figure 6.15 *A schematic representation of a human MHC class I molecule. It is a heterodimeric glycoprotein, composed of one transmembrane α-chain bound noncovalently.*

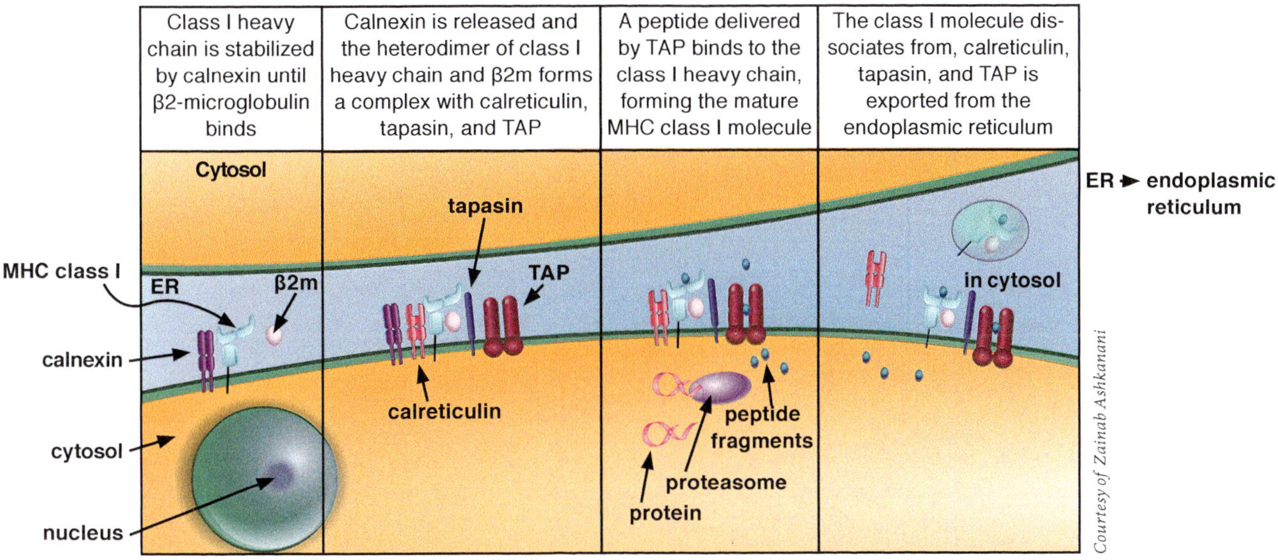

Figure 6.16 *A schematic representation of MHC class I molecule's functioning. MHC class I molecules do not leave the endoplasmic reticulum unless they bind peptides. MHC class I α-chains assemble in the endoplasmic reticulum with a membrane-bound protein, calnexin. When this complex binds β2-microglobulin (β2m), it is released from calnexin, and the partly folded MHC class I molecule then binds to the TAP1 subunit on the TAP transporter by interacting with one molecule of the TAP-associated protein, tapasin. It is retained within the endoplasmic reticulum until released by the binding of peptide, which completes the folding of the MHC class I molecule. Peptides generated by the degradation of proteins in the cytoplasm are transported into the lumen of the endoplasmic reticulum by the TAP transporter. Once peptide has bound to the MHC molecule, the peptide–MHC complex is transported through the Golgi complex to the cell surface.*

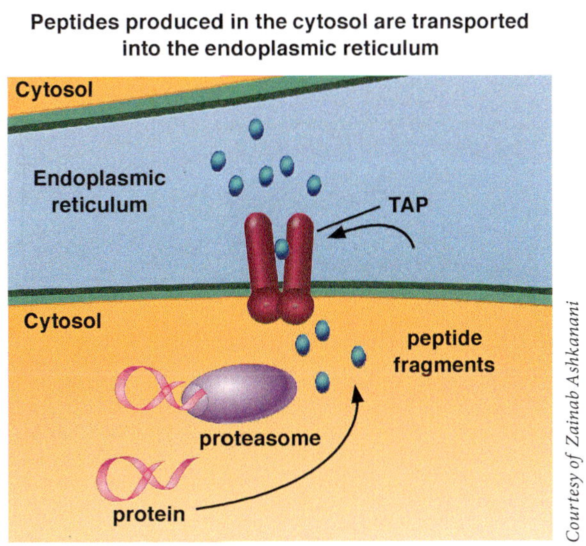

Figure 6.17 *Formation and transport of peptides to MHC class I molecules. Proteasomes break down proteins, resulting in peptide fragments which are transported into the endoplasmic reticulum via the ATP.*

This is illustrating what happens in the case of class I MHC protein assembly and delivery to cell surface (Figures 6.15–6.17). The point of assembly is the endoplasmic reticulum. The assembly process shows that the heterodimer which consists of α_1, α_2, α_3, and β2-microglobulin are synthesized separately and assembled as illustrated. In the illustration, the monomers are produced separately, brought in and held in position by calnexin; a deficiency of calnexin would trigger a disturbed assembly. The subsequent positioning of β2-microglobulin releases calnexin. Calreticulin then functions to make sure that β_2-microglobulin remains in perfect fit. The groups of proteins responsible for transportation of selected and carefully cleaved conserved peptides are transport-associated protein (TAP) and tapasin. The process of cleavage of protein and selection takes place in the proteasomes subsequent to ubiquitin labeling (the process is called ubiquitination). Any peptide that is marked by ubiquitin is sentenced to fragmentation in proteasomes. The MHC molecule is taken to the cell surface with proper fitting peptide and displayed on the cell by exocytosis.

The class II genes are also highly polymorphic, and they code for peptides that usually act as receptors that bind antigen and present them to T cells, helper T cells, thus regulating immune response. Common MHC class II binding proteins include MHC II DM, MHC II DQ, MHC II DR, and MHC DP. They present peptides to $CD4^+$ T cells. The assembly of MHC class II protein is illustrated side by side with MHC class I protein in Figure 6.18. Since antigens here are exogenous, they process by engulfment, degradation, and selection of conserved peptide by professional antigen-presenting cells. The assembly of the MHC protein is also in the endoplasmic reticulum as in the case of class I molecules.

MHC Class II Molecules

- Involved in **Ag presentation to $CD4^+$ T cells.**
- **Peptide Ags** presented are from **extracellular pathogen**, also proteins or **peptides derived from pathogens in intracellular vesicles**, for example, Mycobacterium sp.
- MHC class II molecules are expressed constitutively on **B cells, macrophages, and dendritic cells.**
- MHC class II molecule's expression can be induced principally **interferon-γ**.

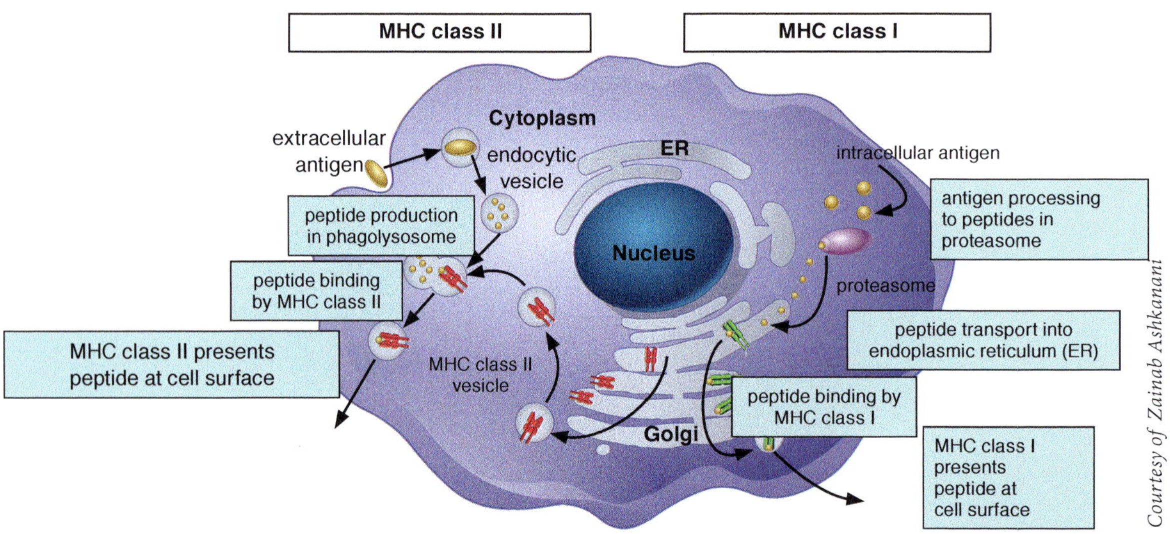

Figure 6.18 *Illustration of assembly of MHC class I and class II protein. Processing of peptide and assembly of MHC class I and II are done in different cellular compartments. MHC class I is loaded largely in the endoplasmic reticulum after proteasomes have already broken down peptides, whereas MHC class II molecule is produced in the ER and the Golgi, and meets a peptide broken down by phagolysosome and moving to the surface in outgoing vesicles.*

The class III genes are uniquely different. They code for proteins that are usually not related to antigen processing and presentation. These proteins are related to complement function, the cytokines of immune signaling, for example, tumor necrosis factor-alpha and heat shock proteins.

USES OF HUMAN LEUKOCYTE ANTIGEN (HLA)

Proteins produced by the MHC genes in humans are called human leukocyte antigens (HLAs). Clinical importance of HLA is summarized as follows:

1. Mostly applied in **organ matching** for transplantation. Better survival is assured when the donor graft and the recipient are closely matched.
2. HLA is used as part of the **genetic profile** in paternity testing. The evaluation of multiple markers help to eliminate falsely accused men. Although it can never be established with absolute certainty that an alleged father is the biologic father, due to the polymorphic nature of HLA and rare genetic recombination, HLA gives a high probability. When combined with other markers, it provides more powerful evidence.
3. HLA gene is used in the **verification of the risk of disease** distribution in a given population. This is described as evidence of high relative risk. It usually involves a positive association of HLA antigen distribution or expression with disease incidence.

SAMPLE QUESTIONS

ANTIGEN PRESENTATION AND MAJOR HISTOCOMPATIBILITY COMPLEX

Answer True or False to the following:

Major histocompatibility complex (MHC)

1. MHC are specialized receptor glycoproteins.
2. Antigens can only be presented between cells when bound to MHC molecules.
3. MHC class III genes code for proteins uninvolved in antigen presentation.
4. MHC genes are located on the long arm of chromosome 12.

MHC class I

5. MHC class I molecules are found on the surface of all nucleated cells.
6. There are three types of MHC class I molecules, Ia, Ib, and Ic.
7. MHC class I is usually recognized by receptors on CD8+ T cells.
8. It is composed of two alpha (α) moieties and two beta (β) moieties.

MHC class II

9. MHC class II molecules are found only on macrophages, dendritic cells, and B cells.
10. MHC class II molecules present antigens to CD 8+ T cells.
11. The expression of MHC class II can be induced principally by TNF-α.
12. MHC class II molecules present peptide antigens from exogenous pathogens.

MHC class I molecule production

13. MHC class I molecules leave the endoplasmic reticulum whether they are bound to an antigen or not.
14. The alpha chains of MHC class I molecules are assembled with the help of a membrane-bound protein, calnexin.
15. TAP transporter shuttles peptide fragments from the cytosol to the endoplasmic reticulum to be bound to MHC class I molecules.
16. Assembled MHC molecules are transported through the Golgi complex to the cell surface.

Uses of HLA

17. The proteins produced by MHC genes in humans are called human leukocyte antigens (HLA).
18. HLA is used clinically to determine tissue match for transplantation.
19. HLA is also used as part of genetic profiling for paternity testing.
20. HLA antigen distribution has not been associated with increased risk for certain diseases.

Suggested Laboratory Practicals

- Case Studies on:

1. Nature of Epitopes
2. Major Histocompatibility Complex
3. Antigen Presentation

- Enzyme-Linked Immunoassays
- Precipitation Reactions
- Ouchterlony Double Diffusion
- Fluorescence Immunoassays

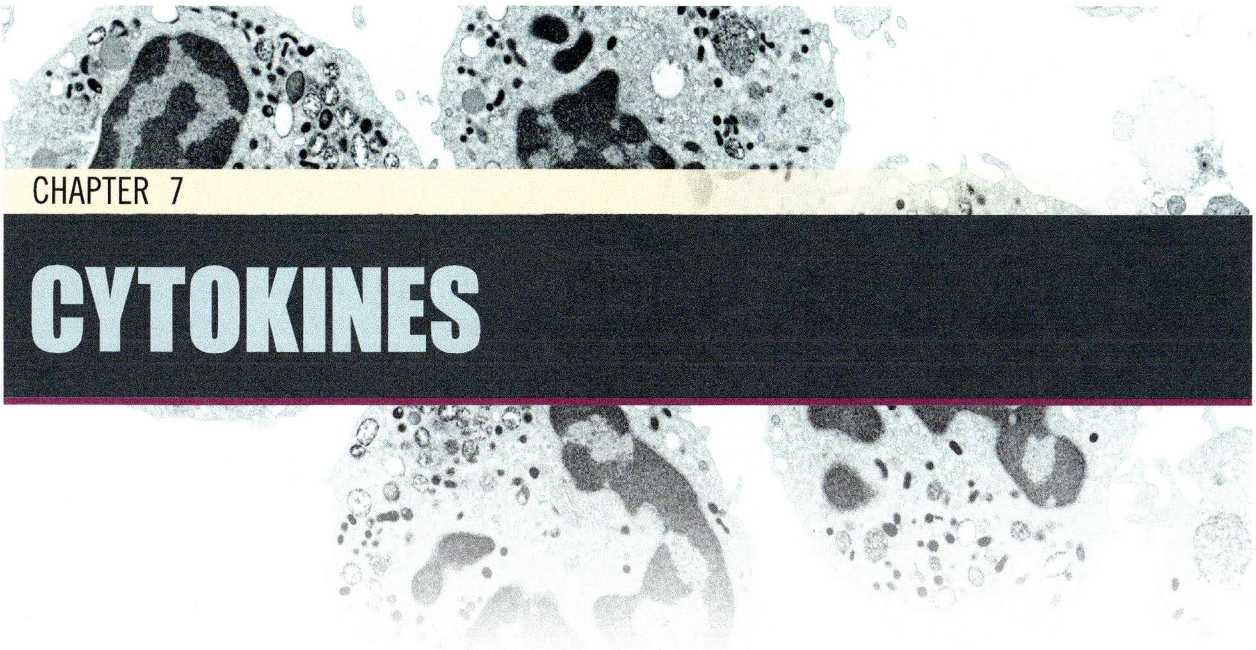

CHAPTER 7

CYTOKINES

- These are soluble substances that regulate immune response.
- They mediate interaction between cells.

There are four main types of cytokines:

- **Colony stimulating factors** (**CSF**): Important in cellular differentiation and propagation.
- **Interferons (IFN)**: **(1)** A protein that can interfere with viral replication. **(2)** Important agents of cellular immunity.
- **Tumor necrosis factor** (**TNF**): Factors from macrophages and some T cells that exert toxic effects on neoplastic cells.
- **Interleukins** (**IL**): Proteins that act between leukocytes. They are growth and differentiation factors.

Cytokines are immune mediators which in their functions relate cells to one another and communicate information between cells during immune response. They are complex proteins (glycoproteins). Although they play a central role in immune responses, their role is not limited to immune responses, but they also play an enormous role in physiologic and developmental processes, such as embryogenesis. In terms of their functions and actions, they are either designated as autocrines—these are the ones that function on the cells that secrete them—or are described as paracrines, in which case their action is on other cells distances away from the secreting cells. It is worth noting that some cytokines can be both autocrines and paracrines in function. Cytokines literally mean proteins that communicate between cells (*cyto* = cells; *kines* = protein). They are also designated in other terms such as lymphokines, meaning proteins produced by lymphocytes, which represents only a group of them. There are some described as interleukins, meaning proteins that act between leukocytes, facilitating communications within leukocytes (white cells). Also, some are described as chemokines. Chemokines are secretions that facilitate the migration of cells toward a particular direction (chemicals that facilitate chemotaxis). There are some interleukins that are also chemokines, such as IL-8. Functionally, the cytokines are broadly classified as colony stimulating factors (these bring about differentiation and proliferation of primitive cells, especially in the bone marrow), the interferons (these interfere with viral replication and bacterial infection), tumor necrosis factors (destroy neoplastic cells), and the interleukins (the proteins that relate leukocytes to each other).

Cytokines are also very important agents of cellular immunity (see Figure 7.1).

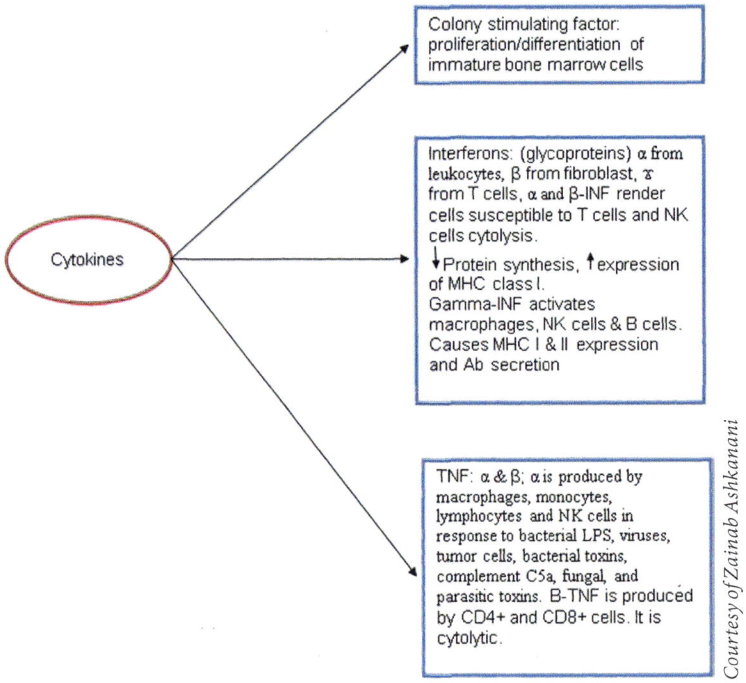

Figure 7.1 *Cytokines and their functions.*

COLONY STIMULATING FACTORS

- Colony stimulating factors cause the proliferation and differentiation of immature bone marrow cell.
  - Granulocyte colony stimulating factor (G-CSF) stimulates the growth of matured granulocytes.
  - Macrophage-CSF stimulates the growth of monocytes/macrophage colonies.
  - GM-CSF (granulocyte/macrophage colony stimulating factor) stimuates the formation of both mature granulocytes and monocyte/macrophage colonies.

Colony stimulating factors act at the level of the bone marrow; they bring about differentiation and propagation of primitive cell colonies in the bone marrow. They are further classified according to their specific function. The granulocyte colony stimulating factor (G-CSF) stimulates the growth and maturation of granulocytes. It causes the bone marrow to be more committed to producing cells that are of the granulocyte series out of the pluripotent stem cells. The macrophage colony stimulating factor (M-CSF) stimulates the differentiation and growth of myeloid cells into monocytes/macrophage colonies. The granulocytes/macrophage colony stimulating factor (GM-CSF) stimulates the differentiation and proliferation of cells from the marrow to the formation of both matured granulocytes and monocytes/macrophage colonies.

TABLE 7.1 CYTOKINES

CYTOKINE	SOURCES	BIOLOGICAL ACTIVITIES
Interleukin-1	Many different cells	Fever, acute immune response, stimulation of neutrophils
Interleukin-10	Activated CD_4^+ and CD_8^+ T_H cells	B and T cell proliferation
Interleukin-11	Bone marrow stromal cells, fibroblasts	Growth factor
Interleukin-12	Macrophages, dendritic cells	T_H cell differentiation
Interleukin-13	Activated T cells, mast and NK cells	IgE synthesis and suppresses inflammation
Granulocyte/macrophage colony-stimulating factor	Many different cells	Growth factor involved in hematopoiesis
Granulocyte colony stimulating factor	Bone marrow stromal cells, dendritic cells	Growth and development of eosinophils
Interferon-α	Cells, macrophages	Antiviral actions
Interferon-β	Fibroblasts, epithelial cells	Antiviral actions
Interferon-γ	Helper and cytotoxic T-cells	Growth and differentiation of B and T cells, macrophages, and NK cells
Leukemia inhibitory factor	Many cell types	Hematopoiesis
Macrophage colony stimulating factor	Many cell types	Growth, differentiation, and survival of macrophages
Oncostatin M	T cells, monocytes	Hematopoiesis
Stem cell factor	Stromal cells	Hematopoiesis
Thrombopoietin	Many cells	Regulates platelet production
TGF-β	Many cells	Inhibits cells growth
Tumor necrosis factor-α	Many cells	Stimulates inflammation
Tumor necrosis factor-β	B and T cells	Mediates inflammation

INTERFERONS

- **Interferons** are **glycoproteins** produced in **response** to **viral infections**, **immune stimulation**, or **chemical stimulators**.
  - **IFN-α** is produced by **leukocytes**.
  - **IFN-β** is produced by **fibroblasts**.
  - **IFN-γ** is produced by **T cells**.
- IFN-α and IFN-β are antiviral proteins. They **inhibit** viral **replication**, **increase** the **expression of MHC** class I molecules on virally infected cells and activate NK cells.
- α and β IFN **inhibit** viral replication by **interfering** with viral **RNA** and ultimately **protein production**.
- The expression of MHC class I molecules on virally infected cells renders them susceptible to NK cells and cytotoxic T cells, since these cells (NK cells and cytotoxic T cells) have receptors to MHC molecules.

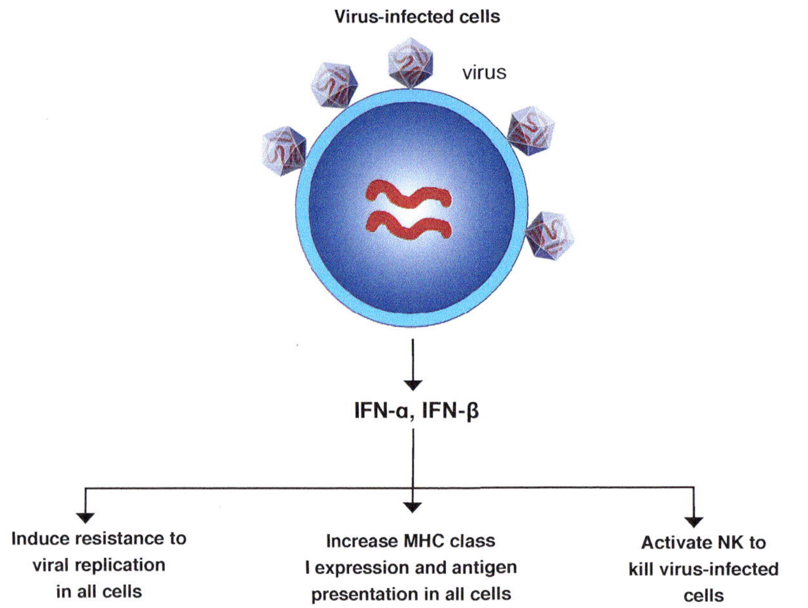

Courtesy of Zainab Ashkanani

Figure 7.2 *Function of type I interferons (α and β). These interferons induce resistance to viral replication in all cells, increase MHC class I expression and antigen presentation in all cells, and finally activate NK cells to kill virus-infected cells.*

The production of IFN-α and IFN-β by virally infected cells and the induction of resistance to viral replication in cells is depicted in Figure 7.2.

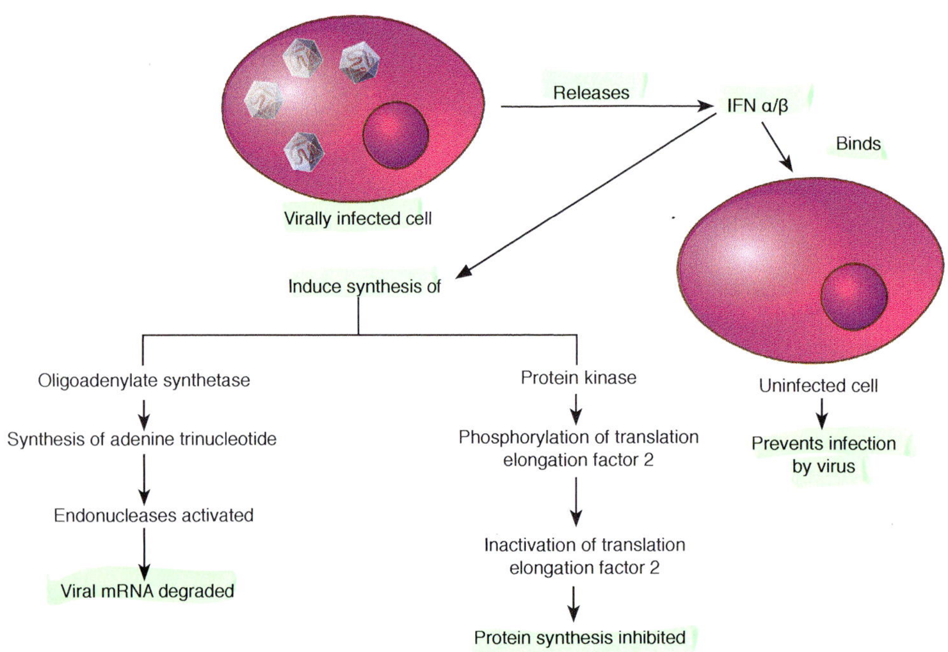

Courtesy of Zainab Ashkanani

Figure 7.3 *The immune system in action: molecular action of interferon in viral infection.*

Interferon protects other cells and impairs the virus from further development by

i. inhibiting the synthesis of proteins through the induction of an initial increase in adenine trinucleotide which enhances the activation of endonucleases, resulting in the degradation of viral mRNA which translates into viral proteins
ii. inactivating translation elongation factor-2, which results in the inhibition of protein synthesis. This is well illustrated in the chart.

- IFN-gamma has antiviral and regulatory effects on specific immune response. For instance,
  - it activates macrophages.
  - causes macrophages to increase the expression of MHC class I and II receptor molecules.
  - it activates NK cells.
  - it activates B cells and causes antibody secretion.

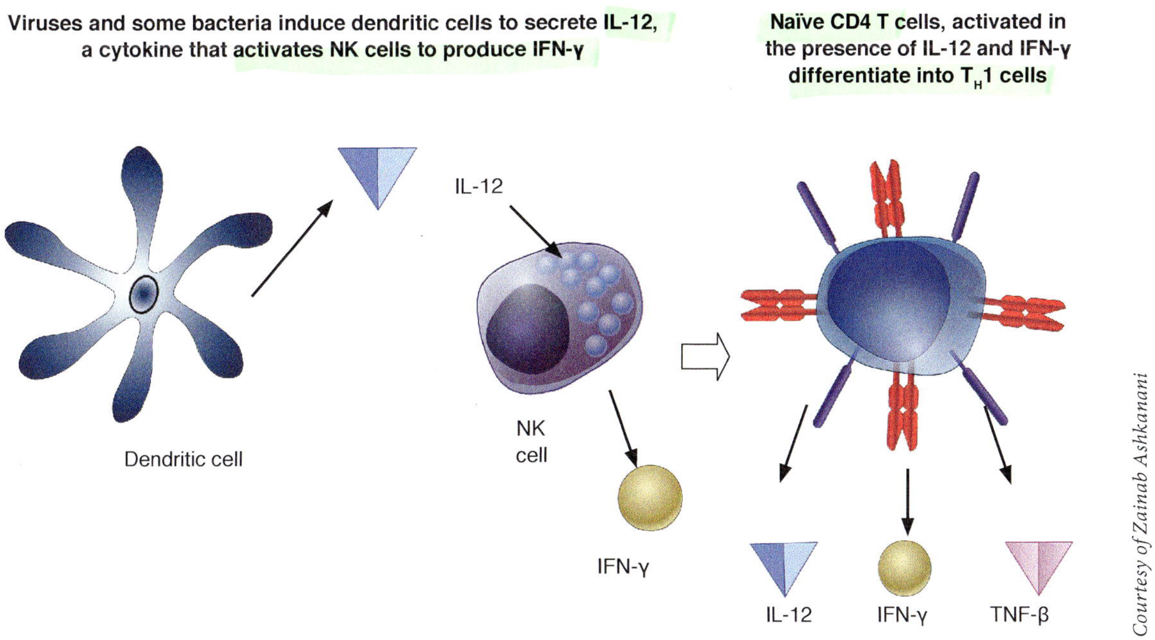

Figure 7.4 *Viruses, as well as some bacteria, induce the production and secretion of IL-12 by DCs, which in turn elicits production of IFN-γ by NK cells. This results in the differentiation of naïve T cells into TH1 cells.*

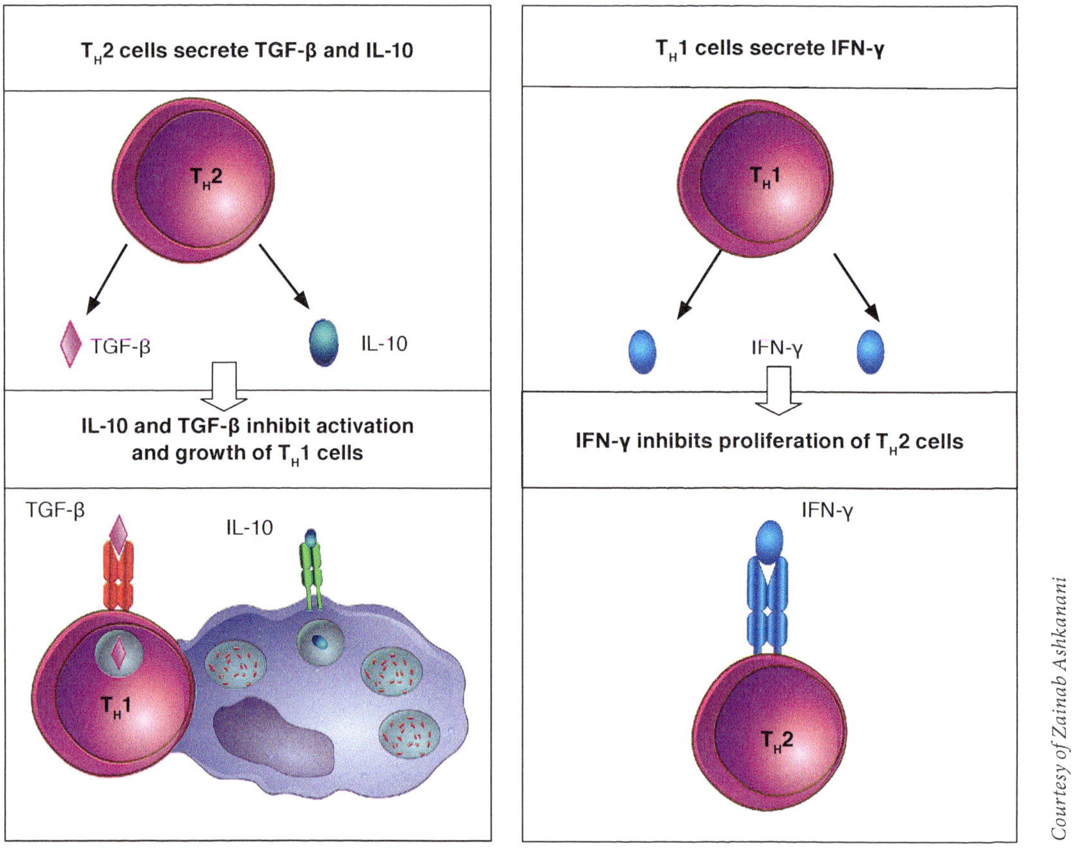

Figure 7.5 *The two types of CD4 cells produce cytokines that inhibit the proliferation and differentiation of the other type of cell. TH2 cells secrete IL-10 and TGF-β, inhibiting activation and growth of TH1 cells. TH1 cells secrete IFN-γ, inhibiting proliferation of TH2 cells.*

And the chart shows how IFN-γ comes to play when viruses and some bacteria induce the production and secretion of IL-12 by dendritic cells, which in turn elicits production of IFN-γ by NK cells, resulting in the differentiation of naïve T cells into TH1 cells (Figure 7.4). This is regulated when transformation growth factors inhibit the activation and growth of TH1 cells (Figure 7.5). Also, the TH1 cells can secrete IFN-gamma, which inhibits the proliferation of TH2 cells, thus heightening the TH1 response.

TUMOR NECROSIS FACTORS

They are macrophages in origin mainly, but some T cells and NK cells also secrete them and they exert toxic effects on neoplastic cells.

- TNF are of two types—**α and β. TNF-α** is **produced** by **macrophages**, **monocytes**, **lymphocytes**, and NK cells in **response** to
  - **bacterial** lipopolysaccharide (**LPS**),
  - **viruses** (or viral protein coat),
  - **tumor cells**,

- **bacterial toxins** (mainly proteins),
- **complement component (C5a)**, and
- **fungal** and **parasitic toxins**.

- TNF-α acts by killing tumor cell lines. It regulates immune response by
  - increasing the production of B and T cells.
  - suppressing the hematologic progenitors.
  - of myeloid and erythroid cell lines.
  - increasing the rate of differentiation of hematologic progenitors already present, causing the onset of anemia.
- TNF-β, previously known as lymphotoxin, is produced by $CD4^+$ and $CD8^+$ cells after exposure to antigen and is directly cytotoxic to selected cells.

Figure 7.6 shows the extensiveness of the action of tumor necrosis factor-alpha. Apart from its role in tumor destruction, TNF-alpha increases muscle cell and hepatocyte catabolism. On adipocyte (fat cells), it inhibits lipid metabolizing enzyme and lipoprotein lipase, which modifies triglycerides and other complex lipids. Its action on neutrophils enhances its phagocytosis capability. It acts on B cells, resulting in enhanced growth and differentiation, and it increases proliferation of fibroblasts. Its action on endothelial cells causes increased intercellular adhesion molecules (ICAM) and IL-1 production.

Tumor necrosis factor-beta (TNF-β), previously known as lymphotoxin, is produced by $CD4^+$ and $CD8^+$ cells after exposure to antigen and is directly cytotoxic to selected cells.

INTERLEUKINS

Produced by leukocytes and affect leukocytes and other cells.

- **IL-1**: Macrophage and fibroblast origin. Suppresses B cells and induces acute phase protein. Activates T cells.
- **IL-2**: CD4+ cell origin; causes T and B cells to proliferate. Increases NK cells, IL-2R expression, and increases B cells antibody production.
- **IL-3**: Increases mast cell production. It is a growth factor for hematopoietic precursors.
- **IL-4**: It increases IgE levels and also increases the proliferation of T, B, and NK cells. Elaboration of IFN- γ, TNF-α and TNF-β.
- **IL-5**: Causes eosinophilia and increases IgE levels.
- **IL-6**: T cells, fibroblast and monocyte origin. Regulates hematopoiesis and Ab production.
- **IL-10**: Is anti-inflammatory, reduces IFN-γ, enhances Ag presentation, and impairs macrophage production of IL-1.
- **IL-12**: Is inflammatory. It activates macrophages, NK cell, and IFN-γ.

Interleukins act as mainly growth and differentiation factors.

IL-1. They are produced by monocytes/macrophages and sometimes by fibroblasts and B cells. They bind to IL-1 receptors on T cells, stimulating T cells to produce IL-2. Interleukin-2 acts on T cells in an autocrine fashion, resulting in the clonal expansion of T-cell clone. This event takes place in B cell (paracrine) and it results in expansion of B-cell clones that have recognized an antigen, thus causing the elaboration of antibodies (Figure 7.6).

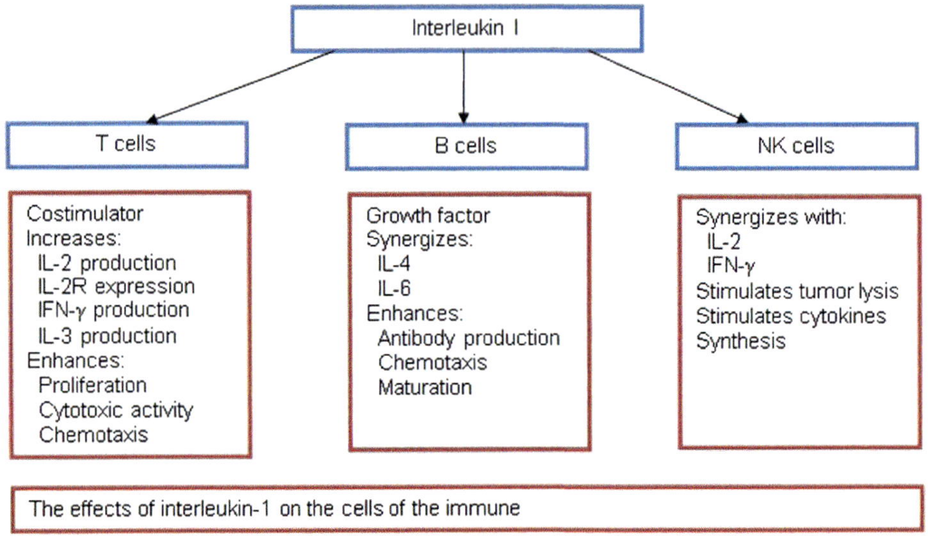

Courtesy of Zainab Ashkanani

Figure 7.6 *Effects of interleukin-1 on the cells of immune system.*

- **IL-1**, produced by **macrophages** and **fibroblast**, it acts as an **initiation** molecule for **immunologic** and **inflammatory responses**.
  - It **activates T cells** and **initiates** the **release** of other lymphokines.
  - It **suppresses B cell** proliferation (if used directly on B cells alone)
  - It **stimulates** bone **marrow** growth in response to colony stimulating factors.
  - It **activates NK cells.**
  - It **activates vascular endothelium.**
  - It induces fever.
  - It increases the synthesis of acute phase protein by the liver.
  - It induces the growth and differentiation of
  - hematopoietic precursors.
- **IL-2** is a glycoprotein produced by $CD4^+$ lymphocytes. It acts by
  - causing the proliferation of T and B cells.
  - increasing the production of NK cells by bone marrow.
  - inducing IL-2 receptor expression.
  - stimulating antibody production by B cells.
  - causing the activation of NK cells.

IL-2. It is of $CD4^+$ cell origin. It initiates T cell and B cell proliferation, increases NK cell proliferation, IL-2 receptor expression, and antibody production.

This is illustrated in Figure 7.6. Interleukin-2 is produced mainly by helper T-cell subpopulation designated as TH1 cells, but other cells such as cytotoxic T cells can also produce them.

- **IL-3** is a glycoprotein produced by activated T cells. It is related to allergy responses. It acts by
  - serving as a growth factor for many hematopoietic precursors.
  - increasing mast cells number in the skin, spleen, and liver.

- **IL-4** is also a **glycoprotein** produced by
  - **activated T cells. In *vivo* function** is **not well**
  - **defined** but there is **indirect evidence** that it
  - **increases IgE levels**.

- *In-vitro* effects include
  - **increasing** the **proliferation** of **T** cells, **B cells**, and **NK cells**.
  - it **suppresses** the **elaboration** of **IFN-γ**
  - **TNF-α** and **TNF-β** production by **T cells**.
- **IL-5** is produced by activated **T cells.** It has effects on **B cells** by stimulating **antibody production.** In mice, it increases **IgE production** and **causes eosinophilia**.

IL-5. The binding of IgE Fc receptor to eosinophil results in the elaboration of histaminases which counteract the actions of histamine. This is an event which is supposed to balance the activation of mast cells which is accompanied by histamine release.

- **IL-6** is **produced** by activated **T** and **B cells as well as monocytes and fibroblasts. It plays a role in**
  - the **regulation** of **hematopoiesis**.
  - **production** of **acute phase** proteins by hepatocytes.
  - **antibody production**.

IL-6. They influence the production of acute phase proteins, which are inflammatory proteins, produced by the liver cells. IL-6 occupies a unique position of being able to activate the antigen-presenting cells. It may suppress B cells when used on it directly, but *in vivo* acting in concert with IL-21 produced by $CD4^+$ cells, it is a promoter of humoral response and antibody production by B cells.

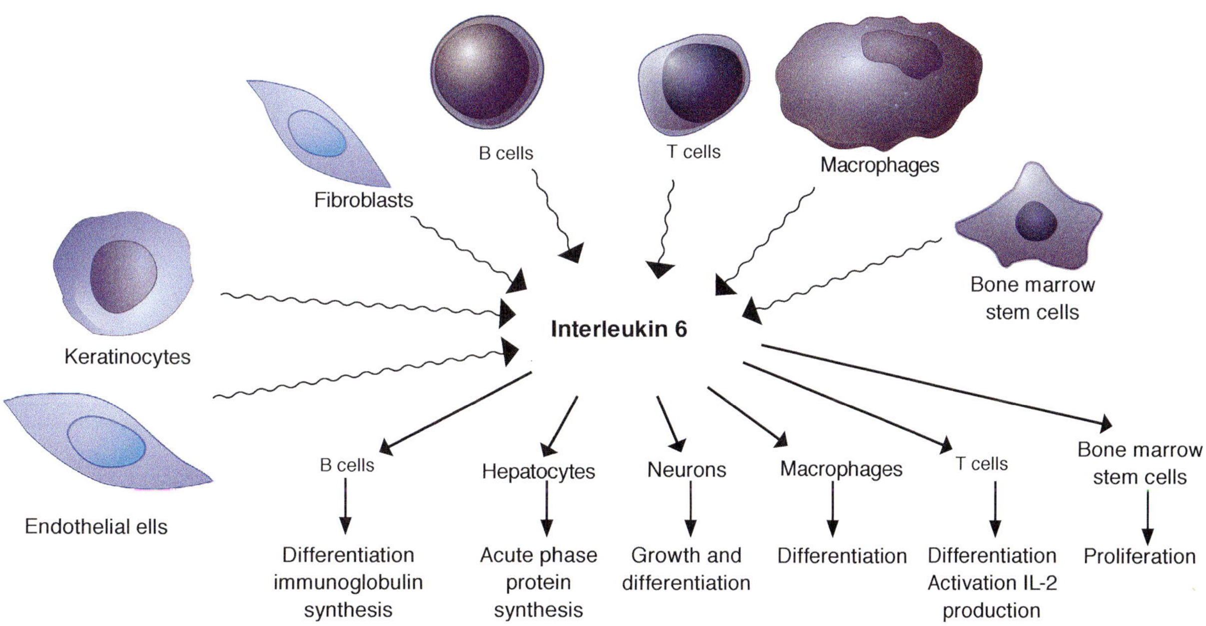

Courtesy of Zainab Ashkanani

Figure 7.7 *The origin and targets of interleukin-6.*

While **IL-10** is **anti-inflammatory**, **IL-12** is **inflammatory**.

- **IL-10**
  - **Inhibits IFN-γ**.
  - **Inhibits antigen presentation**.
  - Inhibits **macrophage production** of **IL-1**.
- **IL-12**
  - **Activates macrophages** and **NK cells**.
  - **Increases IFN-gamma production**.

IL-10. It is anti-inflammatory. It means that most of the response that we have associated with them is a decrease in IFN-γ, because it makes macrophages not react in inflammation. Antigen presentation is decreased, as is the production of IL-1, because IL-1 is actually an inflammatory cytokine.

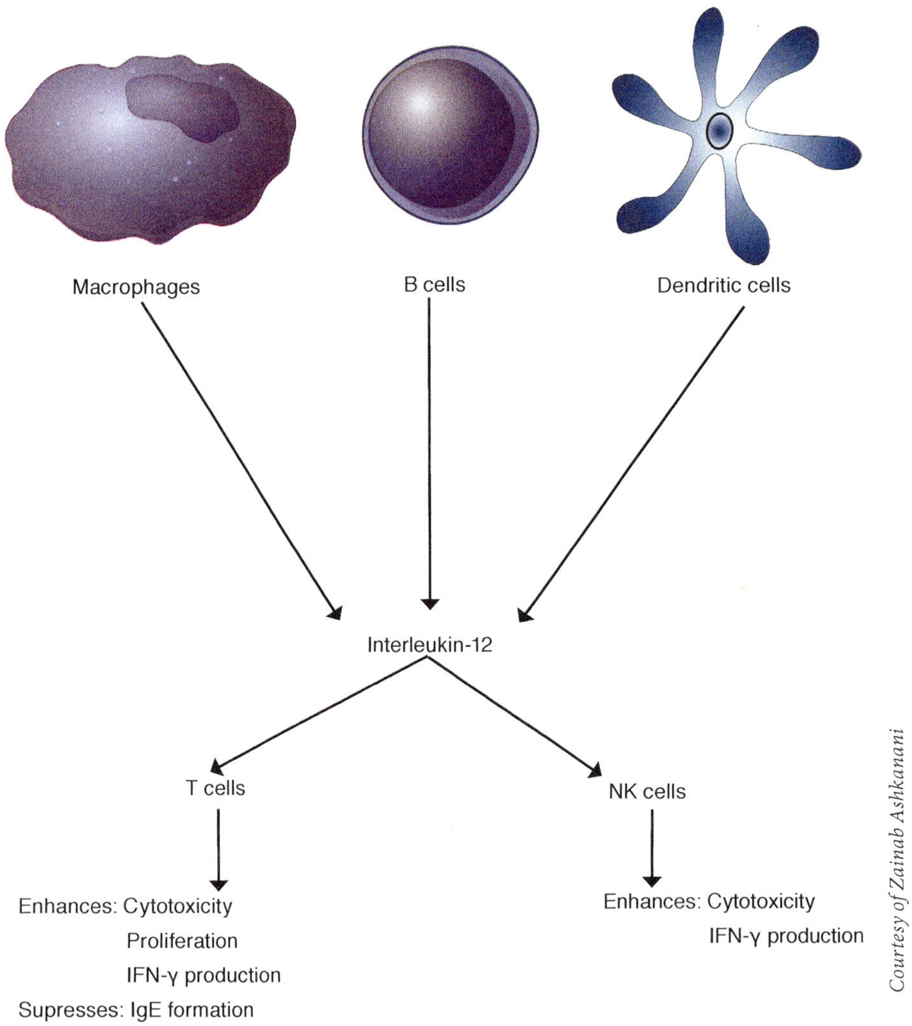

Figure 7.8 *The origin and targets of interleukin-12.*

IL-12. It is the exact opposite of IL-10 in function; therefore, it is inflammatory. It activates macrophages and NK cells and causes IFN-γ elaboration.

This is the summary showing an extensive list of cytokines, their origin, target cells, and impact.

SAMPLE QUESTIONS

CYTOKINES

Answer True or False to the following:

Cytokines

1. Activated neutrophils secrete a range of cytokines.
2. Tumor necrosis factor alpha increases antibody production.
3. Some cytokines act on the hypothalamus resulting in an increase in body temperature.
4. Interferons block the spread of virus to uninfected cells and are hence called antiviral cytokines.
5. Which of the following molecules is classified as a chemokine?
   a. Interleukin-1
   b. Interleukin-2
   c. Interleukin-4
   d. Interleukin-6
   e. Interleukin-8
6. When IL-2 acts on B cells, it stimulates the expression of
   a. IL-3
   b. TGF-β
   c. IL-4
   d. IL-1R
   e. IL-2R
7. Which of the following macrophage products activates lymphocytes?
   a. Interleukin-1
   b. Interferon-α
   c. Granulocyte-macrophage colony stimulating factor (GM-CSF)
   d. Plasminogen
8. Which cytokines released by T cells act primarily upon B cells?
   a. IL-1 and IL-2
   b. IFN-α and IFN-γ
   c. IL-4, IL-5, and IL-6
   d. GM-CSF

Answer True or False:

9. Cytokines are soluble substances that mediate interaction between cells of the immune system.
10. There are four main types of cytokines: colony stimulating factors (CSF), tumor necrosis factors (TNF), interferons (IFN), and interleukins (IL).
11. Interleukins affect only the functions of leukocytes.
12. Interferons can interfere with viral replication.

Answer True or False:

IL-5 and IL-6

13. Both cytokines are produced by activated T cells and B cells.
14. Both cytokines stimulate the production of antibodies.
15. IL-6 also plays a role in the regulation of hematopoiesis.
16. IL-5 causes eosinophilia and increased IgE production in humans.

IL-10 and IL-12

17. IL-10 is pro-inflammatory, while IL-12 is anti-inflammatory.
18. IL-10 inhibits the production of IFN-γ, while IL-12 increases its production.
19. IL-12 inhibits the production of IL-1 by macrophages.
20. IL-10 inhibits antigen presentation.

Suggested Laboratory Practicals

- Case Studies on:
  1. Role of Cytokines in Innate Immune Response
  2. Role of Cytokines in Specific Immune Response
- Erythrocyte Sedimentation Rate
- Immunofixation
- Stimulation of Cell Proliferation

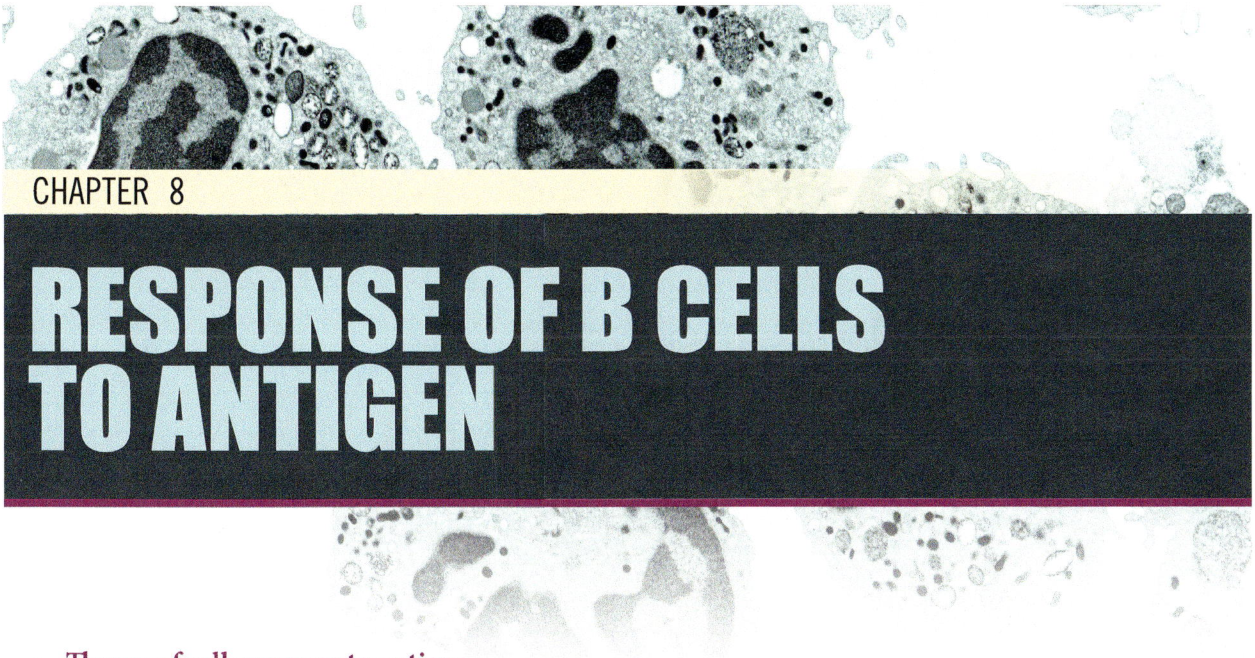

CHAPTER 8

RESPONSE OF B CELLS TO ANTIGEN

- **Theory of cell response to antigen**
- **B cells**
- **Response of B cells to antigen**
- **Plasma cells**
- **Hybridoma**

B cells have some unique aspects to them as they are able to act as an antigen presenter, especially in relation to picking up iccosomes from the dendritic cells. These are also able to recognize antigens, thus exhibiting a dual attribute. The overall result of this is that stimulated B cells give rise to antibody-secreting plasma cells as shown in Figure 8.1.

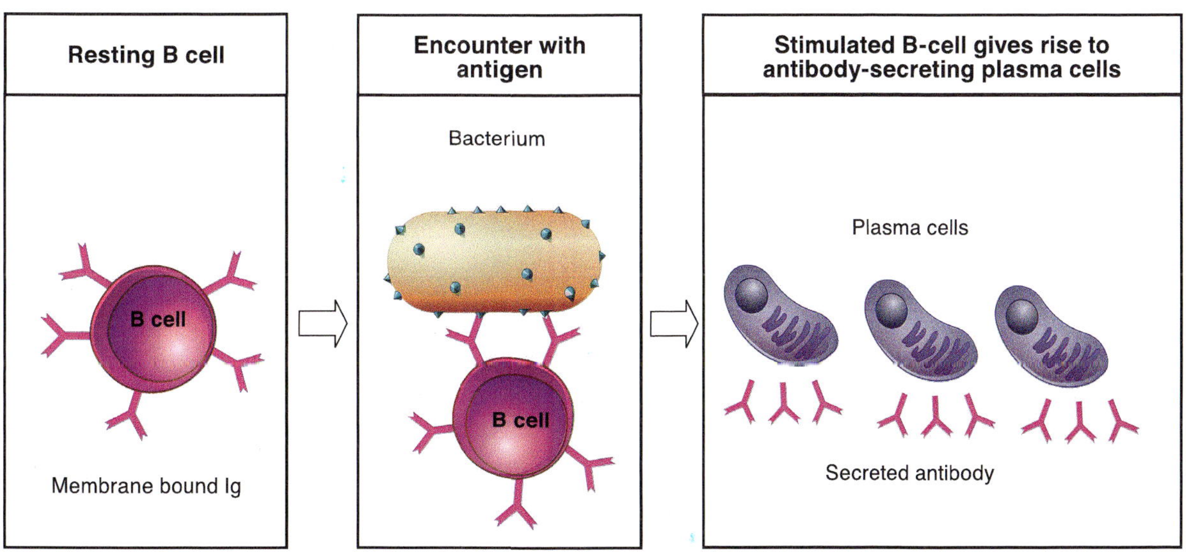

Courtesy of Zainab Asl-kanani

Figure 8.1 *Stimulated by invading bacterium, mature B-cells proliferate into plasma cells which produce antibodies to the same antigen specificity as was encountered by their B-cell precursor.*

Lymphocytes normally develop from primitive cells which are destined to become clones capable of recognizing an antigen. Each clone responds to the recognized antigen by expanding in numbers under the influence of immune mediators.

THEORY OF CELL RESPONSE TO ANTIGEN

The theory of cell response to antigen **is based on clonal selection theory** which can be summarized as follows:

a. Lymphoid stem cells differentiate into clone of lymphocytes and each clone recognizes a single epitope.
b. On binding to Ag, lymphocyte receptors trigger lymphocyte proliferation and differentiation into (i) antibody-producing cells, (ii) effector cells, and (iii) memory cells.

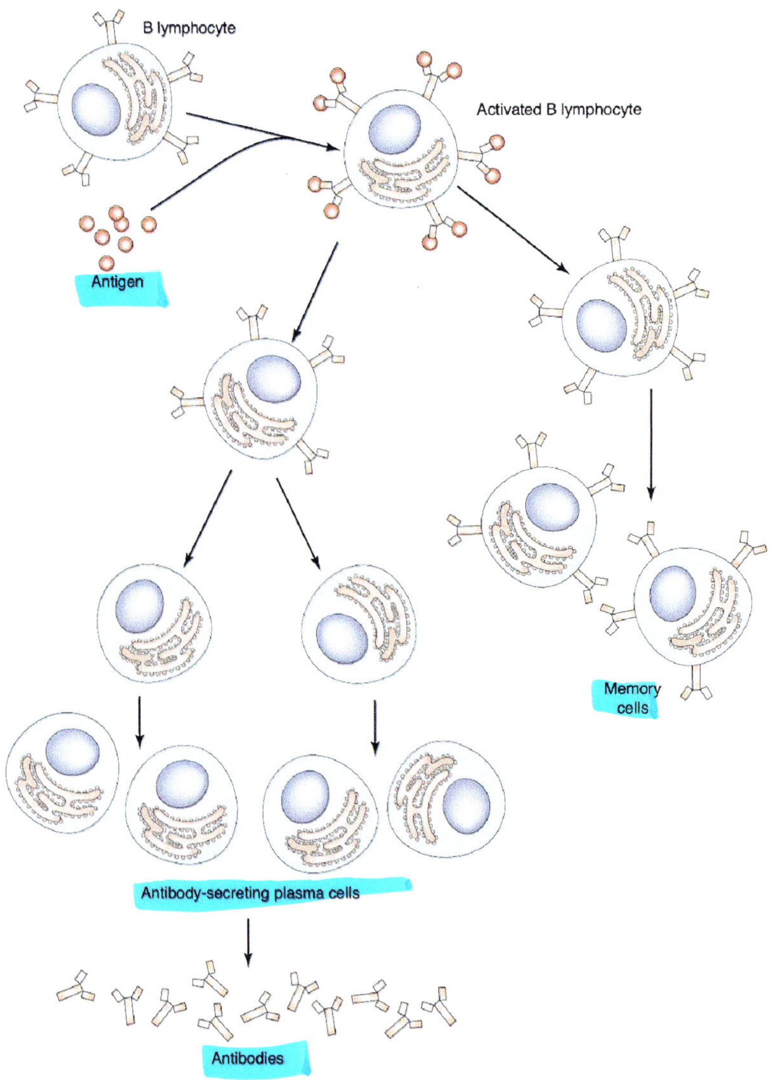

Figure 8.2 *The clonal selection theory. Antigen promotes the growth and differentiation of a B-cell clone (in this case, clone C) responding only to that antigen. As a result, both antibody-producing cells and memory cells specific for that antigen are produced.*

c. Ab specificity is determined by its Ag receptor site.

d. The destruction or suppression of a clone of Ag binding cells causes tolerance. Such Ag binding cells are either B cells (Ab producing) or T cells (cell mediated immune response).

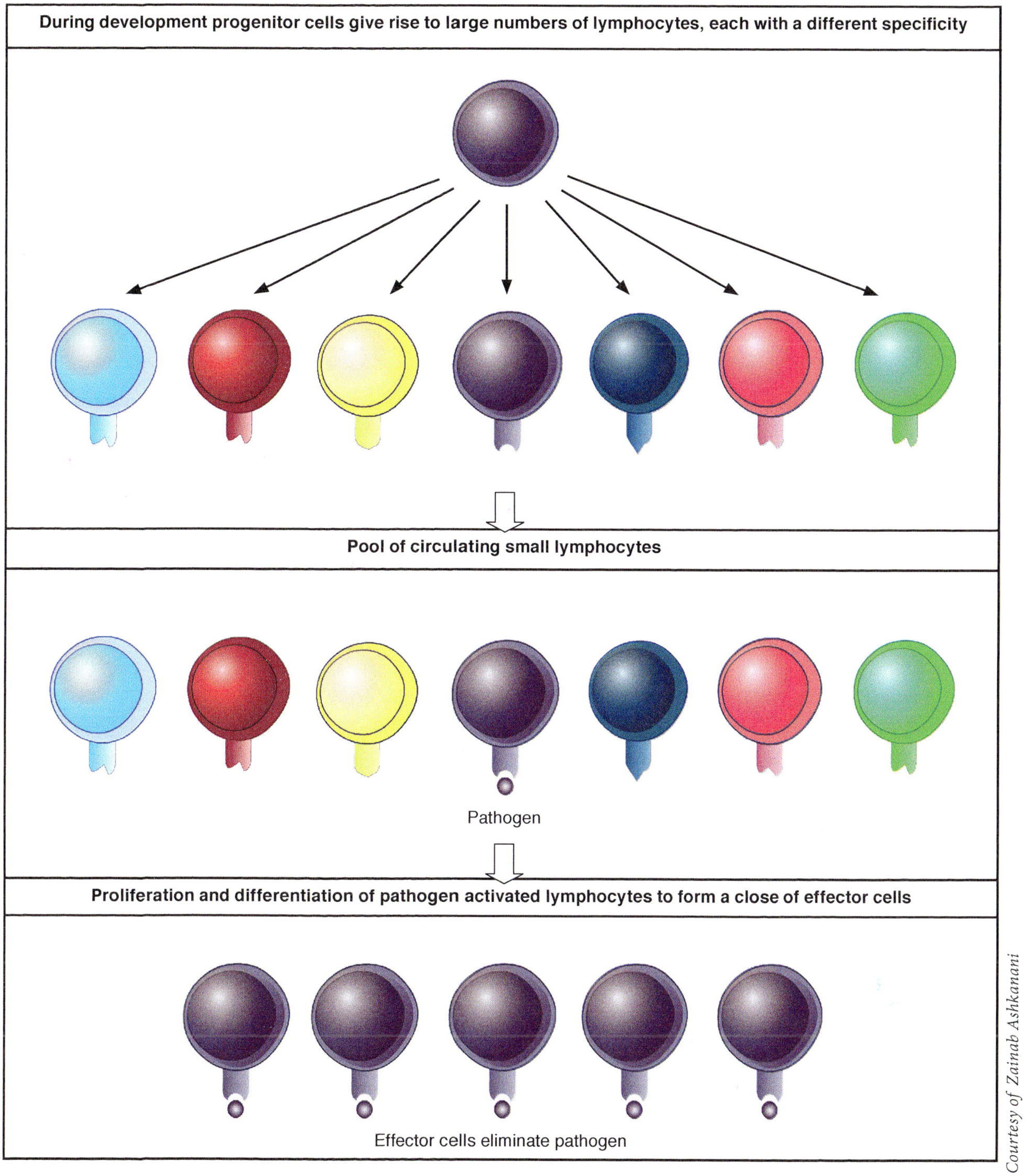

Figure 8.3 *Clonal selection depiction. During development, progenitor cells produce large numbers of lymphocytes all with different specificities and upon a challenge from an invading bacteria, the specific lymphocyte to that bacteria, a clonal expansion arises.*

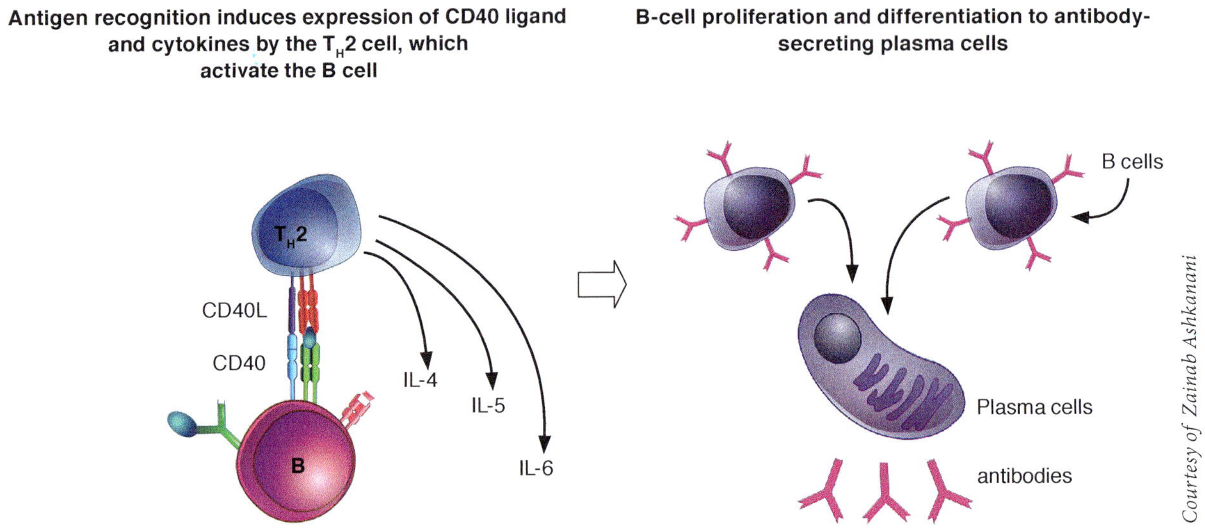

Figure 8.4 *TH2 cells stimulate proliferation and differentiation of B cells into antibody-producing plasma cells.*

In their resting phase, B cells have surface-bound immunoglobulins, which serve mainly as receptors which bind antigens on organized cells such as bacteria. In such an event, they change into plasma cells which secrete antibodies. The mediators of this event are the cytokines; the terminal aspect of this is the formation of a pool of memory B cells, which exhibit accelerated response in terms of antibody production when they encounter antigens to which they have memory. It is important to note that B cells can also present antigen to T cells.

The theory of cell response to antigen is designated as clonal selection theory, and this states:

1. Lymphoid stem cells differentiate into clones of lymphocytes, that each clone recognizes a single epitope (selected conserved peptide).
2. On binding to antigen, lymphocyte receptors trigger lymphocyte proliferation and differentiation. This results in the generation of antibody producing cells (plasma cells), the effector cells that produce cytokines, and the memory cells responsible for memory or anamnestic response (Figures 8.2–8.4).

Antibody specificity (as represented by the paratope) is dependent on the antigenic determinant (epitope); therefore, antibody elaboration by an antibody-producing cell is a specific process. So, the destruction or suppression of a clone of antigen-binding cells incapacitates the immune system when challenged by the antigens for which the clones of cells were destined to act (immune unresponsiveness).

B CELLS

- 10^7 are produced daily by the bone marrow in humans.
- They survive for several months.
- They are found in the cortex of lymph nodes, marginal zone in the spleen, and Payer's patches in the intestine.
- Each B-cell surface is covered by 200,000–500,000 identical Ag receptors (BCR).

FUNCTIONS OF B-CELL RECEPTORS (BCRs)

- Bind antigens.
- Signals B cells to respond when it binds to a ligand.
- Triggers endocytosis of Ag/ligand, leading to proteolysis, processing and expression of peptides associated with MHC class II molecules.
- It is a glycoprotein, expressed as a monomeric IgM
- For effective signal transduction, its transmembrane domains are linked to paired heterodimers (Ig-α/Ig-β)—they have extensive cytoplasmic domains which allow adequate signaling.

About 10 million B cells are produced daily by the bone marrow and they survive for several months. When they leave the bone marrow, they are sufficiently differentiated but become definite in their commitment in the secondary lymphoid tissues (lymph nodes, Payer's patches in the intestine, and the spleen). Each B-cell surface is equipped with 200,000–500,000 receptors. The functions of B-cell receptors (BCRs) include Ag binding and signal transduction in response to ligand–receptor interactions. Subsequent to the binding of BCR to an antigen, there is the internalization of the antigen–receptor complex, leading to the breakdown of protein (proteolysis), processing and expression of peptides associated with MHC class II molecules. The BCRs are glycoproteins expressed as monomeric IgM and sometimes as coupled IgD, so they are cross-linked to result in effective binding to antigen.

Cross-linking of antigen receptors is the first step in B-cell activation. B-cell receptors are physically cross-linked by repetitive epitopes of Ag on the surface of the bacterial cell. Surface IgM binds Ag and signals are transmitted to activate the naïve B cell.

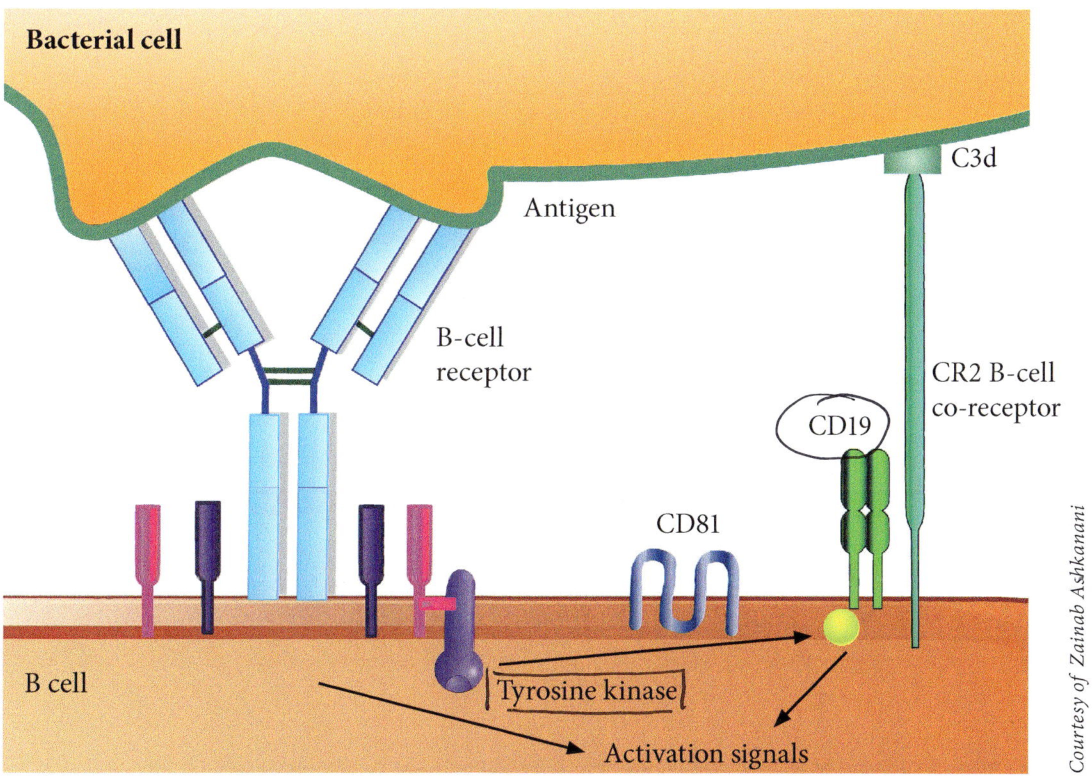

Figure 8.5 *Synergistic signals from B-cell receptor and the coreceptor result in B-cell activation. CR2, a B-cell coreceptor, binds C3d on a bacterial cell to assist in the activation of B cell.*

Immatured B cells have IgM which on maturation are replaced by IgM and IgD, making room for effective binding, that is, immunoglobulin cross-linking.

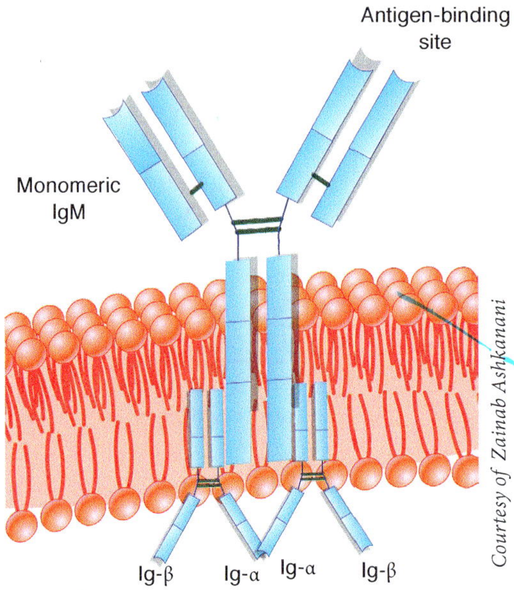

Figure 8.6 *The structure of the B cell antigen receptor. The cell-surface immunoglobulin is linked to two heterodimers with extensive cytoplasmic domains. These serve as signal transducing molecules.*

So, for signal transduction to be effective there is need for extension of signals from the transmembrane domain into the cytosolic domain. This is illustrated in Figures 8.5 and 8.6 above.

RESPONSE OF B CELLS TO ANTIGENS

1. **Cell–cell interaction:**
   - Helper T cells are involved.
   - CD4+ T cells memorize peptide sequence on MHC class II molecules of antigen-presenting cells (including B cells) and activate a set of B-cell population to produce antibodies.
   - Also, B cells can independently recognize antigen and antigen sequence on memory T cells.
   - While B cells recognize **intact molecules**, T cells recognize **processed epitopes**.

Cell–cell interaction occurs in the lymph node.

2. **Activation of cytokines:**
   - Depends on the effect of helper T-cell subpopulation on B cells.
   - Helper T cells are of TH1 or TH2 subpopulation.

- TH1 and TH2 produce different cytokines. While TH1 is optimized for cell-mediated immune response, TH2 is optimized for antibody production.
- TH1 cells secrete IL-1, 2, and IFN-γ which do not stimulate antibody production but promote B-cell proliferation.
- TH2 cells secrete IL-4, 5, 6, 10, and 13, enhancing IgG, IgA, and IgE production.

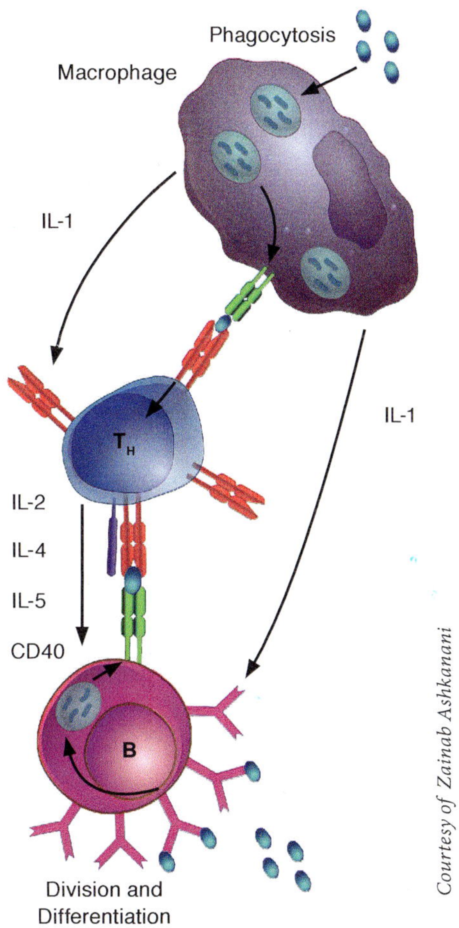

Figure 8.7 *An outline of the cell interactions that occur when a B cell responds to antigen. Macrophages present antigen to a helper T cell and costimulate it with interleukin-1. The B cell is stimulated by free antigen and responds to it under the influence of IL-2, IL-4, and IL-5. B cells may also present antigen to T cells.*

Cytokines also have effect on B cells facilitating their proliferation (Figure 8.7). The capacity of secretions from TH1 to heighten cell-mediated immune response by suppressing antibody production while TH2 exerts an opposite effect is depicted in Table 8.1.

TABLE 8.1 THE AMOUNT OF IMMUNOGLOBULIN CLASSES/SUBCLASSES PRODUCED BY B CELLS IN THE PRESENCE OF EITHER TH1 OR TH2 CELLS.

CLASS	TH2 CELL (NG/ML)	TH1 CELL (NG/ML)
IgG_1	21,600	<8
IgG_{2a}	39	14
IgG_{2b}	189	<8
IgG_3	354	<8
IgM	98,000	248
IgA	484	<1
IgE	187	<1

Note: Adapted from Coffmann et al. Immunol. Rev., 102.5, *1988. With permission from the author and Munksgaard International Publishers Inc.*

3. **B cell response:**
   - **Ab production by plasma cells.**
   - The **earliest recognizable cells** when **B cells** are **activated** to become plasma cells are **plasmablasts found in 2° lymphoid tissue** cortex, usually in the area of T- and B-cell cooperation.
   - Plasma cells are ovoid, 8–9 μm in diameter (Figures 8.8 and 8.9). They have round eccentrically placed nucleus, their cytoplasm is abundant and rich in endoplasmic reticulum. At the termination of I° response, B cells undergo apoptosis.

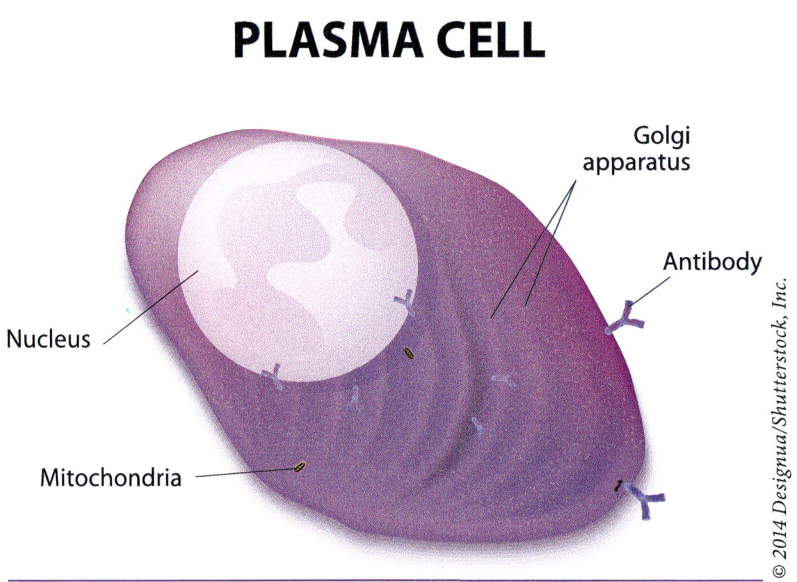

Figure 8.8 *The major structural features of a plasma cell.*

B-lineage cell	Property					
	Intrinsic			Inducible		
	Surface Ig	Surface MHC class II	High rate Ig secretion	Growth	Somatic hypermutation	Isotype switch
Resting B cell	Yes	Yes	No	Yes	Yes	Yes
Plasma cell	No	No	Yes	No	No	No

Courtesy of Zainab Ashkanan

Figure 8.9 *Comparison of resting B cells and plasma cells.*

- Other B cells that are left after primary response differentiate into memory cells. This happens under the control of bcl-2 gene. Expression of bcl-2 gene makes a cell escape from apoptosis. Over expression of this survival gene can cause lymphoma.

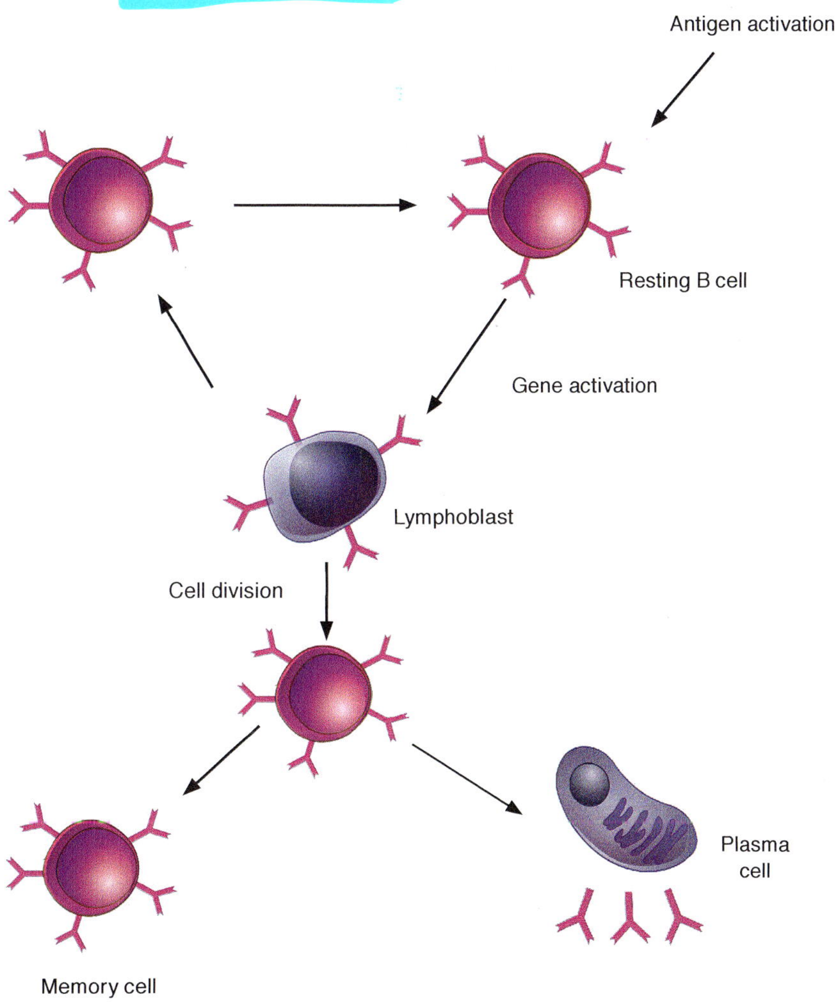

Courtesy of Zainab Ashkanan

Figure 8.10 *Activation of B cells leads to cell division and differentiation into memory cells and plasma cells.*

LABORATORY PRODUCTION OF MONOCLONAL ANTIBODIES (HYBRIDOMA TECHNOLOGY)

HYBRIDOMAS

- Plasma cell tumor is known as myeloma. Under this condition, homogenous immunoglobulin called myeloma proteins are produced.
- Hypergammaglobulinemia is the condition of increased gammaglobulin in blood seen in myeloma.
- Hypergammaglobulinemia is described as gammopathy. There are two types:
  - Monoclonal gammopathy.
  - Polyclonal gammopathy.
- Electrophoresis is used to show the difference between monoclonal and polyclonal gammopathy.
- In gammopathies, fragments of immunoglobulin, especially light chains, are recovered in urine because light chains are filterable in the kidney. However, they are toxic to the kidney; they destroy the glomerulus, causing kidney failure, resulting in nephrotic syndrome, glomerulonephritis, sand so on.
- Myeloma cells can grow in tissue culture indefinitely.
- The Abs produced are random. However, if normal plasma cells that make specific Abs are fused with a myeloma cell, then a hybrid is formed—Hybridoma.
- This hybridoma will make specific Abs indefinitely.

The tumor of plasma cells is called myeloma. Under this condition, there is the production of monoclonalimmunoglobulin and fragments of immunoglobulin moieties called myeloma proteins. Sometimes, light chains or heavy chains alone are produced. Usually, the condition is characterized by hypergammaglobulinemia (increased gammaglobulin in blood). Hypergammaglobulinemia is often described as a gammopathy. There are two types:

i. Monoclonalgammopathy: Produces immunoglobulins in high concentrations of one clone, monoclonal.
ii. Polyclonalgammopathy: In this case, you have more than one clone.

Myeloma cells can grow in tissue culture indefinitely, but they elaborate immunoglobulin fragments and other random antibodies. However, if a normal plasma cell that makes specific antibodies is fused with a myeloma cell, then a hybrid is formed called a hybridoma (Figure 8.10). The hybridoma makes a specific antibody indefinitely. Advantage is taken of this capability of the hybridoma to produce specific antibodies indefinitely in the manufacture of monoclonal antibodies (Figure 8.11).

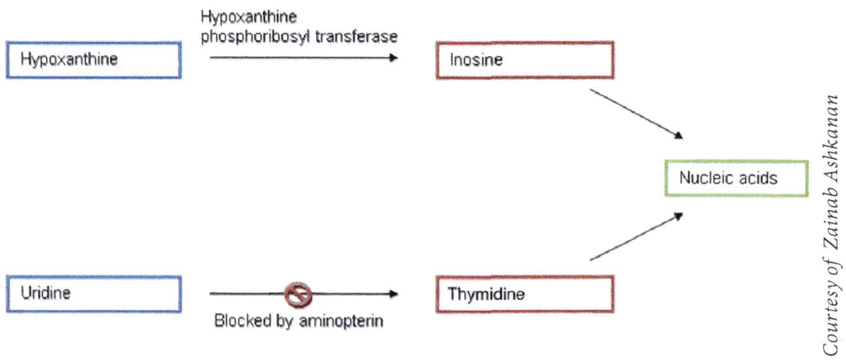

Figure 8.11 *A highly simplified diagram showing the two pathways involved in nucleic acid synthesis, Myeloma cells used in hybridoma formation lack hypoxanthine phosphoribosyl.*

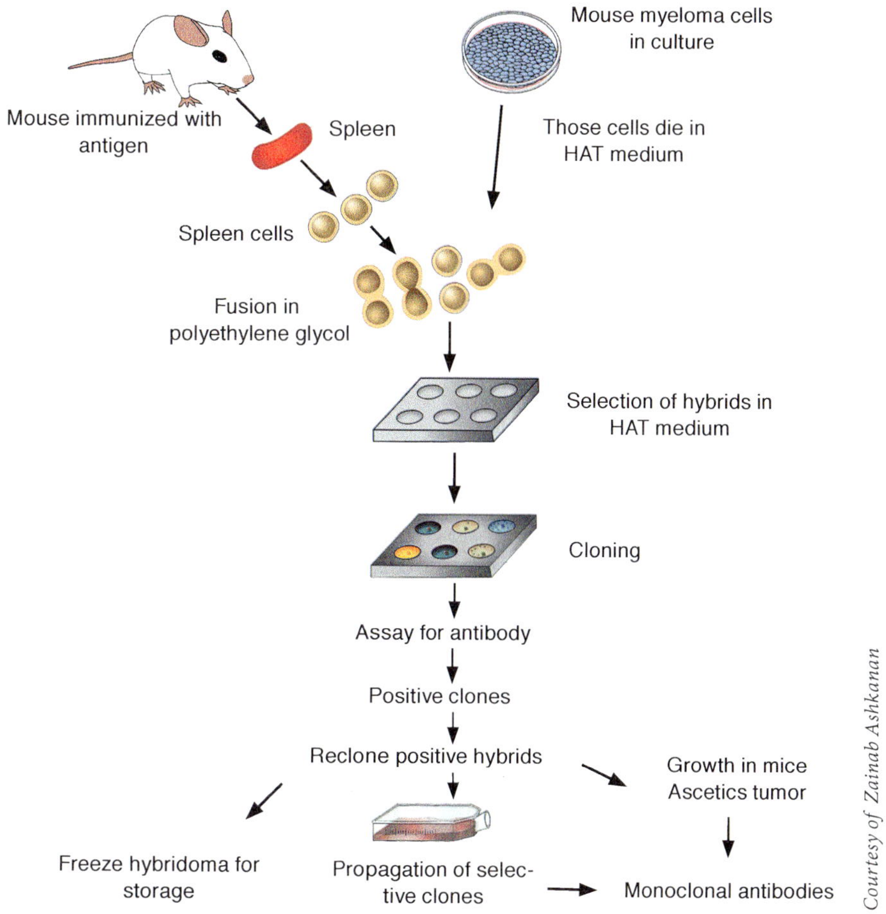

Figure 8.12 *The production of monoclonal antibodies from clone hybridoma cells (HAT medium is hypoxanthine, aminopteridine, and thymidine). The hybrids are generated by fusing spleen cells with myeloma cells in the presence of polyethylene glycol.*

The fusion of myeloma cells and the specific antibody-producing plasma cells is achieved in the medium polyethylene glycol. Also, care is taken to produce a pure system that is devoid of all myeloma cells after fusion. To do this, advantage is taken of the fact that myeloma cells cannot synthesize DNA as normal cells do. Instead, it adopts a salvage pathway. This pathway can be blocked after the fusion process, without affecting the product of the fusion. In this process, pure hybrid of myeloma–plasma cell is produced. The process is illustrated in Figure 8.12. It involves the use of HAT medium (hypoxanthine, aminopteridine, and thymidine medium). The hypoxanthine content of the medium is a source of inosine, which is a nucleoside. The enzyme required for producing inosine from hypoxanthine is hypoxanthine phosphoribosyltransferase. This enzyme is not present in myeloma cells. However, myeloma cells go through a salvage pathway involving the conversion of uridine to thymidine to make nucleic acids. Aminopteridine content of HAT medium blocks this salvage pathway, thus ensuring the death of myeloma cells. The thymidine content of HAT medium is low but sufficient to allow successful fusion. The specificity of the fused myeloma–plasma cell is determined by the nature of the antigen used to stimulate the animal. The specificity resides in those B cells which are found in the spleen or other secondary lymphoid tissue. When the mouse is sacrificed, the spleen is squashed through gauze to produce free spleen cells (splenocytes) which are very rich in B cells (antibody-producing cells). These cells are committed to producing antibodies, but they are not long-lived, so they are conferred with immortality by conjugating them with the myeloma cells in polyethylene glycol medium. The hybrid of myeloma cells and spleen cells or B cells that are produced, elaborate specific antibody indefinitely. The supernatant of this culture is rich in the specific monoclonal antibodies. They can be stored in the –80°C freezer, and then transferred into liquid nitrogen tank. They can also be stored in mice.

SAMPLE QUESTIONS

RESPONSE OF B CELLS TO ANTIGEN

Answer True or False to the following:

B cell activation upon antigen encounter

1. Once a naïve B cell encounters a specific antigen, the antigen is bound by the antigen binding site of IgG.
2. Cross-linking of BCR is required for naïve B cell activation.
3. Tyrosine kinases phosphorylate CD19.
4. Combined signaling produces tenfold stronger stimulation.

T-cell-dependent activation of B cells

5. Combined signaling from the B-cell receptor and the coreceptor is only sufficient to activate naïve B cells stimulated by thymus-independent antigen.
6. B cells, antigens, and helper CD4 T cells are brought together in the secondary lymphoid tissues.
7. IL-4, IL-5, and IL-6 are secreted by CD4 T cells and induce B cell proliferation and differentiation.
8. Most antigens are thymus-dependent; therefore, CD4 T lymphocyte help is not needed to activate the B cell.

CD4 T helper cells

9. Naïve CD4 T cells become activated when their receptors bind to specific antigenic peptides presented in the context of MHC class I molecules.
10. Activated B cells can deliver a costimulatory signal to activate naïve CD4 T cells via CD28 interaction with B7 molecules.
11. Resting B cells do not express B7 molecules.
12. Bacterial products activate B cells and induce expression of B7 molecules.

Somatic Hypermutation and Affinity Maturation

13. CD8 T cell cytokines are essential for somatic hypermutation.
14. B cells with a range of affinities to the specific antigen are produced due to hypermutation.
15. Competition between B cells that have undergone hypermutation leads to the selection of cells bearing BCR with the highest affinity to the specific antigen.

Suggested Laboratory Practicals

- Case Studies on:

1. Monoclonal Antibody Production
2. Multiple Myeloma
3. Interrelationship between B Cells, T Cells, and Macrophages/Dendritic Cells during Antigen Presentation and Recognition

- Demonstration of B-Cell Surface Markers
- Differences between B-Cells and Plasma Cells

CHAPTER 9

COMPLEMENT

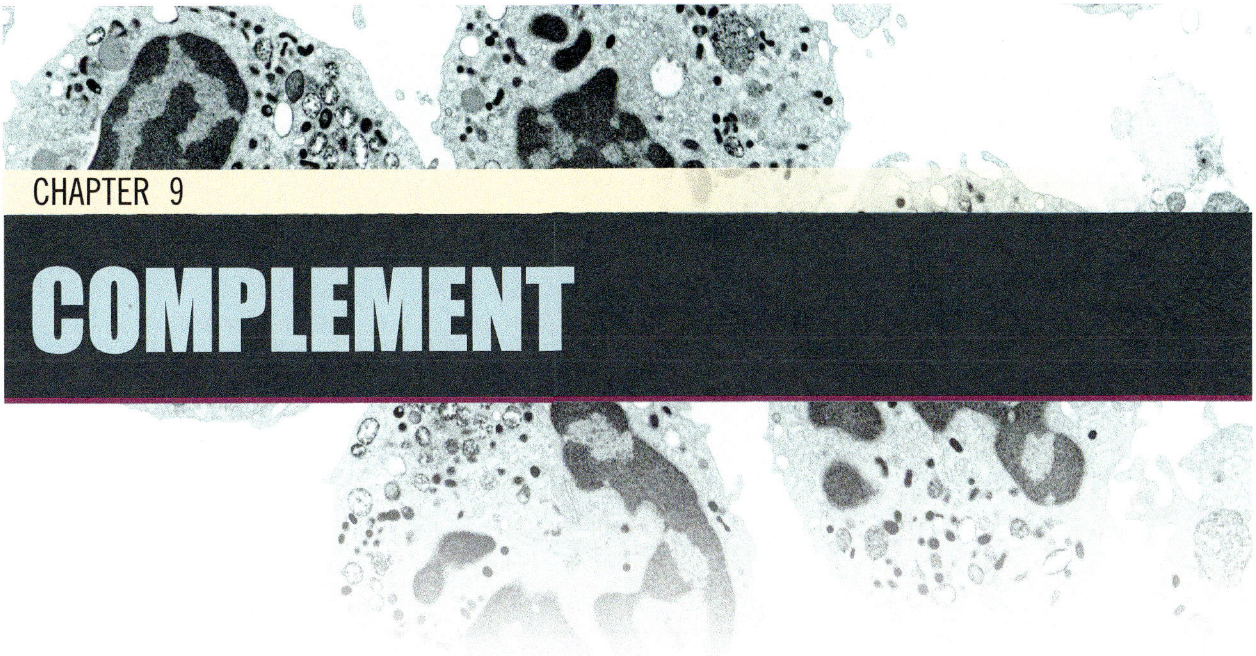

One of the impacts of antigen–antibody interaction is the activation of complement cascade, resulting in the eradication of the challenge. The relevance of the binding of antibody to an antigen to trigger the activation of antibody is that this process exposes the complement binding site on the antibody. This complement reactive site is situated on the constant region of the heavy chain of the antibody, which is usually concealed by the flapping down of the heavy and light Fab chains. So, when the Fab region which normally masks the Fc region binds to an antigen, the shape of the molecule changes and the Fc region is exposed, thus becoming functional. It is important to note that multiple binding of antigen to antibody will amplify the number of exposed sites, therefore, enhancing complement activity.

The complement system consists of a group of proteins that are closely related; they are found in normal fresh serum. They are thermolabile and deteriorate with the aging of the serum. They play a critical role in immune defense in the body and function in association with antibodies and the cells of the immune system.

THE COMPLEMENT SYSTEM

It consists of a family of proteins which play a critical role in the defense of the body in association with antibodies and the cells of the immune system. We shall study the following:

- How the system is turned on and leads to the destruction of invading microbes.
- The regulation of this complex system.
- Their role in chemotaxis, opsonization, and inflammation.
- Complement system dysfunction
- The use of complement in diagnostic test.

It is intriguing to note that the switching-on of the complement system leads to the destruction of invading microbes. However, this process can also bring about the destruction of the host cell system; therefore, it is a tightly regulated process. The complement components, especially the protein fragments generated during the activation process, have a role in chemotaxis, resulting in the drafting of immune cells to the site of activity. They play enormous roles in opsonization and the localization of immune response (inflammation). There is, therefore, a serious consequence arising from complement dysfunction.

COMPLEMENT

- A chain of enzymes whose activation leads to the disruption of cell membrane and cell death.
- There is sequential activation of the enzymes in a manner that each product catalyzes the next reaction.
- It is carefully regulated, because uncontrolled activation can lead to massive cell destruction.
- There are at least 19 protein components of the complement system, designated as C1, C2, C3, etc. and B, D, P, etc. Together they constitute 10% of the globulin fraction of serum.
- Complement proteins are synthesized mainly by the liver and macrophages. For example C3, C6, C8, and B are of liver origin, while C2, C3, C4, C5, B, D, P, and I are of macrophage origin.

  B, C4, and C2 are coded for by genes located in the MHC class III region.

The chain of enzymes of the complement cascade is activated in a sequential manner, with the ultimate result leading to the disruption of cell membrane and cell death (Figure 9.1). Each protein is a proenzyme which upon activation acts as an enzyme for a subsequent step.

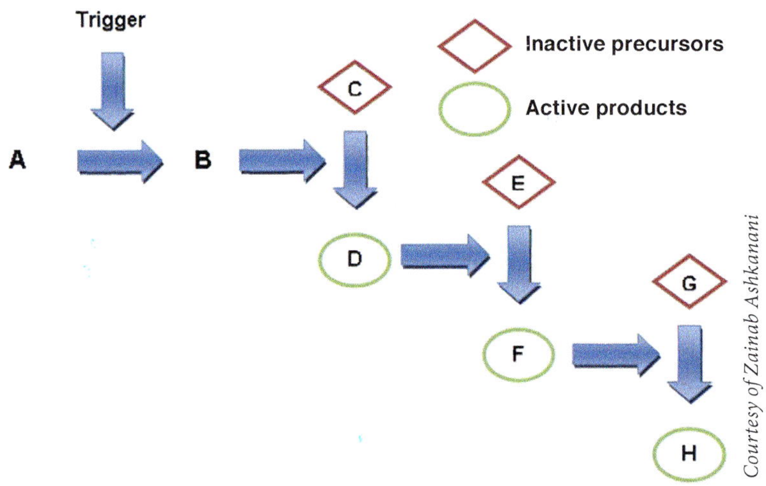

Figure 9.1 *Cascade reactions: The process is started by a trigger that initiates the conversion of an inactive proenzyme A to an active enzyme B. Enzyme B acts to convert proenzyme C to active enzyme D, enzyme D in turn converts proenzyme E to active enzyme F, and so on. The net effect is a very rapid acceleration of these reactions.*

There are three complement pathways: the first is the classical pathway, the second is the alternate pathway, and the third is the terminal pathway. There is the "fourth" pathway, known as the lectin pathway, which is activated by the capacity of mannose-binding protein to bind on to mannose on the pathogen surface; it is linked to the classical and alternate pathways.

The diagram below illustrates the activities in the three pathways that finally lead to the terminal pathway (Figure 9.2).

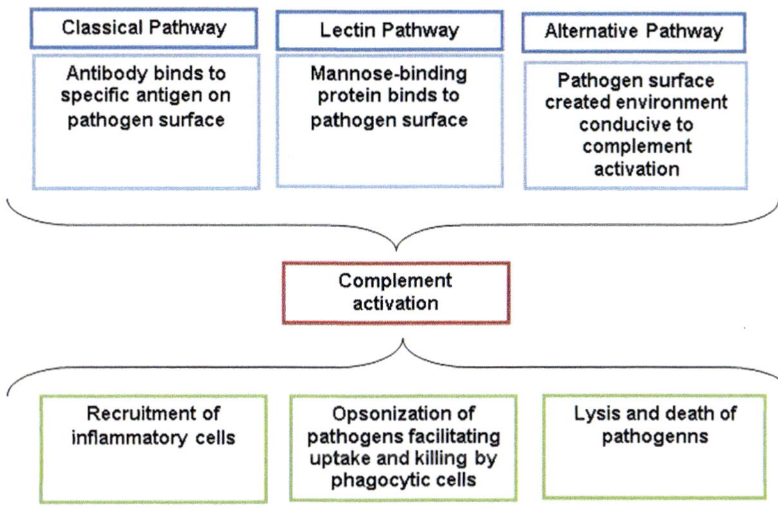

Courtesy of Zainab Ashkanani

Figure 9.2 *Schematic overview of the three pathways of complement activation, classical, lectin, and alternate, all result in complement activation.*

THE CLASSICAL PATHWAY

The initiation of the process is triggered by the activation of C1 complement component (see Figure 9.3). The C1 component has three protein moieties, namely, C1q, C1r, and C1s, held together by a calcium-dependent bond. The binding of C1q to the exposed complement-binding site on an antibody results in the release of C1r and C1s, and their subsequent conversion from inactive to active forms. The released C1r is active and it initiates the cleavage of C1s to an active form. The active form of C1s is a proteolytic enzyme which cleaves C4 into C4a and C4b. The C4b moiety has a site that has affinity for C2; the binding between C2 and C4b modifies C2 and presents it in a more vulnerable form to the enzyme C1s to produce C4b2a and C2b. It is important to note that C4b2a is a very active enzyme described as a C3 convertase.

THE CLASSICAL COMPLEMENT PATHWAY

- The first protein of the pathway is C1. C1 consists of C1q, C1r, and C1s subunits held together by a Ca^{2+}-dependent bond.
- Complement C1q does not bind free immunoglobulin probably because of the masking by Fab regions.
- Activation of C1 in normal serum is prevented by a protein C1 inhibitor (C1-INH).
- C1-INH acts by binding C1r and C1s, thereby preventing their removal from the complex (Figure 9.4).
- Immune complexes overcome this inhibitory effect.

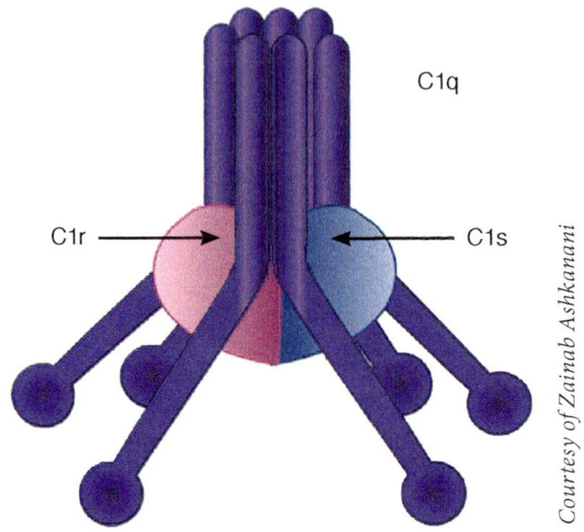

Figure 9.3 *Complement component C1.*

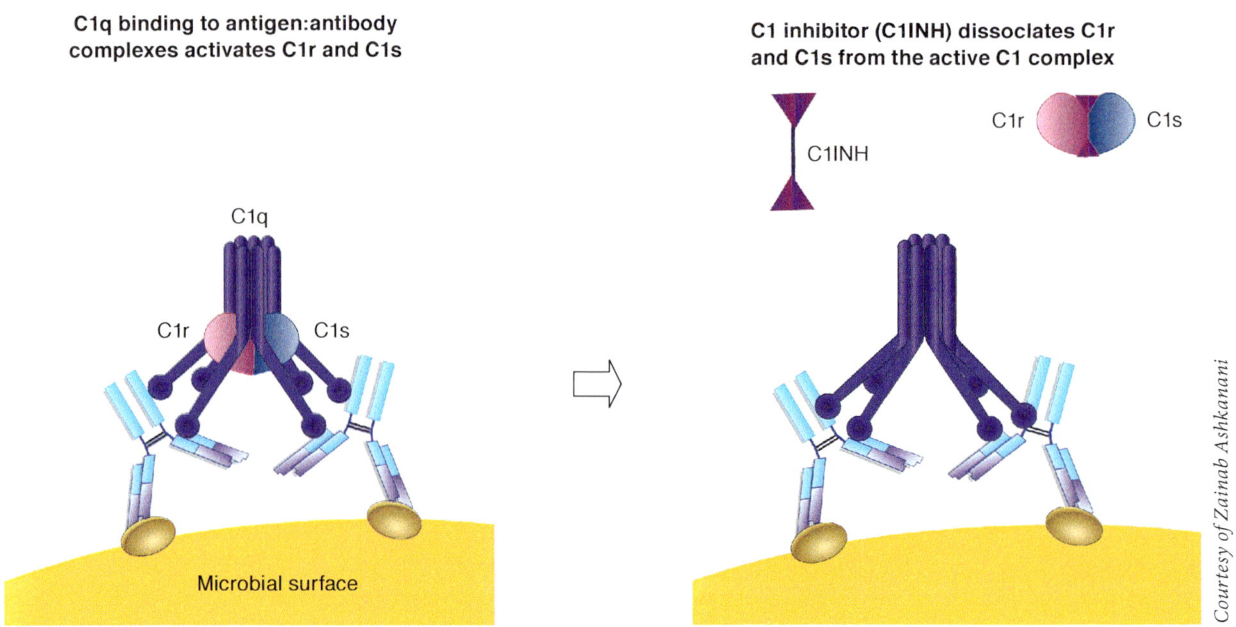

Figure 9.4 *C1-INH blocks the first steps of the classical activation pathway.*

- The stimuli that activates C1 include
  - single-antigen bound molecule of IgM or paired antigen bound molecules of IgG.
  - surface proteins of some viruses or bacteria (*Escherichia coli* and *Klebsiella pneumoniae*).
- Although complement proteins are numbered, they do not act in numeric order, for example, activated C1 acts on C4 and C2. C4 and C2 act on C3.
- Some of them are synthesized as proglycoprotein, for example, C4 is synthesized as pro-C4 and converted to C4 by plasmin.
- In some cases, binding occurs between an active form of an enzyme and another substrate in order for the substrate to be susceptible to its active enzyme (substrate modification). This confines activities to the target under attack.

Note that:

- The C1 complex consist of C1q, r, and s held together in a Ca^{2+}-dependent bond.
- The binding of C1q to immunoglobulin leads to the release of C1r and C1s and their conversion from zymogen state to active enzyme state.
- The activation of C1r causes the cleavage of C1s to the active form.
- The proeolytic activity of active C1s leads to activation of C4 and C2 to generate C4b2a which is a C3 convertase.
- Apart from its role in the regulation of C1 activity in the classical complement pathway, C1-INH also inhibits serine proteases of clotting and kinin systems. The importance of C1-INH is seen in hereditary angioneurotic edema (HANE), suffered by persons with one normal and one defective copy of the C1-INH gene.
- These patients have bouts of swelling, called edema of the skin, gut, and airways, usually triggered by some forms of physical or mental stress. In this situation of relative lack of C1-INH, there is (i) excessive production of C2a which is a kinin and causes fluid to enter tissue from blood resulting in edema, (ii) there is overproduction of bradykinin, a vasoactive peptide, the main product of kinin system, also contributes to the edema.

The stimuli that activate C1 include

- single-antigen bound molecule of IgM or paired antigen molecules bound to IgG. The reason for that is also clear because IgG would need to bind 2, at least a pair, but IgM is a pentamer.
- surface proteins of some viruses, or bacteria like *E. coli*, *Listeria*, *Klebsiellap neumoniae*, and others.

The capacity of C4b2a to cleave C3 into C3b and C3a is a committed stage in the classic complement pathway. In a substrate modulation fashion, C3b binds to C5, thereby making C5 vulnerable to C4b2a to form C3b5b and C5a. The complex C3b5b can be seeded into the terminal pathway to generate membrane attack complex (Figure 9.5).

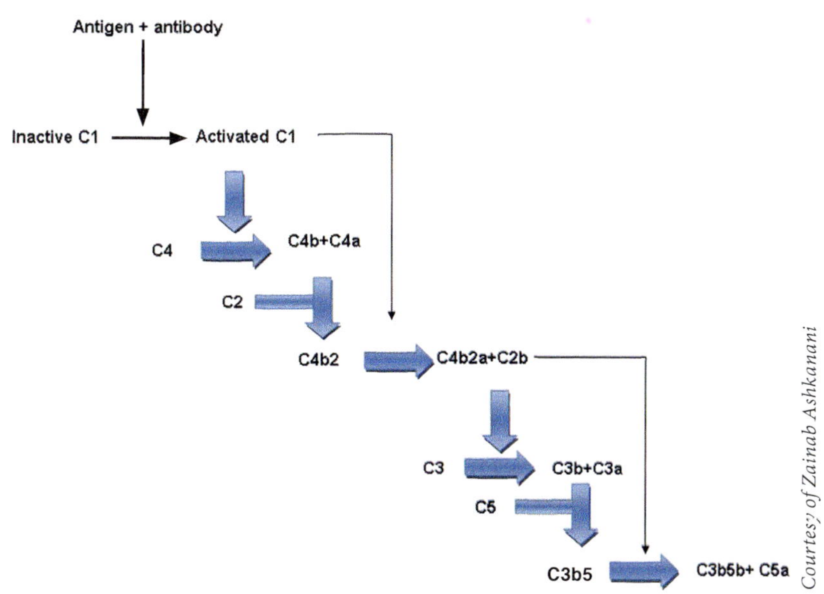

Figure 9.5 *The classical complement pathway. The pathway is activated by antigen binding to a single IgM molecule or two closely spaced IgG molecules. C4b2a is the classical C3 convertase.*

It is important to note that complement protein fragments may have very significant bioactivity outside the complement cascade. It is known that C4a is a peptide mediator of inflammation and C2b is a precursor of C2 kinin. C3b binds covalently to the pathogen surface and acts as an opsonin; it also initiates the alternate pathway, while C5a and C3a are peptide mediators of inflammation.

The phenomenon of substrate modulation is very important, and is well illustrated below (Figure 9.6).

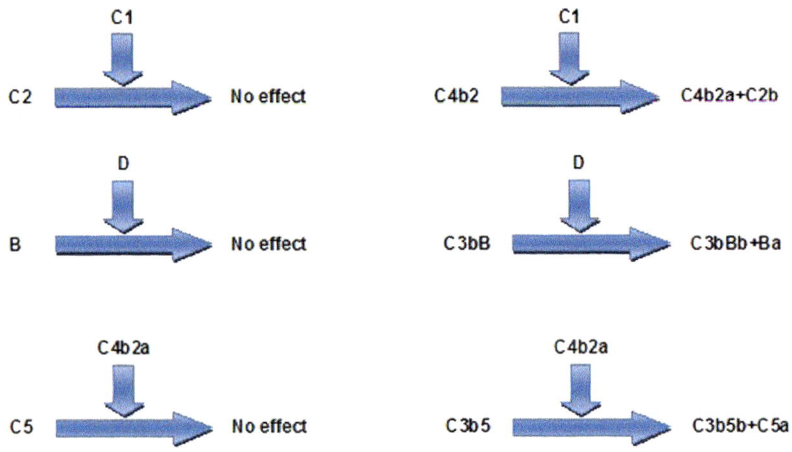

Courtesy of Zainab Ashkanani

Figure 9.6 *Depicted is the phenomenon of substrate modification. The enzymes C1, D, and C4b2a cannot act on their substrates unless the substrates are first bound to another molecule.*

The C3 complement component is very important; it is seeded into all the pathways as a central player. It is heterodimeric, consisting of α (120 kDa) and β (70kDa). It is synthesized in the liver and macrophage and has the highest concentration in serum of all complement proteins. C4b2a is the classical C3 convertase which acts by splitting C3 into C3a (a 6 kDa protein) and C3b. C4b2a can activate as many as 200 molecules of C3. C3b has an exposed carboxyl group which enables it to bind to the cell surface. C3a has anaphylatoxic activity.

THE ALTERNATIVE COMPLEMENT PATHWAY

This is so called because it is an alternative pathway for metabolizing C3, one of the very important protein components. Since this complement component repeats itself in all the pathways, it is a very useful tool for assessing the complement system's effective function. While the classic pathway produces C4b5b that is seeded into the terminal pathway and C4b2a that is a C5 convertase (also a C3 convertase) which is also useful in the terminal pathway, the alternate pathway produces C3bBb, which is a C5 convertase, and C3bBbP, which can be lytic to the cell.

THE ALTERNATIVE COMPLEMENT PATHWAY

- This is the alternative route of the third complement component.
- Spontaneous breakdown of C3 to C3b occurs in small amounts and the thioester bond on C3b enables it to bind to the nearby cell surface. Such cell-bound C3b may be inactivated or may initiate the alternative pathway.
- The fate of C3b depends on the affinity of C3b for a protein called H factor and the nature of surface.
- The state of H factor affects its affinity for C3b. When H factor interacts with sialic acid or other anionic polysaccharides, it then binds strongly to C3b. In so doing, it makes C3b more susceptible to hydrolysis by factor I (esterase).

- On the other hand, surfaces deficient in sialic acid do not enhance C3b and H protein interaction.
- Since most mammalian cells are heavily glycosylated, thus rich in sialic acid, they therefore do not trigger the alternative pathway.
- In contrast, bacteria polysaccharides, nucleic acid, viruses, aggregated immunoglobulin, and foreign particles such as asbestos have their sialic acid removed by means of neuraminidases and so do not enhance interaction between H protein and C3b, therefore, allowing C3b to act.
- Abs may initiate the activation of alternative complement pathway by masking sialic acid on cell surfaces.
- Bacteria such as some strains of *E. coli* that have abundant sialic acid may evade this pathway.

Thus, the alternate pathway leads to cell lysis and death of pathogens (Figure 9.7). It is through the alternate pathway that the lectin pathway enters the complement system. Ordinarily, in normal serum, C3 is dissociated into C3a and C3b spontaneously. C3b has a carbonyl group that makes it bind to membranes, it's a thioester bond. The fate of the cell to which C3b is bound is dependent on other factors, resulting in C3b becoming either active or inactive. Under normal circumstances, it is inactivated. In circumstances of infections or challenges that have brought about the conversion of C3 to C3b, it is activated. The factors interacting in these circumstances are factors H and I on the one hand and factor B, D, and P on the other. Under normal conditions, the host cell is heavily glycosylated, thus endowed with sialic acid and therefore has a high affinity for factor H. When factor H binds to sialic acid, it is oriented in a way that it interacts with C3b already bound to membrane to form C3bH. C3bH is susceptible to factor I, an esterase. Thus, the decay of all C3b bound to normal cell is assured and does not progress along the path of the alternate pathway. However, on the other hand, if the surfaces are deficient in sialic acid, then C3b persists because factor H will not bind and there will be no decay of C3b. The surfaces that will facilitate a prevention of such decay include those with bacterial polysaccharide, nucleic acid, viruses, aggregates of immunoglobulin, and foreign particles such as asbestos. Antibodies may initiate the activation of alternative complement pathway by masking the sialic acid, when this occurs, then it may be possible for the C3b to still remain viable and not bind to factor H. Bacteria such as some *E. coli* strains that do have a lot of sialic acid on their surfaces can evade the alternate pathway but this is prevented through such antibody clouding.

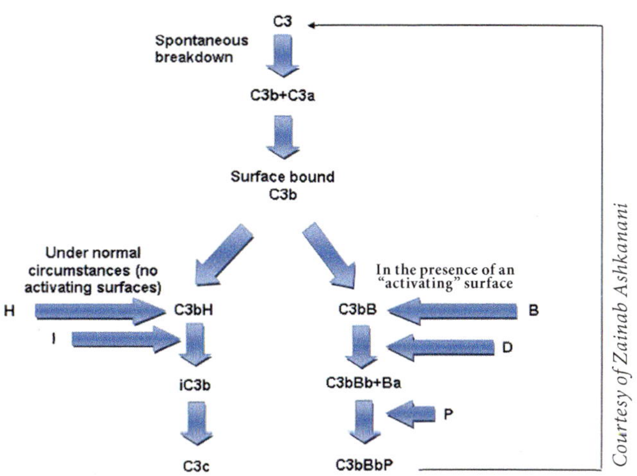

Figure 9.7 *The alternate pathway of complement activation. C3b may bind either factor B or factor H. Binding of factor B leads to the progressive activation of the alternate pathway. Binding to factor H leads to inactivation of C3b.*

- In the presence of an activating surface, C3b binds to factor B magnesium dependently to form C3bB.
- Bound factor B is cleaved by an enzyme factor D into Ba and Bb. The complex C3bBb has potent C3-convertase activity. Factor B is of liver and macrophage origin. Its synthesis is facilitated by IFN-γ.

Table 9.1 shows a summary of complement proteins in the alternate pathway

TABLE 9.1 PROTEINS OF THE ALTERNATIVE PATHWAY OF COMPLEMENT ACTIVATION

COMPONENT IN SERUM	ACTIVE FRAGMENTS	FUNCTION
C3	C3b	Binds covalently to pathogen surface and acts as opsonin. Binds B, which is then cleaved by D. C4b2a is C3 convertase and C3bBb is C5 convertase.
Factor B (B)	Ba	Small fragment of B, no known function
	Bb	Active enzyme of the C3 convertase C3b, Bb and C5 convertase C3b, Bb
Factor D (D)	D	B cleaves to Ba and Bb when it is bound to C3b

Courtesy of Zainab Ashkanani

So, in the presence of favorable circumstances where there is no activity of factor H and I, C3b will bind to factor B, and it orients B in a way that it becomes vulnerable to factor D, then C3bBb and Ba are formed. This complex C3bBb combines with factor P, properdin, and makes C3bBbP, which is a very efficient membrane disruptor.

Factor D is a serine esterase. It cleaves factor B into Ba and Bb and acts on factor B after it is bound to C3b; this is another example of substrate modulation. Factor D is synthesized by monocytes, its synthesis is facilitated by IFN-γ.

TERMINAL PATHWAY

The C5 convertase generated in the classical pathway, C4b2a (also designated C3 convertase), and the C5 convertase of the alternative pathway, C3bBb, can both act in the terminal pathway. Through these processes, C5 is split into C5a and C5b (Figure 9.8).

TERMINAL COMPLEMENT PATHWAY

- Both classical C3 convertase and the alternate C3 convertase act on C3 to cleave off C3a and generate surface-bound C3b.
- C3b acts as the initiator of the terminal complement pathway by binding to C5 and rendering C5 susceptible to C4b2a or C3bBb—thus, these enzymes are also C5 convertases.
- Through the above processes, C5 is split into C5a and C5b.
- C5b binds to C6 to form a complex C5b6.
- C7 (a 120 KDa protein) can bind C5b6 to form C5b67. Unbound C5b67 is unstable and decays rapidly. It, however, acts as a chemotactic agent. Bound C5b67 has affinity for C8 (a 163 KDa protein), causing a conformational change in C5b67 that penetrates membrane.

The C5b so formed then binds to C6 to form C5b6 complex. C5b6 orients itself in a way that it binds to C7. The complement component C7 is itself a 120 kDa protein. When it binds to C6, it forms C5b67. This is accompanied by the addition of C8, and then a polymerization process occurs. So, the entire C5b67 induces polymerization of C9 that creates a complex that is called membrane attack complex (MAC). The membrane attack complex is able to probe the transmembrane aspect of the membrane such that there is a pouch through the membrane and an accompanying osmotic lysis results. Although C8 is added to C5b67, it also requires the C5b67 complex to induce polymerization, but C8 has hydrophobic area that inserts into membrane bilayer (Figures 9.9 and 9.10)

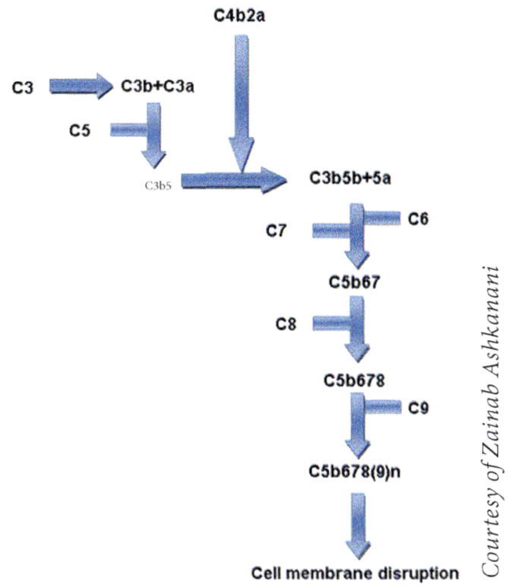

Figure 9.8 *The terminal complement pathway. Initiated by C3b, it terminates in the production of polymerized C9 and cell-membrane lysis.*

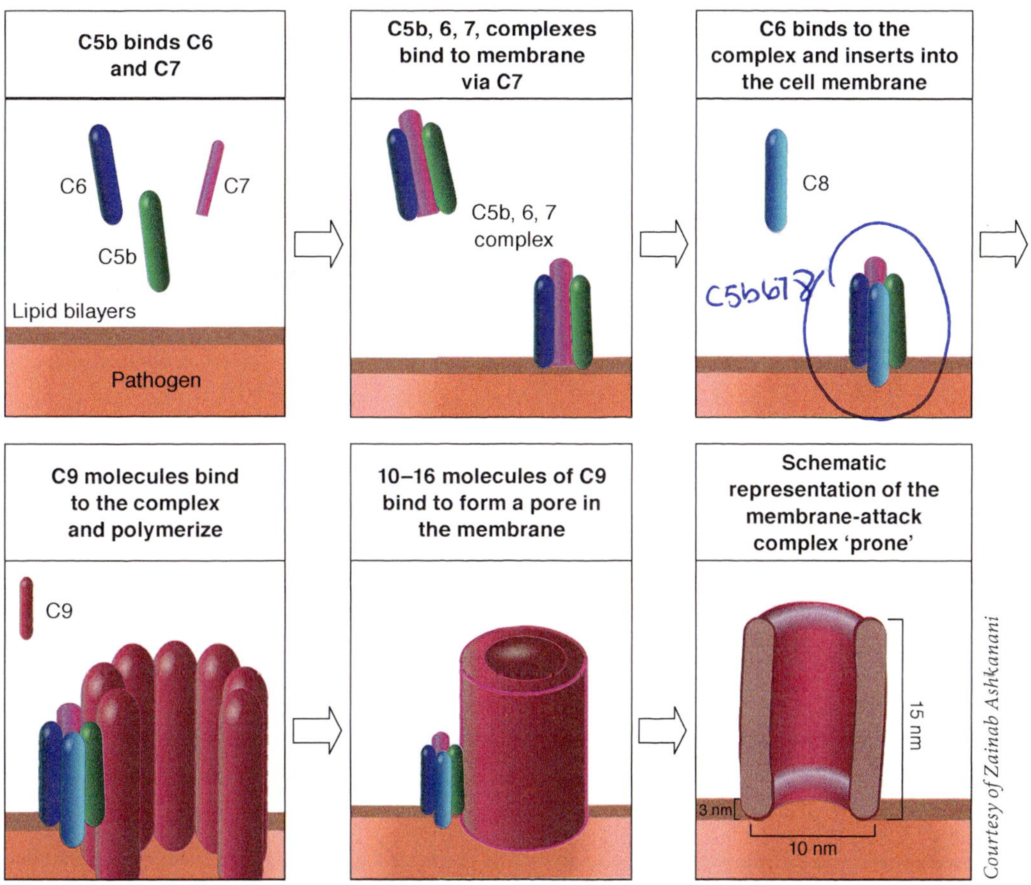

Figure 9.9 *Membrane attack complex (MAC) formation. C5 binds to C6 and C7, followed by binding to the pathogen membrane. C8 then binds to the complex followed by C9 binding and polymerization, forming a pore on the membrane of the pathogen.*

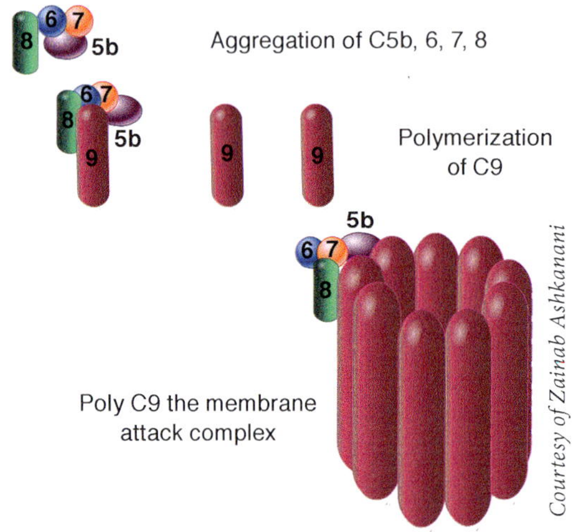

Figure 9.10 *The structure of poly C9, the membrane attack complex together with a photomicrograph of human (and rabbit) poly C9 on a red cell surface.*

MANNOSE-BINDING PROTEIN (LECTIN PATHWAY)

The principle is that the bacterial cell wall has mannose as a principal sugar. The proteins that can bind to the cell's mannose are abundant in host blood. They act as opsonins and complement is activated. Mannose-binding proteins (MBPs) are produced by the liver, thus are inflammatory proteins, just as C reactive proteins are also inflammatory proteins. They are produced when IL-1, IL-6, and TNF-α, all macrophage derived, stimulate the liver. So, MBP activates the complement via the alternate pathway. It is important to note that mannose-binding protein alone will not activate complement; it needs to act in concert with a serine protease, which is usually abundant in the serum.

CONTROL AND REGULATION OF THE COMPLEMENT SYSTEM

Since the complement system is very effective in killing bacteria and other challenges, it must be tightly regulated and controlled. The deleterious potentials are averted by controls in all the pathways. The controls are represented in the charts below (Figures 9.11 and 9.12).

REGULATION OF COMPLEMENT SYSTEM

- Needs an efficient control because of its potentially deleterious effect.
- Most important regulator of classical pathway is C1- inhibitor. It controls the assembly of C4b2a (C3 convertase) by blocking C1.
- Effect of H and I factors in C3b already discussed.
- C4 binding protein (C4-bp). It binds C4b and inhibits formation of C4b2a.

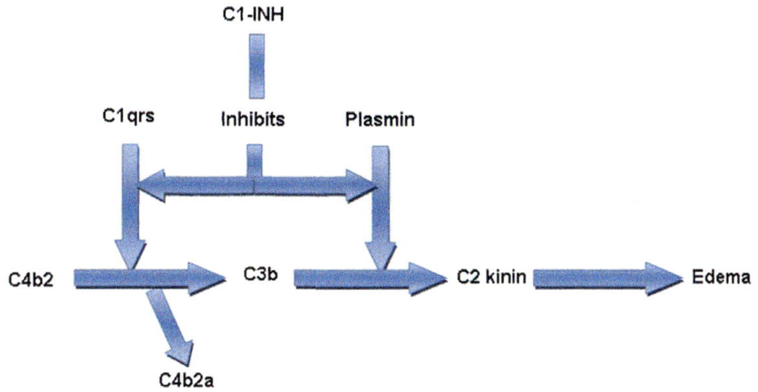

Courtesy of Zainab Ashkanani

Figure 9.11 *The site of action of C1 inhibitor and the pathogenesis of hereditary angioedema.*

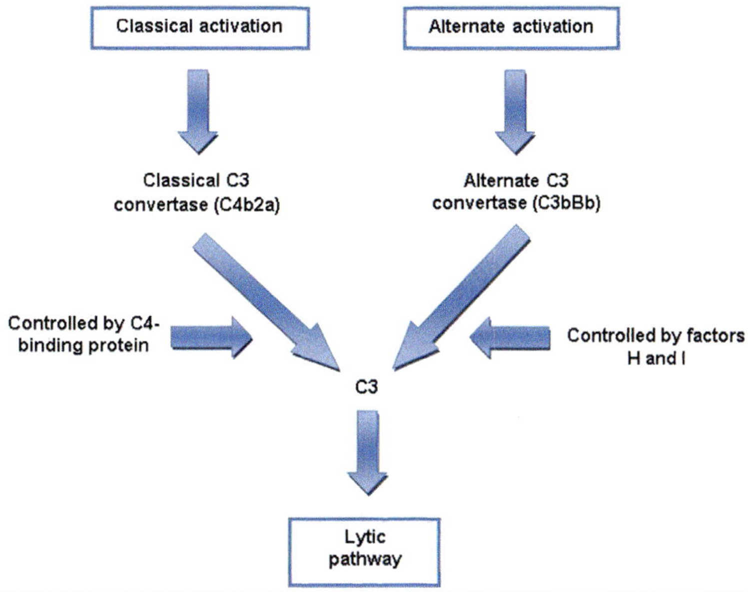

Courtesy of Zainab Ashkanani

Figure 9.12 *The lytic pathway.*

The deficiency of C1 inhibitor causes overaccumulation of C2b and C2a, which increase blood vessel permeability, causing edema. If that efflux of fluid from blood vessels into the tissue were to occur in the blood vessels of the larynx, it will cause choking. The disease is called angioedema.

RECEPTORS THAT CONTROL COMPLEMENT ACTIONS

The CD55 is a receptor on cells, it is a 70 kDa glycoprotein and it is common on cells such as erythrocytes, neutrophils, lymphocytes, platelets, and endothelial cells. It is a C3 convertase decay accelerating factor, that is, it makes C3 convertases (C4b2a and C3bBb) to decay fast. This is because an accelerated decay of C3 convertases is protective to the cell by terminating the alternate and classical pathways.

RECEPTORS

- CD55, a 70 KDa glycoprotein, is common on the membrane of red blood cells, neutrophils, lymphocytes, platelets, and endothelial cells; it is a C3 convertase decay accelerating factor. It has a protective effect on membrane by binding to their C4b2a (C3 convertase) of the classical pathway or C3bBb (C3 convertase) of the alternate pathway and accelerating their decay.
- Deficiency of CD55 causes the accumulation of C3b on red cell surfaces resulting in complement-mediated lysis seen in paroxysmal nocturnal hemoglobinemia.
- CD59, also called protectin, protects leukocytes, red cells, and endothelial cells from lysis by acting at the final stages of membrane attack complex. It competes with C9 for binding site on C8. It blocks C5b678 insertion into the cell membrane and so inhibits C9 polymerization.
- CD46 is a membrane cofactor protein, which functions as a receptor for C3b or iC3b, it controls C3 turnover on cells by acting as a cofactor for the cleavage of C3b or C4b by factor I.
- The control of the C5b6789 complex is mediated by two adhesive glycoproteins: vitronectin and clusterin. Three molecules of vitronectin and one molecule of clusterin can bind C5b67, render them soluble, and stop membrane binding.
- Finally, MAC can be removed by endocytosis.

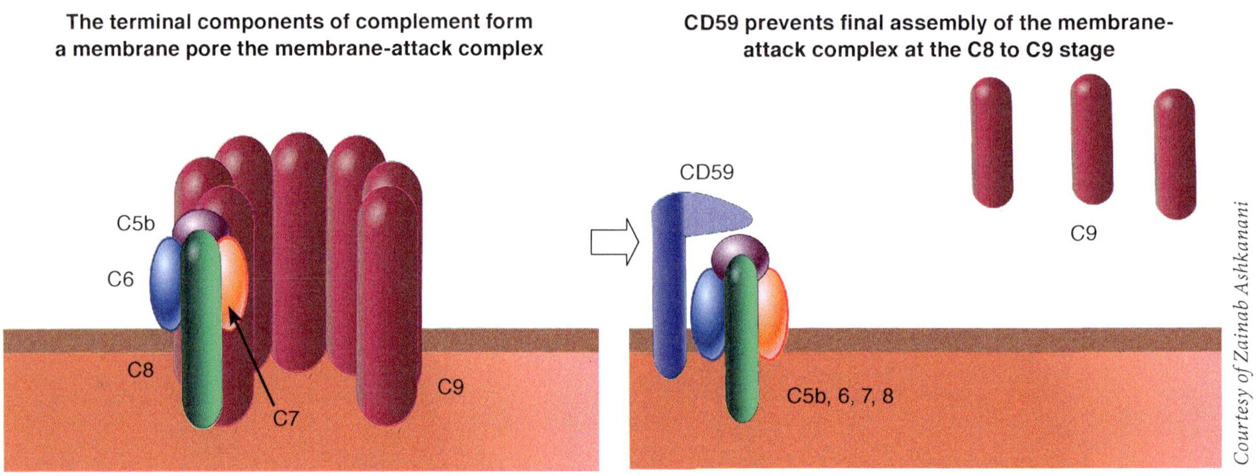

Figure 9.13 *CD59 blocks formation of the MAC and inhibits destruction of cells by this mechanism.*

The paroxysmal nocturnal hemoglobinuria, which is night-time alternate hemoglobinuria, occurs because it takes a while for MAC to accumulate enough on red cells to result in observable lysis of erythrocytes, hence the paroxysm.

Another cluster of differentiation receptor is CD59, also called protectin, because it protects leukocytes, red cells, and endothelial cells from lysis by acting at the final stages of membrane attack complex. It competes with C9 by binding to the C8 site, blocks C5b678 insertion into the cell membrane, and inhibits C9 polymerization, so the MAC will not form (Figure 9.13).

CD46 is a membrane cofactor protein which functions as a receptor for C3b or the inactivated C3b (iC3b) and because it functions as a receptor, it controls the turnover of C3b on cells by acting as a cofactor for the cleavage of C3b or C4b by factor I.

The control of C5b6789 complex is mediated by two adhesive glycoproteins: vitronectin and clusterin. Three molecules of vitronectin and one of clusterin can bind C5b67, and when this happens, they become soluble and it stops their binding to membrane.

Finally, membrane attack complex can be removed by endocytosis, nonreceptor-mediated endocytosis.

BIOLOGICAL CONSEQUENCES OF COMPLEMENT ACTIVATION

- **Complement**-mediated **opsonization**: This arises from the presence of FcR and CR1 causing antibody and complement-coated cells to be phagocytosed.
- **Removal** of **immune complexes**: It helps in the uptake of immune complexes by phagocytosis. Complement deficiency causes the accumulation of immune complexes in the kidney and results in tissue damage.
- **Complement** mediated **immune regulation**: B cells but not T cells have CR1; these receptors can bind C3b. C3b blocks B cell differentiation. C3a is immunosuppressive, blocking helper T-cell activity and inhibiting NK cell activity. In contrast, C5a stimulates T- and B-cell responses by enhancing IL-1 production by macrophages.
- **Complement**-mediated **cytolysis**: This is achieved through MAC formation and C9 (perforins) activity.
- **Complement**-mediated **chemotaxis**: Activation of complement cascade generates chemotactic proteins such as C5a, C5b67, C3a, and Bb.
- **Complement**-mediated **inflammation**: C3a and C5a are anaphylatoxins, which cause smooth muscle spasms and function with leukotrienes.

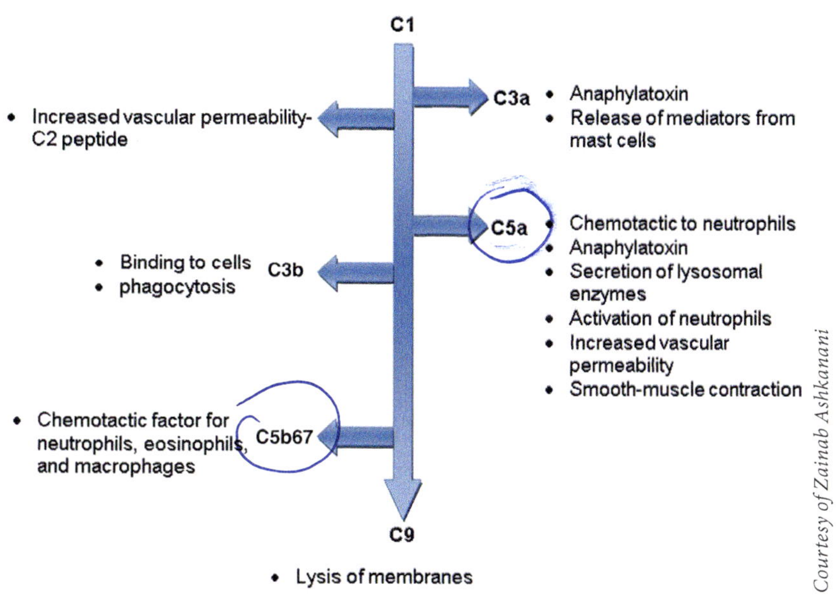

Figure 9.14 *The Biological consequences of complement activation.*

One of the biologic consequences of complement activation is the mediation of opsonization by the complement. Complement fragments C5a and others are opsonins as already stated, thus enhancing engulfment by the professional phagocytes (Figure 9.14). Another consequence of complement activation is the removal of immune complexes. The immune complex is formed when an antigen and antibody interact, which exposes the complement fixation site, and this whole complex is easily removed by professional phagocytes. This prevents the destruction of the kidneys and other tissues by these immune complexes.

The immune process is regulated by complement components; those proteins that are produced during complement activation, for instance, C3b can block B cell differentiation. Complement component C3a is also immunosuppressive. If there is no control of the hydrolysis of C3 to C3a and C3b, then impairment in B-cell differentiation or immunosuppression in general can occur. C3a is immunosuppressive; it does this by blocking helper T-cell activity, and inhibits NK cell activity. In contrast, C5a stimulates T- and B-cell responses by enhancing IL-1 production by macrophages.

Activation of complement-mediated cytolysis has a direct action *in vivo* in the destruction of cells of challenges to the body by the formation of membrane attack complex. Also, complement mediates chemotaxis, so C5a, C5b67, C3a, and Bb are chemotactic agents. Complement also mediates inflammation; this is the localization of immune response. The fact that complement components are chemotactic agents implies that they localize immune response. C3a and C5a are anaphylatoxins, they cause smooth muscle spasm. It becomes more pronounced when they function with slow acting substances like leukotrienes, which are products of fatty acid metabolism.

COMPLEMENT FIXATION TEST

It is an application of membrane attack complex in the laboratory to detect the presence of antibodies to pathogens in host system (Figure 9.15).

- Complement activation causes the generation of MAC which disrupts cell membrane.
- If MAC is generated on red cells, then hemolysis occurs. This is the basis of CFT.
- It is widely used in viral disease diagnosis. The test is of two parts.
- First part: Ag (from kit) and Ab (serum under test, deprived of complement by heating at 56°C) are incubated in the presence of normal guinea pig serum (source of potent complement). If serum contains Abs, then Ag–Ab complex will fix complement. When SRBC (an indicator) is added, they will remain intact since there is no complement to lyse it. This is a positive result for the Ab.
- However, if antibody is absent, complement will not be fixed, so on addition of SRBC + anti-SRBC (hemolysin), lysis occurs. This is a negative result for antibody.
  - Sheep red blood cell (SRBC) serves as indicator.
  - When SRBC is exposed to anti-SRBC (hemolysin) and the complex formed is reacted with free complement, there is lysis of SRBC.
  - When complement is fixed, thus not available, SRBC is not lysed.
- Cytotoxicity Test: Involves the use of nucleated cells to detect the presence of antibodies in serum. Cell + serum (Ab) → Ab-coated cells. Then, add complement and observe for lysis. Count remnant cells using trypan blue exclusion studies.

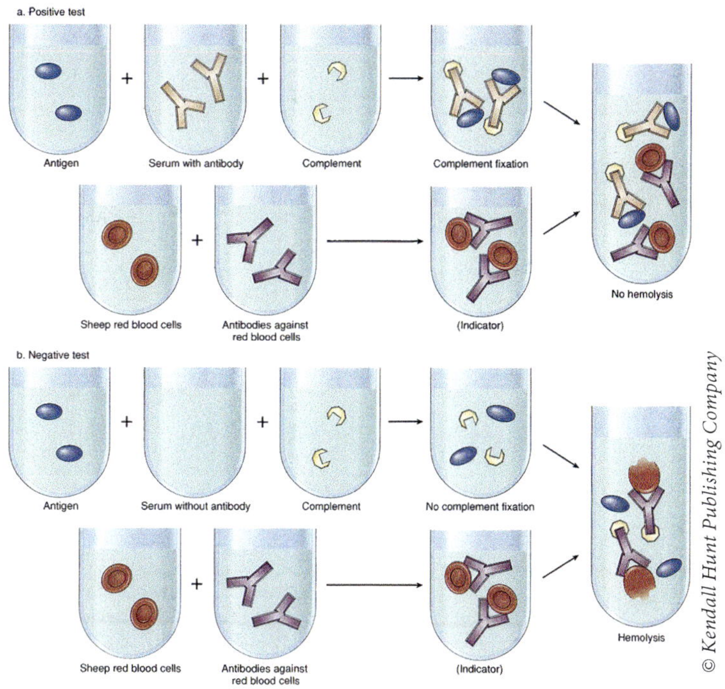

Figure 9.15 *The principle of the complement fixation test. Complement-fixed (activated) by antigen and antibody is unavailable to lyse the indicator system. In the absence of an antibody, the complement will remain unfixed and available for lysis of the indicator system.*

Whenever an antibody interacts with complement, the complement will not be effective *in vitro*. If one is interested in an infectious agent, then the antigen to the agent is fixed on a microtitre plate and the fluid sample from the patient (serum, usually inactivated of complement by heating at 56°C) is added. After the required incubation period, the excess patient sample is washed off and complement from guinea pig serum is added, followed by another incubation period and washing. The sheep red blood cells are added. If there is no antibody to the antigen in the patient sample, then complement will remain unbound and free to lyse the sheep red cells. There will be no free noticeable sheep erythrocytes because they have been lysed. This is a negative result for the pathogen being tested. However, if the host has the antibody to the pathogen, in which case, the host has been exposed or has an ongoing infection, then the antibodies that have reacted with the antigen bound to the plate will remain after the wash and will react with complement. Thus, after the second wash, there will be no free complement to lyse the added sheep erythrocytes. This is the positive result for the pathogen.

THE CYTOTOXICITY ASSAY

There is a second assay for which you use complement. It is called the cytotoxicity assay. This one is useful for nucleated cells. In this assay, sample is added and incubated for the desired period. This is then washed to remove excess sample from cells. If there are antibodies in serum, they will all adhere to the cell; they cluster around the cell and react with the specific receptors. Complement is added, incubated, and washed. If there is any antibody in the sample, it reacts with the complement because the antibody complement-biding sites are exposed. On counting of cells using trypan blue exclusion studies, there will be comparatively the same number of cells as those previously enumerated at the beginning of the experiment. However, if the sample is devoid of any antibody, then the process will result in cell lysis and there will be comparatively fewer numbers of cells compared to the numbers enumerated at the commencement of the experiment.

SAMPLE QUESTIONS

COMPLEMENT

1. Which complement component produces an anaphylatoxin?
   a. C1
   b. C2
   c. C3
   d. Properdin
   e. Immunoconglutinin

2. Complement used for serological tests is usually derived from
   a. horses
   b. guinea pigs
   c. sheep
   d. cattle
   e. rabbits

3. Activation of the classical complement cascade requires interaction of antigen with
   a. at least two IgG molecules
   b. five IgG molecules
   c. an IgA molecule
   d. a single IgG molecule
   e. at least two IgA molecules

4. Which autoimmune disease appears to be provoked by a deficiency of C4?
   a. Thyroiditis
   b. Systemic lupus erythematosus
   c. Rheumatoid arthritis
   d. Myasthenia gravis
   e. Multiple sclerosis

5. Which complement component has the highest concentration in serum?
   a. C1q
   b. C1r
   c. C3
   d. factor B
   e. C9

6. The alternative complement pathway is inhibited by
   a. factor H
   b. factor B
   c. factor D
   d. factor P
   e. factor F

7. C9 is a member of which family of proteins?
   a. Immunoglobulins
   b. Acute phase proteins
   c. Cytokines
   d. Addressins
   e. Perforins

8. Which complement component has chemotactic properties?
   a. C1a
   b. C2a
   c. C4a
   d. C5a
   e. C6a

9. What is the major ligand for CR1?
   a. C1
   b. C2
   c. C3b
   d. C5
   e. C7

10. Which of the following is coded for by MHC class III genes?
   a. C3
   b. Properdin
   c. C9
   d. Factor B
   e. C5a

Suggested Laboratory Practicals

- Case Studies on:
  1. Formation of Membrane Attack Complex and Complement System Controls
  2. Biologic Consequences of Complement Activation and Complement Deficiencies
- Complement Fixation Test
- CH50 Hemolytic Assay and AH50 Assay
- Enzyme-Linked Immunoassay of Individual Complement Components

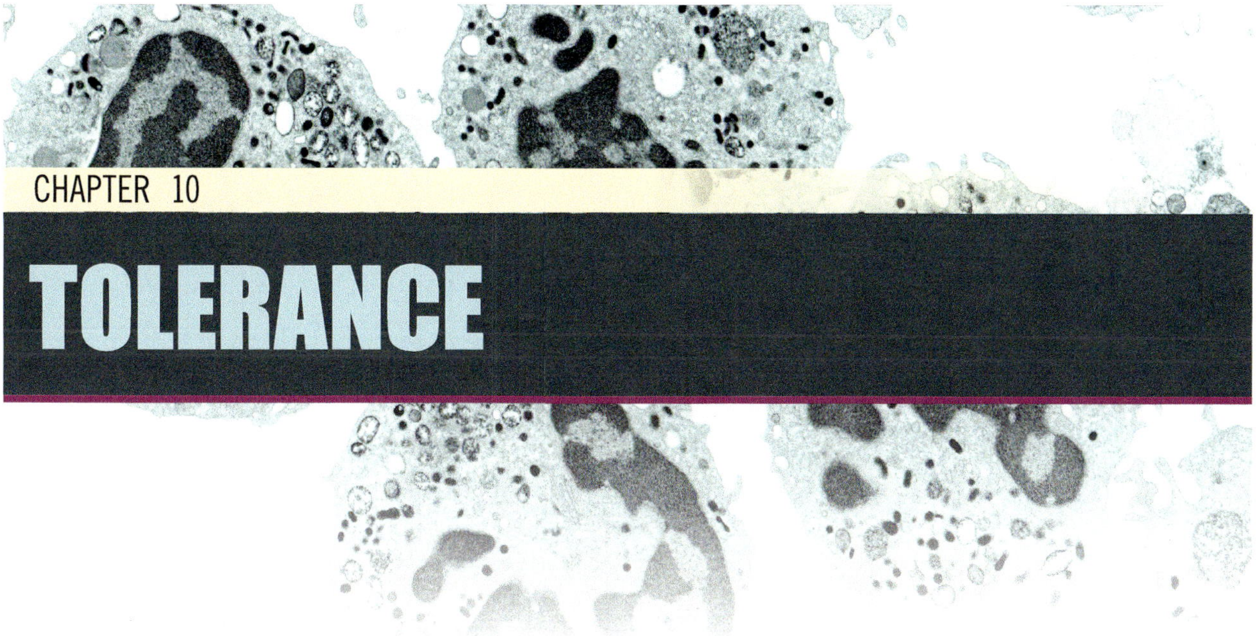

CHAPTER 10

TOLERANCE

The conventional wisdom of antigenic challenge is that a clone of antibody-producing cells is generated and usually results in the resolution of the infection. In the event that such clone of cells is deleted, the individual becomes susceptible to infection. This is ordinarily described as tolerance to such infection (immune unresponsiveness). In a physiologic sense, tolerance is the development of the capacity to discriminate between self- and nonself-cells. This capacity protects the host from self-destruction.

SOME POINTS ON TOLERANCE

- Tolerance of infection (immune unresponsiveness): (i) Acquired immune deficiency syndrome and (ii) Congenital immune deficiency syndrome.
- Tolerance of transplant, as seen in compatible transfusion and tissue transplants.
- Physiological aspects of tolerance (selection and deletion).

The development is an integral part of T- and B-cell development. It is important to note that T cells usually need further education leading to their functional commitment and initiation to the performance of specific effector functions in the thymus, while in the case of B cells, they are partially committed to perform their function at the point of emergence from the bone marrow with marginal further development in the secondary lymphoid tissues.

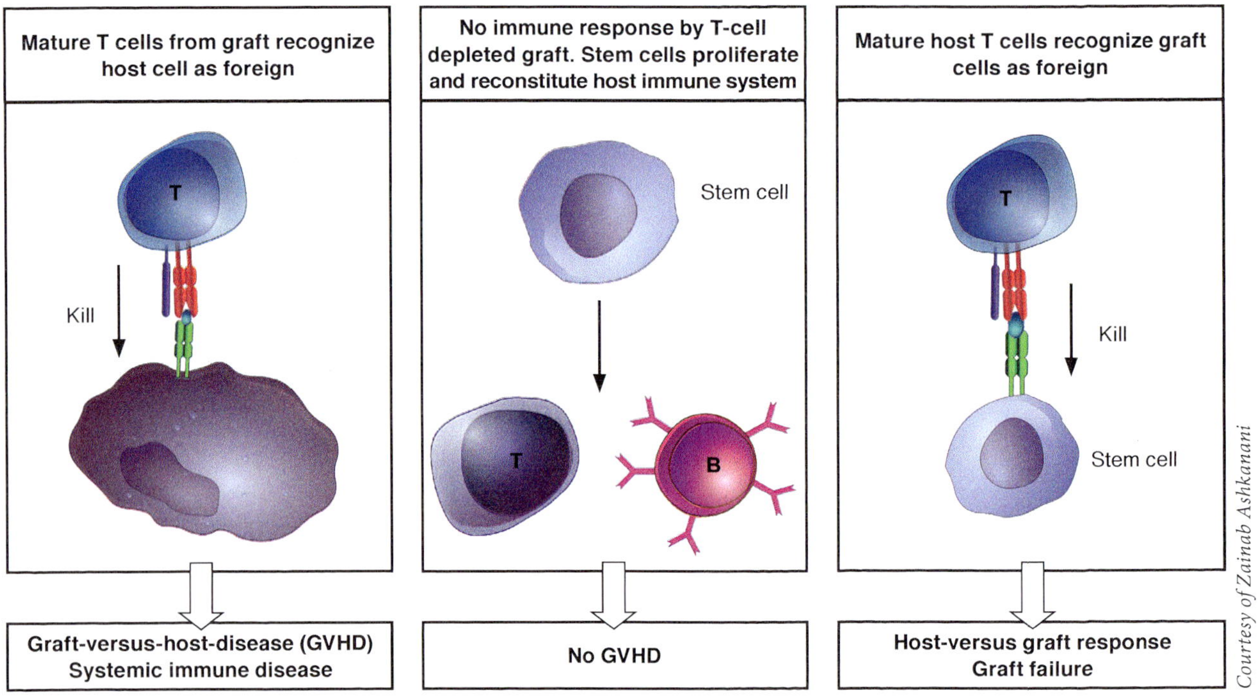

Figure 10.1 *Alloreactions by either donor or recipient lymphocytes can cause graft rejection.*

An important aspect of tolerance development is in the application of tolerance in transplant medicine. The type of rejection that accompanies transplantation may be of donor or recipient origin. In an event of absence of graft rejection, then the recipient system is gradually educated about the graft in a manner suitable for the host stem cells resulting in the acceptance of such compactable graft. The outcome of this process is the emergence of B and T cells that carry receptors acceptable to the graft. This usually marks the effective reconstitution of the graft.

- The suppression or **destruction** of a **clone** of **lymphocytes** (B or T cells) initiates **tolerance**.
- It is a process by which the body ensures that **immune responses** are **directed against foreign Ags** and **not** against **self-Ags**.

The events attending to the tissue rejection process is marked by the infiltration of T lymphocytes all around various arterioles. The suppression of the lymphocytes through therapeutic intervention is helpful in the restoration of normalcy.

- Specific immunological unresponsiveness of an individual to an Ag depends on the stage of development of Ag-sensitive cells when they first encounter the Ag.
- Persistence of tolerance depends on continuous presence of Ag.
- There is disparity in the susceptibility of T and B cells to tolerance induction. T cells develop tolerance rapidly and easily within 24 hours and remain in such state for more than 100 days. B cells develop tolerance much more slowly (about 10 days) and return to normal within 50 days.

The selection process of making lymphocytes tolerant of self-cells affects both B and T cells. The selection process of T cells occurs in the thymus, the T cells whose receptors will not bind self-antigen (recognize self-antigen), and the T cells whose receptors can recognize self-major histocompatibility complex are selected (positive selection). T cells that cannot recognize self-major histocompatibility complex are deleted by apoptosis. This process is accompanied by a second selection process in which the strength of recognition is considered (Figure 10.2). Those cells that strongly recognize the self-major histocompatibility complex are deleted (negative selection).

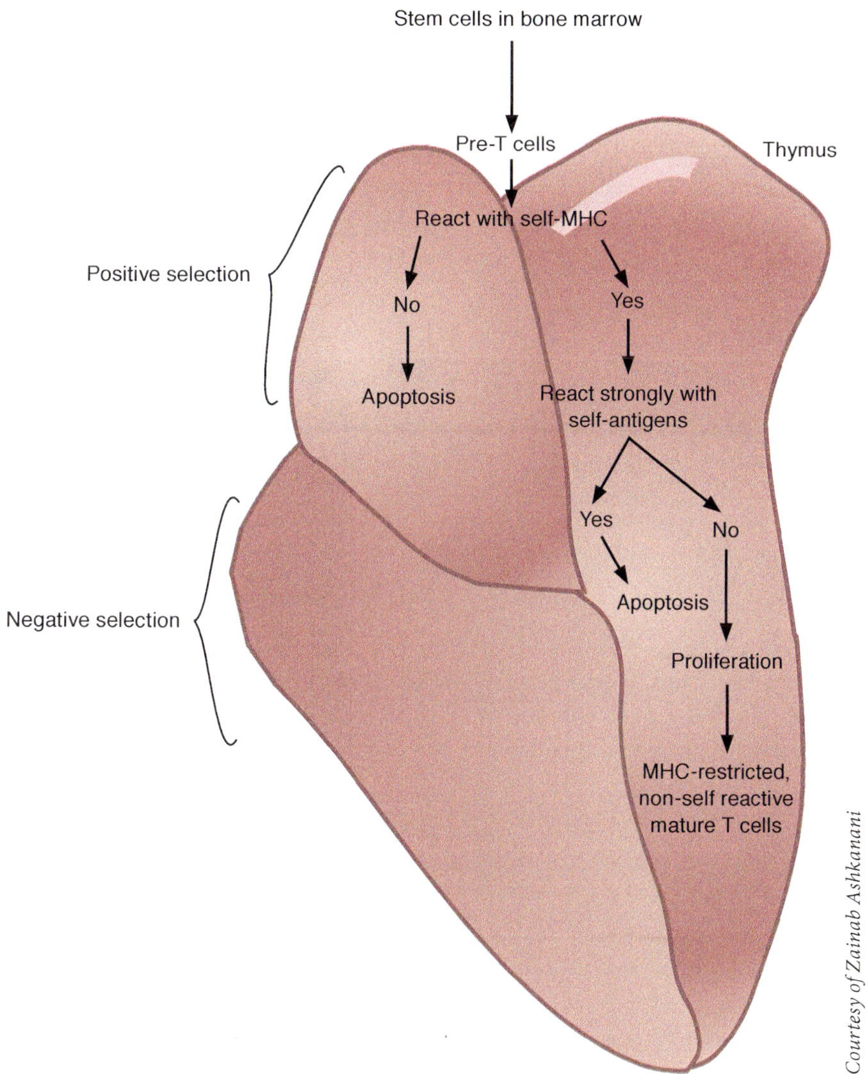

Figure 10.2 *The Tcell repertoire in the developing animal is determined by sequential positive and negative selection in the thymus. This ensures that only MHC-restricted, nonself reactive T cells reach maturity.*

Persistence of tolerance depends on continuous and early presence of antigen. This can explain some of the problems associated with autoimmune diseases.

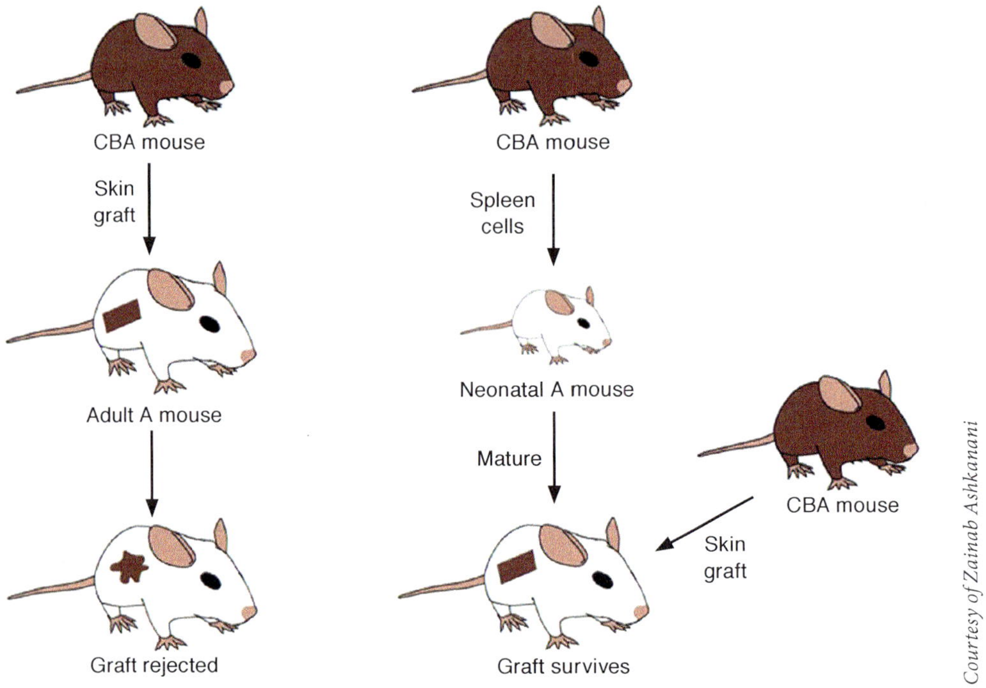

Figure 10.3 *Medawar's tolerance experiment. He succeeded in making a CBA skin graft survive on a strain A mouse by injecting the recipient at birth with CBA strain spleen cells. Thus, the strain A animal was fully tolerant to CBA cells.*

There is a disparity in the way T and B cells become susceptible to induction of tolerance. While T cells' tolerance comes rapidly, and remains for a longer period of time, B cells are slower and shorter, and for this reason, most of the problems with T cells appear protracted. So, problems with T-cell tolerance manifest rapidly and remain sustained (Figures 10.3 and 10.4).

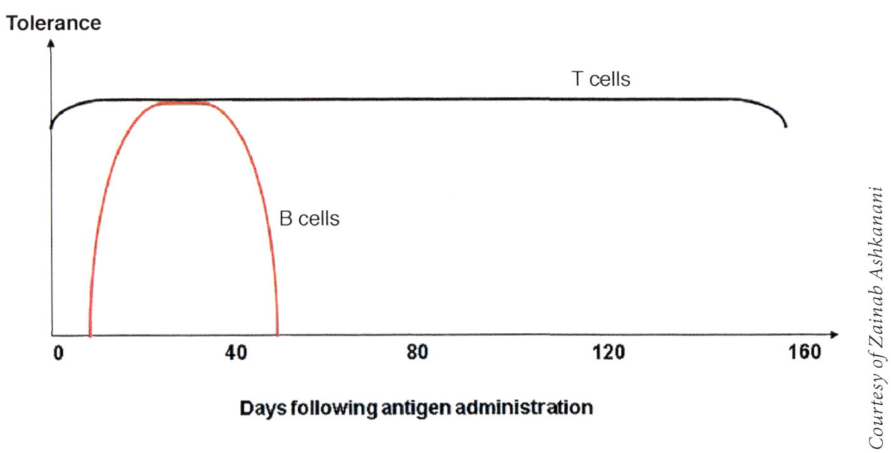

Figure 10.4 *The duration of tolerance in T and B cells in mice. T cells develop tolerance rapidly and it lasts for a long period. In contrast, B cells can only be made tolerant for a short period. This probably results from the continuous production of B cells with specificity for the inducing antigen as a result of somatic mutation.*

When T cells leave the bone marrow, they are not committed yet, so they have primitive markers. When they enter the thymus, the first test that they confront in terms of tolerance is the selection in relation to major histocompatibility complex as stated above; the reason for this is that the antigens that may compound immunologic tolerance will be displayed later by the major histocompatibility complex. Thus, the body's way of handling a process that is still naïve is to rely on the major histocompatibility complex (see Figures 10.5–10.7).

T-CELL TOLERANCE

- **Tolerance** of T cells to a specific **Ag occurs** when there is **lack** of **receptors** to the **Ag**. Theoretically, T-cell receptors are any of the following combinations of alpha/beta (**α/β**) or delta/gamma (**δ/γ**). When thymocyte progenitors **arrive at** the **thymus from** the bone **marrow**, they express **no** receptors. In the **thymus**, they first express (**δ/γ**), then **two days later** (**α/β**) are expressed.
- The underlying principle of T-cell tolerance is the selection of cells that have the capacity to **recognize self-MHC** molecules and **allow** these to **expand** in **population**. This is **positive selection**.
- Those that do not recognize self-MHC molecules are negatively selected and passed through apoptosis (**clonal deletion**).
- T cells that evade self-tolerance induction in the thymus are taken care of through **functional tolerance**. This involves T-cells exposure to free Ag, that is, nonmacrophage bound. This is **clonal anergy**. Also, high or low dose of Ag can cause **immune paralysis or clonal anergy**.

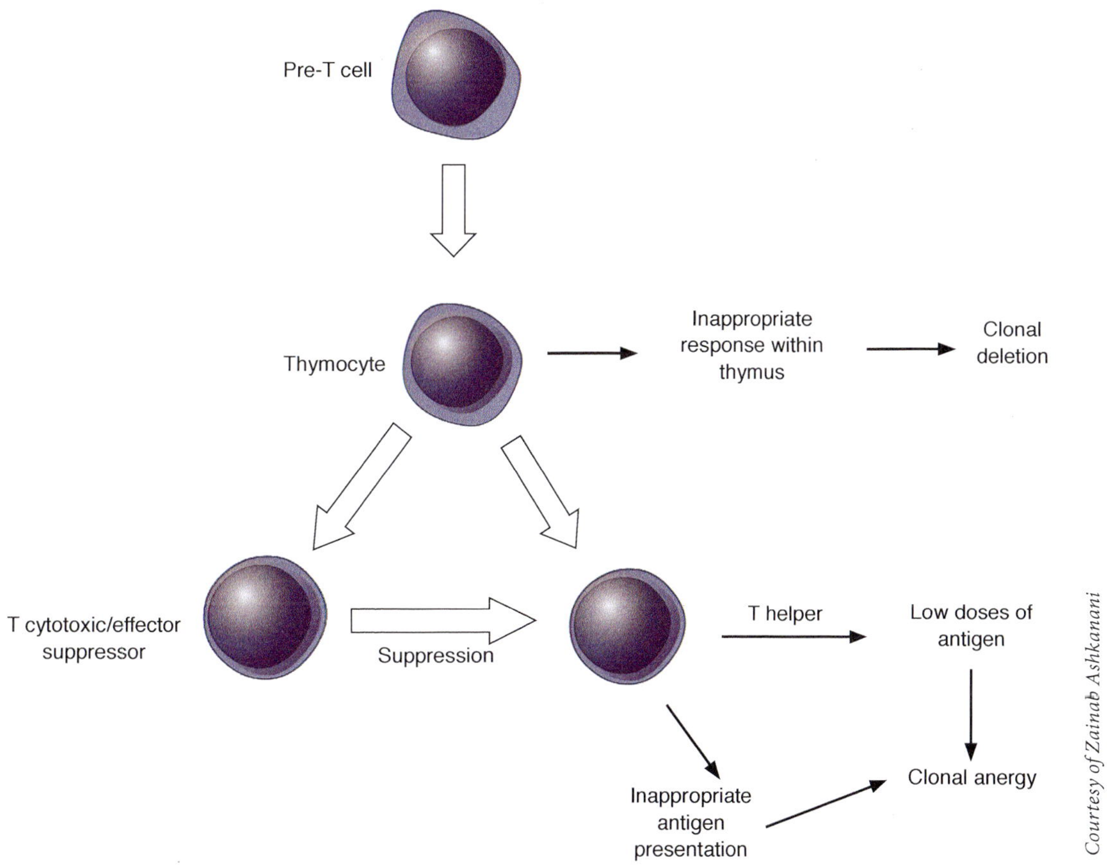

Figure 10.5 *Some of the mechanisms of induction of tolerance in T cells.*

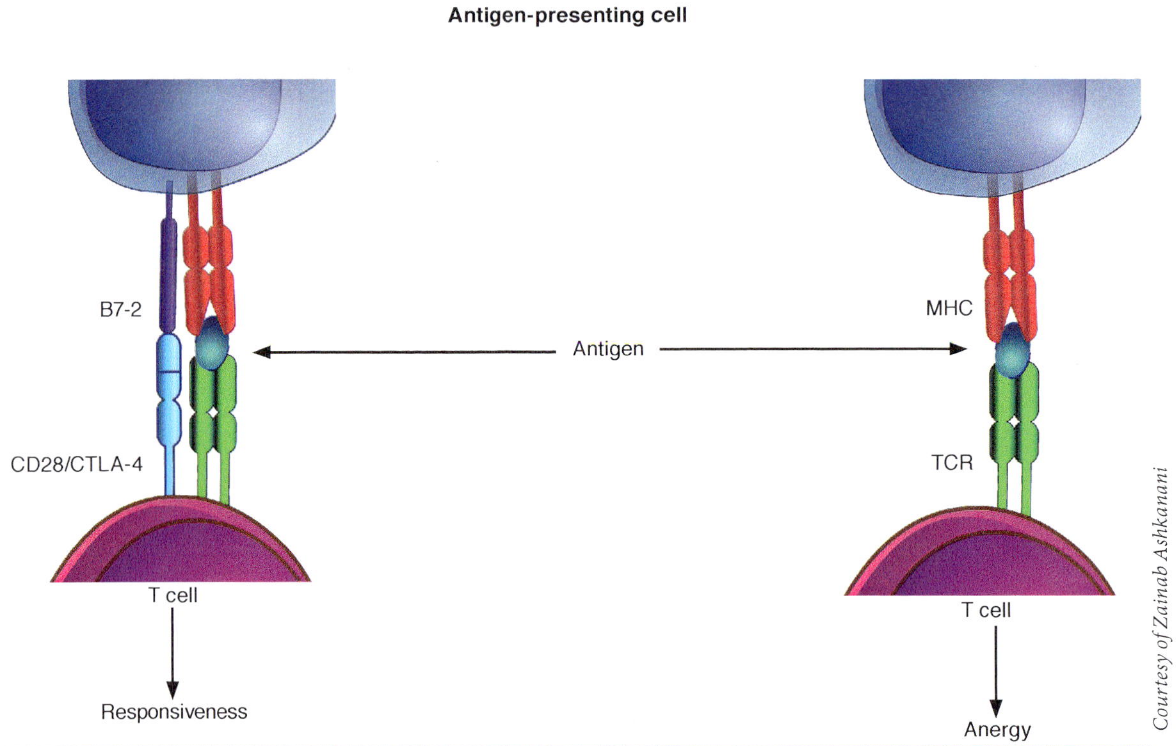

Figure 10.6 *T cells will only respond to processed antigen, when they receive a stimulus from another receptor such as CD28 or CTLA-4, in the absence of this costimulus, anergy and tolerance result.*

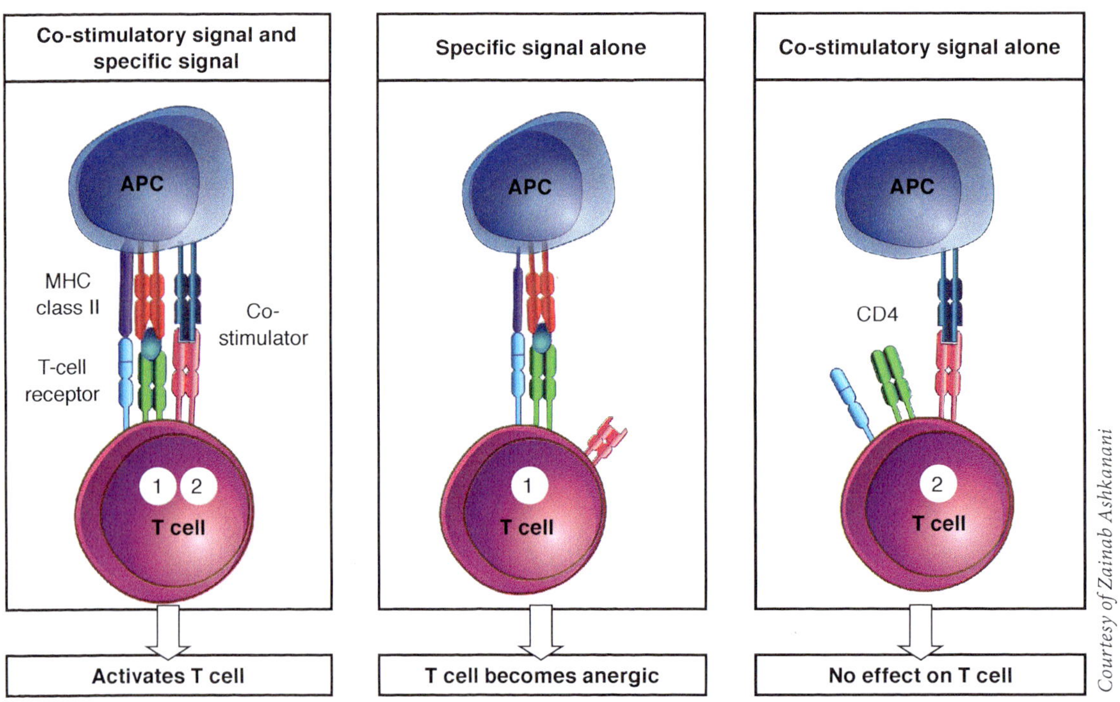

Figure 10.7 *T-cell tolerance. T-cell activation can be achieved only by an APC carrying both a specific peptide: MHC complex and costimulatory molecules on its surface. This combination results in the T cell receiving signal 1 from the TCR and signal 2 from the costimulator. If either of these signals is absent, no activation results.*

The process of selection may not be a perfect process; some of the cells may not recognize self-major histocompatibility complex and thus some of the T cells may escape. It is thought by some researchers in the field of autoimmune diseases that the activation of this escaped small pool of cells in the thymus (cells unable to recognize self-MHC) may resume proliferation at a stage in the life of some individuals and account for the initiation of autoimmune diseases. The escape is controlled by the body by antigenic underdosing or overdosing of such cells, because such cells, generally, will have the opportunity to be exposed to their corresponding antigens over time. When they are exposed, it would not be in an optimal sense, but in a low- or high-dose sense. That kind of exposure will bring about clonal anergy or immune paralysis (Figure 10.8).

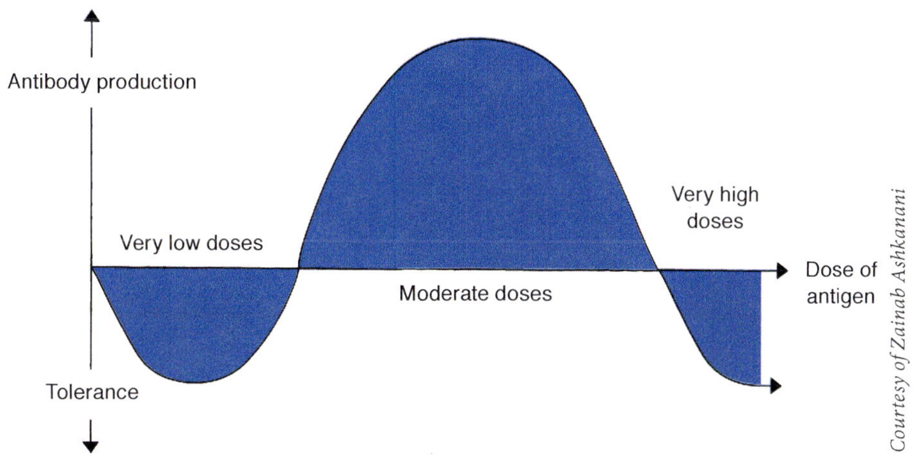

Figure 10.8 *High and low zone tolerance. Both low and high doses of antigen will cause tolerance. Moderate doses induce a conventional immune response.*

Unfortunately for those who end up with autoimmune diseases, there is this postulate that this aspect does not occur in them.

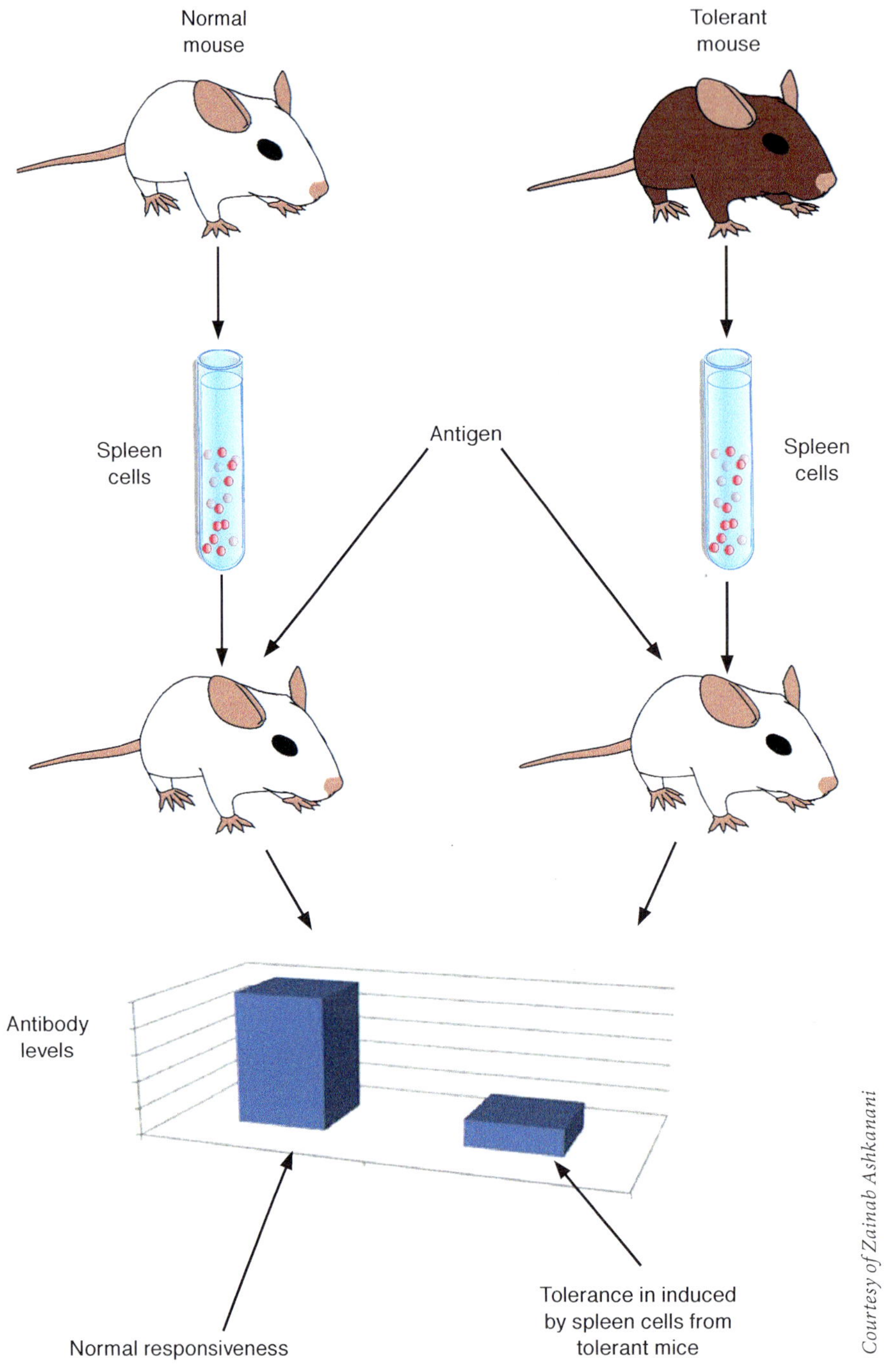

Figure 10.9 *Evidence for the existence of suppressor T cells. Spleen cells from a tolerant mouse will produce a suppressed immune response when adoptively transferred to recipient animals. Treatment of the spleen cells from tolerant animals with anti-Thy-I reversed the suppressive effect in recipient animals. It is, of course, possible that TH2 cells producing IL-10 could have a similar effect.*

There is the evidence that suppression or tolerance can be transferred (Figure 10.9). This can be conferred on an animal by infusion of spleen cells from tolerant animals into normal ones which subsequently develop tolerance. If it is done at an early age, tolerance becomes greater.

B CELL TOLERANCE

B cells are affected by the state of helper T cells. This collaboration between B cells and helper T cells means a lot, even at the level of development of tolerance. The mechanisms involved are discussed as follows:

Clonal Abortion.

In this case, it takes place when B cells arrive at the secondary lymphoid organs such as the lymph nodes; they encounter unique antigens at the follicular sites resulting in the germinal transformation. They encounter unique antigen early in their development in the marrow and sometimes in the spleen. Some of these cells acquire self-reactivity and as a result are deleted.

Clonal Exhaustion.

This occurs as a result of repeated subjection of B cells to exhaustive antigenic stimulation. They develop into short-lived plasma cells; since they do not have memory of the exposure, the effect only ends with antibody production. If the B cells carry memory, then a subsequent exposure to antigen will rapidly bring about proliferation of those memory cells into effector cells that will become plasma cells again and heightened antibody elaboration will occur. The postulate about a small collection of B cells that may have escaped this process also applies here, and B cells can later become activated to produce antibodies that are associated with autoimmune diseases.

Blockage of B Cell Receptors.

This is another aspect of B-cell tolerance in which polymeric antigens such as pneumococcal polysaccharide can bind to B-cell receptors and effectively freeze them, on such grounds, they do not respond further.

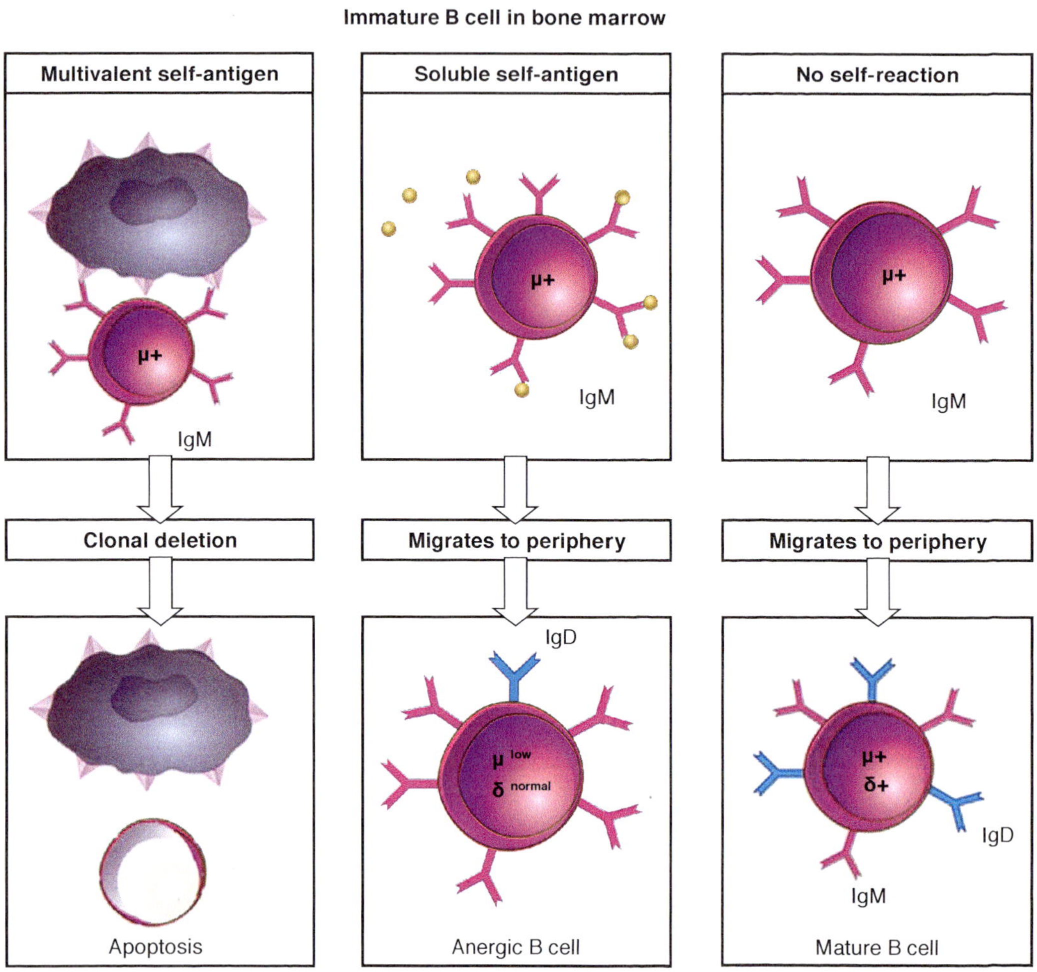

Courtesy of Zainab Ashkanani

Figure 10.10 *Ability to bind to self-antigen in the bone marrow possibly leads to inactivation or deletion of immature B cells. If immature B cells bind to self-antigen, clonal deletion will occur, and if no reaction is seen, maturation can continue normally.*

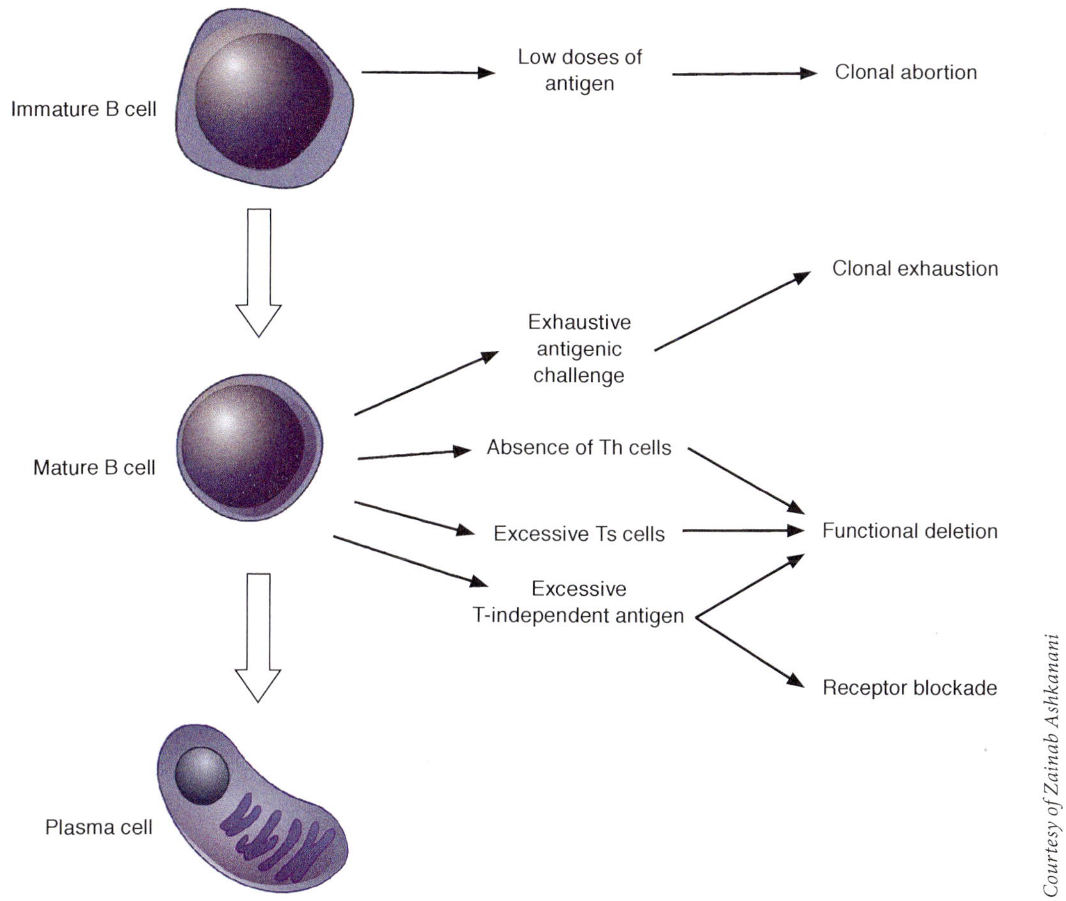

Figure 10.11 *The mechanisms of induction of tolerance in B cells.*

It is important to note that when B cells pass through this process of clonal abortion, a whole clone of B cells that are exposed to antigens that may impact self-cells negatively are deleted (Figure 10.10 and 10.11). Also, repeated stimulation of B cells by antigen can make them exhausted and go into deletion. Finally, there is the case of the blockage of their receptor sites.

The ability to bind self-antigen in the bone marrow will possibly lead to inactivation or deletion of immature B cells. If immature B cells bind to self-antigen, clonal deletion will occur and if no reaction is seen, maturation can continue normally. Since this is in the marrow, binding will involve primitive markers and multivalent self-antigen. The multivalent antigen-binding receptor is the primitive marker μ (IgM). Mature B cells that have escaped this process and still go on to maturity can be taken care of by exhaustive antigenic stimulation (clonal exhaustion). The problem is that in some individuals, a development can occur in which a small pool of B cells that can develop into plasma cells may reside in the secondary lymphoid tissue and keep targeting self-antigens. Activating agents in this instance are diverse and may include infectious and environmental agents.

SAMPLE QUESTIONS

TOLERANCE

1. What cell types can be made tolerant?
   a. T cells alone
   b. B cells alone
   c. NK cells alone
   d. T and B cells
   e. Macrophages

2. The central paradigm of the immune response is called
   a. somatic mutation
   b. antigen presentation
   c. MHC restriction
   d. clonal selection

3. Where does the major step in inducing T-cell tolerance occur?
   a. Spleen
   b. Bone marrow
   c. Bursa of Fabricius
   d. Thymus
   e. Payer's patches

4. The elimination of self-reactive T cells in the thymus is called
   a. negative selection
   b. positive selection
   c. clonal selection
   d. apoptosis
   e. clonal anergy

5. T cells of lpr mice fail to undergo apoptosis because of a defect in the
   a. *lck* gene
   b. *ras* gene
   c. *myc* gene
   d. *fos* gene
   e. *fas* gene

6. When a T cell is made tolerant by receiving insufficient or inappropriate costimulation, this is called
   a. negative selection
   b. clonal anergy
   c. clonal selection
   d. positive selection
   e. receptor blockade

7. Very high doses of antigen induce
   a. negative selection
   b. clonal selection
   c. immune paralysis
   d. receptor blockade
   e. T cell suppression

8. Clonal abortion is a mechanism of inducing tolerance in
   a. T cells
   b. B cells
   c. NK cells
   d. TIL cells
   e. LAK cells

9. Which antigen can cause B-cell tolerance by blocking receptors?
   a. Interleukin
   b. Endotoxin
   c. Gamma globulin
   d. Serum albumin
   e. Pneumococcal polysaccharide

10. Which treatment may hasten the fading of tolerance?
   a. Immunosuppression
   b. Immunostimulation
   c. Low-dose radiation
   d. High-dose radiation
   e. Complement depletion

Suggested Laboratory Practicals

- Case Studies on:
1. Clonal Selection Theory
2. Positive and Negative Selections

- Polyacryl Gel Electrophoresis (PAGE)
- Agarose Gel Electrophoresis
- Demonstration of Markers on T Cells
- Enumeration of T Lymphocytes

CHAPTER 11

VACCINES AND VACCINATION

The hallmark of immune response is the elicitation of antibody production. However, the production of antibodies does not necessarily represent an efficient and effective immune protection. In all instances, a protective response is marked by sufficient specific response involving specifically primed cells of the immune system, immune mediators, and antibodies. The role of antibodies is very paramount, it includes such roles as the opsonization of infecting agents which renders them easy to engulf by professional phagocytes, the prevention of the entry of viruses into cells by antibody binding of important viral site needed for cell receptor attachment, and the neutralization of toxin by antitoxin antibodies. An important feature of specific immune response by antibody production is the possibility of heightened response following secondary exposure to an agent to which there was a previous exposure (anamnestic response). It is in line with this enormously important process of specific immune response associated with antibody elaboration that vaccine production and vaccination process are modeled.

The persuasion is that any immunocompetent agent that is nonpathogenic can be used to protect against identical agents of infections. Louis Pasteur called this process vaccination, after *vacca*, cow, in honor of Edward Jenner. The earliest understanding of vaccine production has to do with attenuation, stepping down the disease-causing capability of the microbe and using this to protect the individual. However, the major flaw here is that the agents that were thought to have lost pathogenic capability may suddenly revert to virulence. Thus, on the basis of reversion to virulence, attenuation of microbes by culture in unusual medium was found to be unreliable in some instances; instead, attenuation by genetic modification is preferred.

VACCINES

- Agents of immunity.
- Major diseases that plague humanity have been controlled. Such diseases include smallpox, rabies, tetanus, cholera, diphtheria, measles, and so on.
- Immunization involves giving out **antigens** of infectious agents to the host so as to elicit an immune response—**active Immunity**. When preformed **antibodies** are given, it is **passive immunity**.

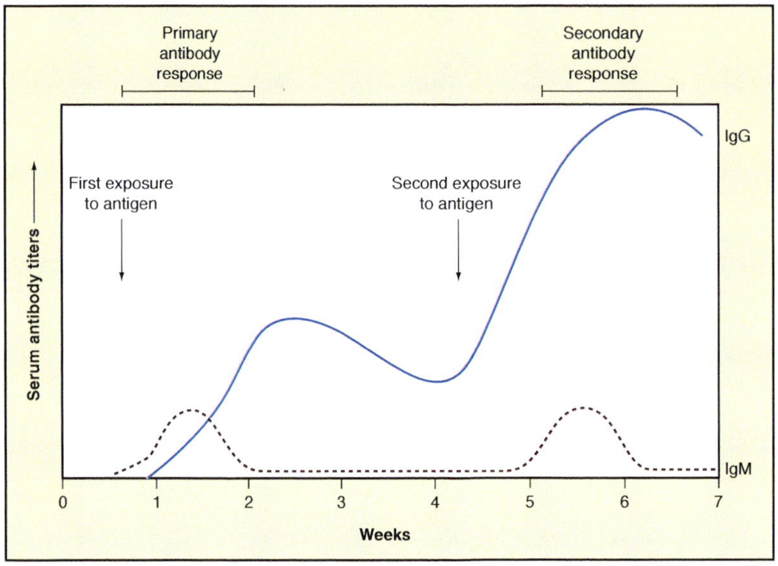

Figure 11.1 *Comparison of primary response and secondary response. Upon infection, a lag phase follows, lasting 3–4 days. After this, a response is seen, lasting about 20–25 days before subsiding. Upon a secondary exposure of the initial challenge, no lag phase is seen and substantially more antibody is produced, and the result is more long lasting.*

CRITERIA FOR IMMUNIZATION

- Absolute identification of cause of disease.
- It must be established that an Immune response is possible, for example, *Haemophilus influenza* type B capsular polysaccharide protects only ages 18 months and above. Younger children do not respond to unconjugated carbohydrates.
- Minimal risk: risk from vaccination should be less than that from the actual infection with the organism, for example, smallpox can cause encephalitis, so vaccination must be given to normal individuals.

TYPES OF IMMUNIZATION PROCEDURE

Passive immunity: Produces **temporary resistance**; it involves the transfer of **preformed antibodies** to susceptible individuals. The antibodies are catabolized and **susceptibility resumes**.

- Examples include

i. tetanus injected into horse to produce **antisera**—antitetanus serum (ATS) and

ii. clostridia toxin rendered nontoxic with formaldehyde (toxoids). The toxoid is injected into the horse to produce antibodies, this is antitetanus toxoid.

Active Immunity: It stimulates the immune system to respond actively

- Examples include

i. BCG (Bacillus calmetteguerrin) attenuated TB bovis vaccine—produced by 13 years culture in bile medium. Attenuation of bacteria is by prolonged growth of the organism in a medium other than that in which it normally grows.

ii. Fowl cholera—aged culture as prepared by Pasteur.

- Response in active immunity is not immediate, but it is long lasting.

PROBLEMS OF HORSE ANTIBODIES

- They are rapidly cleared.
- They suppress response to active immunization
- Immune complex (due to presence of animal serum) causes anaphylaxis (serum sickness).

TABLE 11.1 REPORTABLE CLASS OF VACCINE-PREVENTABLE CHILDHOOD DISEASES IN THE UNITED STATES

DISEASE	MAXIMAL NO. OF CASES (YR)	2013	% CHANGE
Diphtheria	206,939 (1921)	0	–100.0
Measles	894,134 (1941)	0	–100.0
Mumps[1, 2]	152,209 (1968)	0	–100.0
Pertussis	265,269 (1934)	0	–100.0
Poliomyelitis (paralytic)	21,269 (1952)	0	–100.0
Rubella[3, 4]	57,686 (1969)	0	–100.0
Congenital rubella syndrome	20,000 (1964–1965)	0	–100.0
Tetanus	1,564 (1923)	0	–100.0

Note: Data for the "Maximal numbers of cases (yr.)" are from the *New England Journal of Medicine, 327*, p. 1795, 1992.

[1]Data are from Orenstein.
[2]Mumps first becomes a reportable disease in 1968.
[3]Projected number of vaccine-associated cases, 5 to 10.
[4]Rubella first becomes a reportable disease in 1966.
[5]Data for 2013 incidence are from WHO vaccine-preventable diseases: monitoring system. 2014 global summary.

TABLE 11.2 WHOOPING COUGH VACCINE: RISKS VERSUS BENEFIT

	RISK OF OCCURRENCE AFTER	
PROBLEM	**VACCINATION**	**DISEASE**
Seizures	1:1,750	1:25–1:50
Encephalitis	1:110,000	1:1,000–1:4,000
Severe brain damage	1:310,000	1:2,000–1:8,000
Death	1:1,000,000	1:200–1:1,000

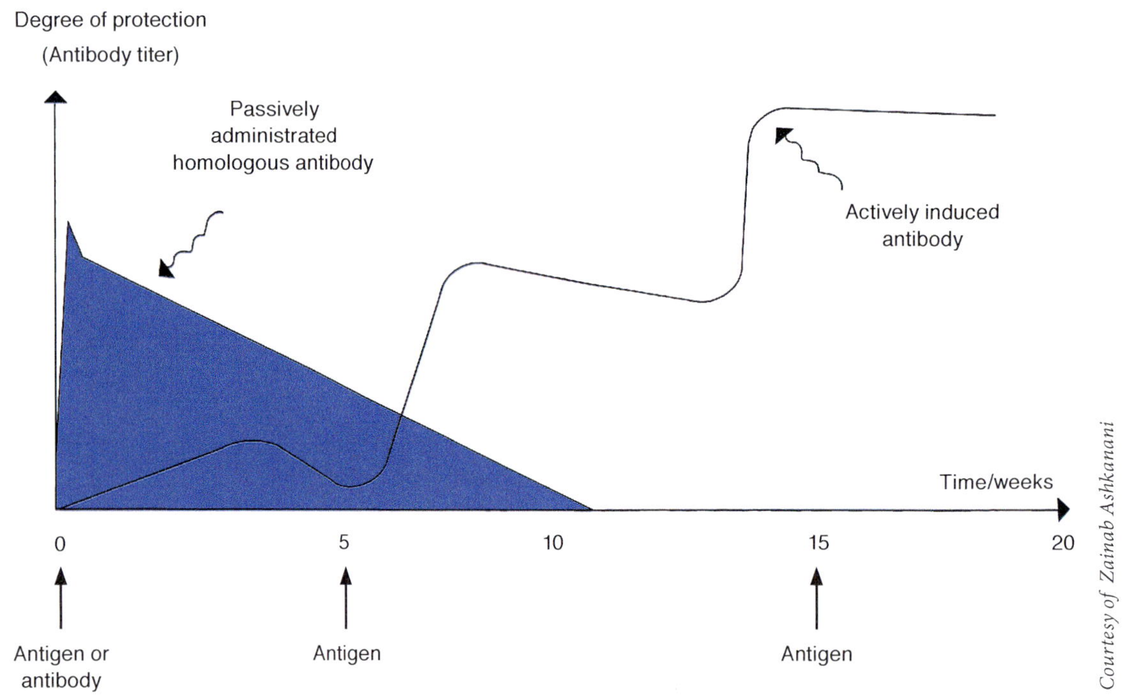

Figure 11.2 *A comparison of active and passive immunization. Passive immunization gives rapid onset but relatively short-lasting immunity. Active immunization in contrast develops slowly but gives prolonged immunity and can be readily boosted.*

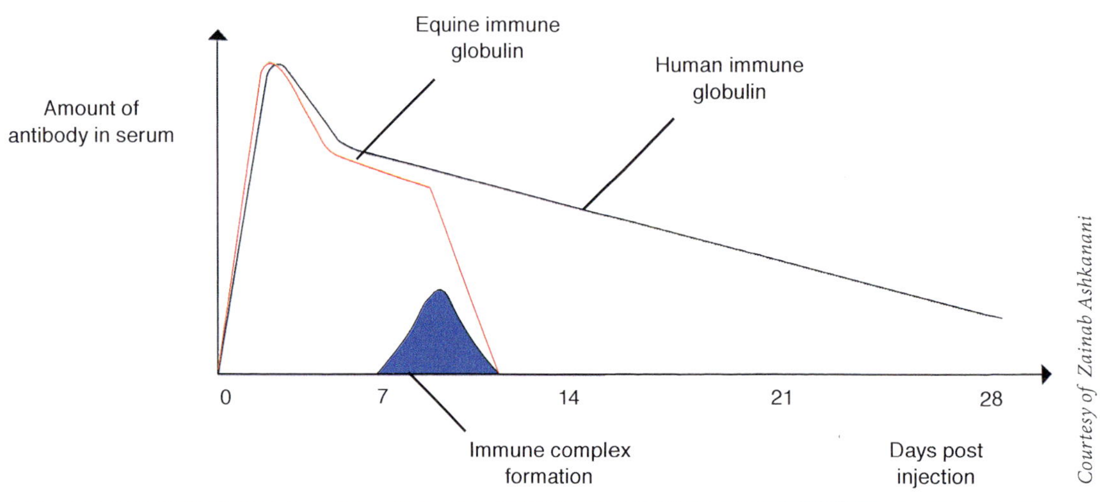

Figure 11.3 *A comparison of the fate of human immune globulin and equine immune globulin when injected into a human. The equine immune globulin is antigenic and is rapidly removed once the host mounts an immune response. Immune complexes form when the foreign antigen is being removed by antibody.*

- The advantage of an attenuated vaccine is that it is accompanied by the production of interferon, but a disadvantage is that it is not good in the case of AIDs patients as they cannot respond to infection.
- Agents of active immunity other than the attenuated vaccines are vaccines obtained from killed organisms. Chemical killing using formaldehyde, ethylene oxide or β-propiolactone can be done.

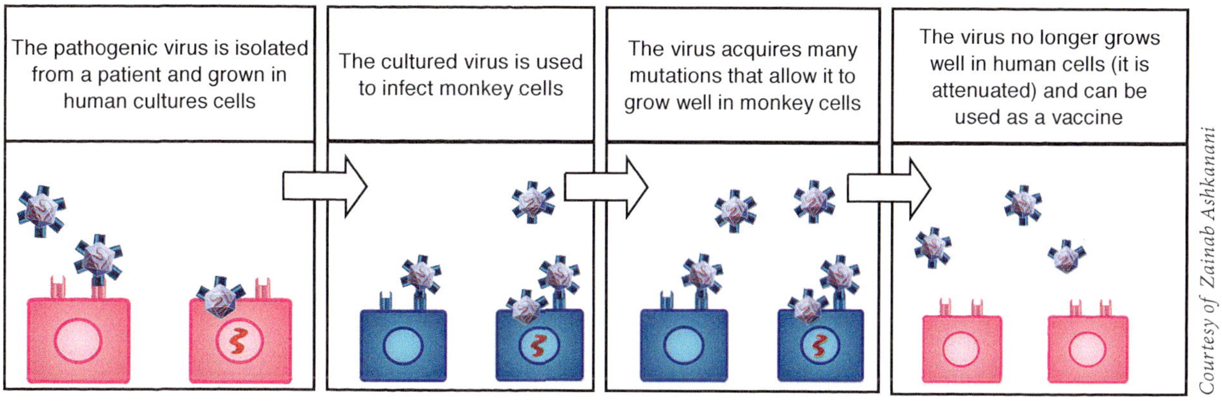

Figure 11.4 *Attenuated viruses are selected by growing human viruses in nonhuman cells.*

VACCINES

They are simply described as agents of immunity. Through them, the major diseases that plague humanity have been effectively controlled, such diseases include smallpox, rabies, tetanus, cholera, diphtheria, measles, and so on (see Tables 11.1 and 11.2).

CRITERIA FOR IMMUNIZATION

- There is need to absolutely identify what the cause of the disease is; so, if there are smallpox-like symptoms or smallpox-like disease in an environment, it may not necessarily be smallpox.
- There is need to establish that immune response is possible. For instance, the bacterium *Haemophilus influenza* has capsular polysaccharide, which because of insufficient complexity does not stimulate the immune system. A conjugated protein that consists of protein and carbohydrate parts would be a better antigenic agent than a simple polysaccharide.
- It is important to weigh the risk of vaccination versus that of the natural course of the disease. For instance, the smallpox vaccine may cause encephalitis (inflammation of the covering of the brain), but this affects only a small percentage of vaccinated individuals; it is, therefore, preferred to vaccinate rather than allowing the disease to run its course.

TYPES OF IMMUNIZATION PROCEDURES

Immunization involves giving of the antigen of the infectious agent, either as an antigen or as a component of the whole organism, to the host to induce an immune response. When the administered agent challenges the immune system, it is considered an active immunization. But there are circumstances in which the immune system is incompetent or there is insufficient time for proper response, then passive immunization involving the administration of preformed antibodies is the method of choice.

Passive immunization has an immediate effect, but it can work only for a short period. The other problem is that these antibodies are easily cleared by the system because they are foreign, so they soon wane and susceptibility will resume. There is also the possibility of developing serum sickness, arising from immune complex formation due to the fact that the antibodies were raised in an animal of a different species. An example is the case of the bacterium *Clostridium tetani*, described in the plates above (Figures 11.2–11.4).

The major problem of active immunization is that the response is not immediate, there is a lag period, but during this period the innate immune response is supposed to be in play. The major advantage is that the protection lasts longer.

VACCINE PRODUCTION

- Genetically modified (genetically stable and lacks disease-causing ability).
- Recombinant vaccine (useful for production of protein Ags, using recombinant DNA).
- Synthetic peptide (chemical synthesis of epitope, that is, antigenic moiety).
- Naked DNA (injection of viral DNA into host).
- Anti-idiotype vaccine (Ab against idiotype is the same conformation as epitope, thus can serve as Ag).

VACCINE PRODUCTION BY GENETIC MODIFICATION

The objective here is to produce genetically stable agents that will not cause a disease. This is because attenuation may not achieve this nondisease causation because of reversion to virulence, so there is the need for a deliberate modification of the genes of the organism that will render them effectively and irreversibly attenuated (Figure 11.5).

GENETICALLY MODIFIED ORGANISMS

The objective is to produce a genetically stable agent that will not cause disease. Attenuation may not achieve this because of the reversion to virulence, thus deliberate modification of the gene of organisms can render them effectively and irreversibly attenuated.

1. **Example 1.** Peudorabies: a pig disease caused by herpes virus. It is neurotropic and needs the gene thymidine kinase (TK) for neuronal cell infection.
2. **Example 2.** Influenza virus and *Vibrio cholerae*: have segmented genome, so gene segment reassortment can cause genetic modification (resulting in the loss of the disease-causing capability).
3. **Example 3.** Insertion of missense gene (resulting in temperature sensitive mutant, thus unable to cause disease).

An example is the pseudorabies. It is a disease that afflicts pigs; it is very important since pork is a source of protein. This virus is a herpes virus that causes pseudorabies. It is neurotropic (grows along neuronal cells). The protein that is required for neuronal colonization and infection is coded in the thymidine kinase gene (TKgene). The careful deletion of the thymidine kinase gene from the herpes virus genome leaves the virus with the ability to propagate but without a disease-causing capability. Another example is the influenza virus. In this case, the virulent gene is deleted and the modification makes the virus non disease causing. Also, the bacterium *Vibrio cholerae*, has genome that is segmented, so that a careful reassortment of the gene or relocation of a gene segment (genetic reassortment) results in loss of disease-causing capability. It is also possible to achieve the same effect by inserting a missense gene, the kind of missense gene that will make the final product temperature sensitive and compromise the capacity to cause disease.

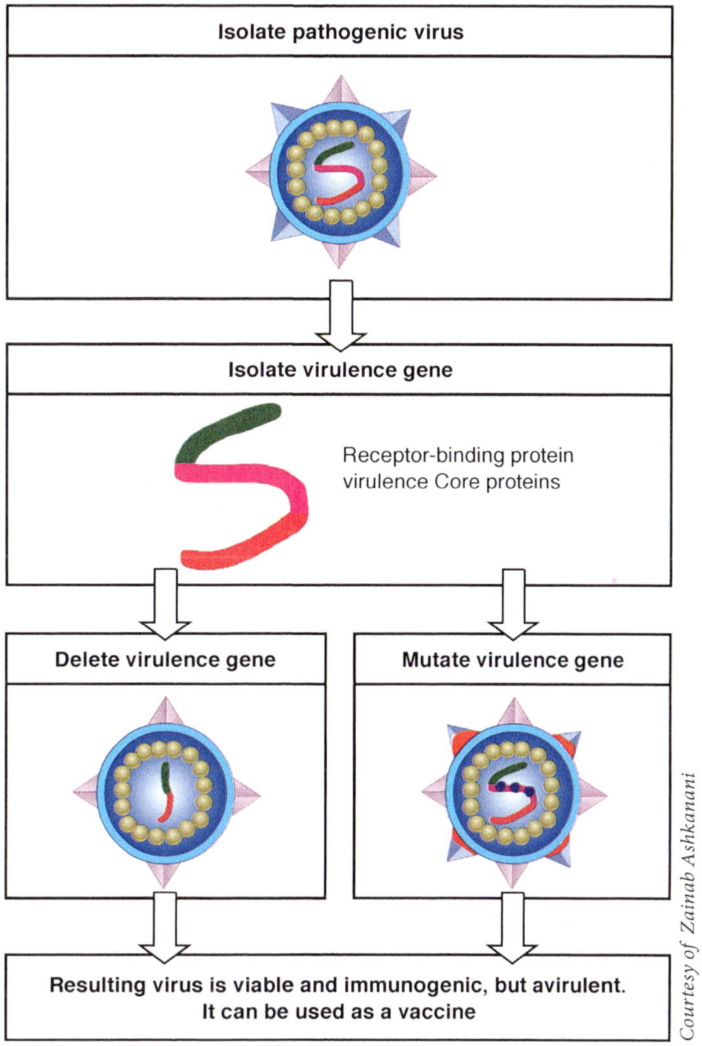

Figure 11.5 *Production of live-attenuated viral strains by genetic modification. Deletion of the virulent gene of the virus can render it nonpathogenic.*

RECOMBINANT VACCINE

The recombinant DNA technology is applied in the production of protein antigens used as vaccines. It involves the isolation of the gene that codes for that antigen that is of interest and this is inserted into a bacterium DNA or a piece of DNA (plasmid), the plasmid is subsequently inserted into an organism that can easily grow. The growth of the organism that was transfected with the isolated gene results in the elaboration of the vaccine candidate protein into the culture broth. An example is the foot-and-mouth disease. The causative agent of this disease is an RNA virus. The isolated RNA virus is transcribed to DNA using reverse transcriptase, the DNA so produced is treated with restriction endonucleases that can remove sections of DNA nucleotides, in this instance of foot-and-mouth disease, the VPI protein gene (Figure 11.6). The gene is inserted in plasmid and transfected into *Escherichia coli*. The propagation of *E. coli* is accompanied by the elaboration of the VPI protein which is harvested and used as vaccine.

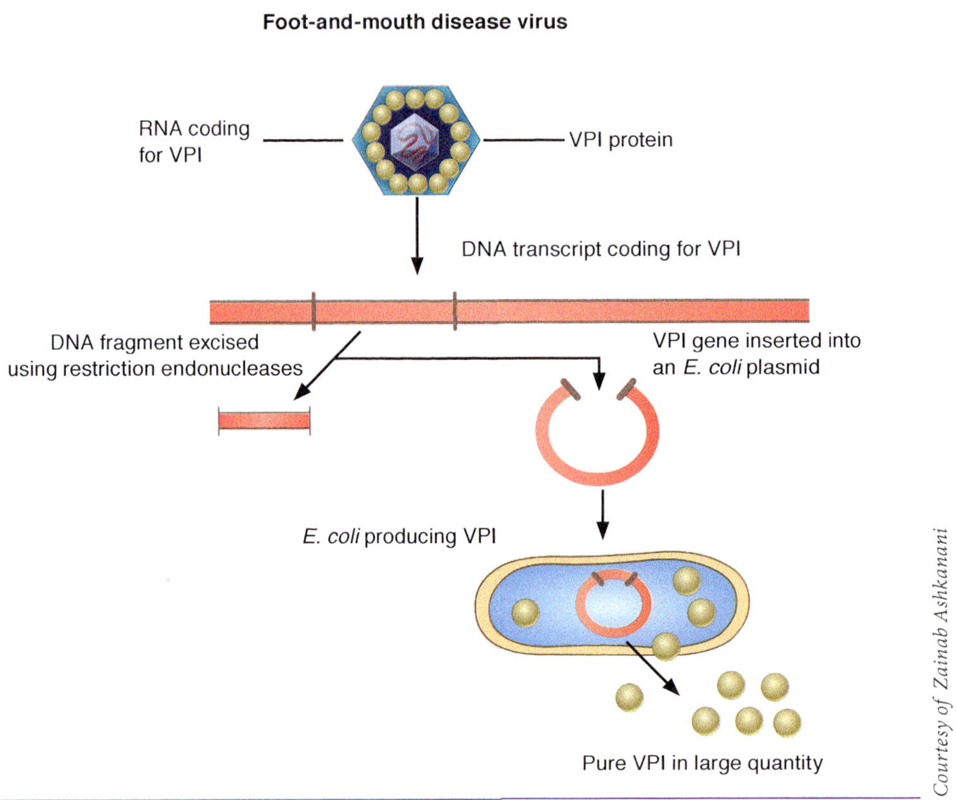

Figure 11.6 *The production of large quantity of VPI antigen from the foot-and-mouth disease virus by the use of recombinant DNA technique. The purified VPI derived from bulk culture of E. coli may be used in foot-and-mouth disease vaccine.*

This is how hepatitis vaccine is also made because it is not easy to culture hepatitis.

SYNTHETIC PEPTIDES

- Since only a few peptide sequences on an Ag constitute the epitope, it is a limited component of the Ag molecule that elicits protective immune response. This peptide sequence may be chemically synthesized and used. Synthetic peptides are safe but expensive.
- Experimental synthetic vaccines are available against several viruses, including hepatitis B and influenza A.

NAKED DNA

- It involves the injection of a viral DNA into the host. DNA encoding for the nucleoprotein of influenza virus can be attached to a plasmid.
- The plasmid is then injected into the muscle of a mouse; the mouse will elicit an immune response in the form of antibody production against nucleoproteins.

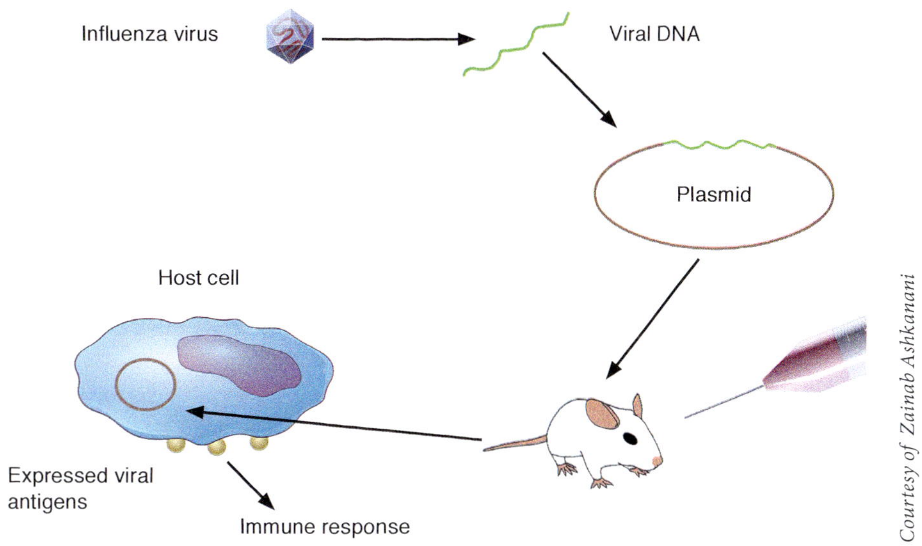

Figure 11.7 *Viral DNA incorporated into a plasmid can cause the formation of viral antigens in host cells in the same way as the original virus. The endogenous antigens are admirably suited to provoke a protective immune response.*

It would be purer if the nucleoprotein was made outside the host system and injected into the host, but then there is the problem of some proteins being very susceptible to degradation by some enzymes found in body fluids (Figure 11.7).

ANTI-IDIOTYPE VACCINES

- The binding site of the immunoglobulin is the **idiotype**. It binds to the antigenic epitope.
- It is induced by an antigenic epitope. An antibody to the idiotype is the **anti-idiotype**.
- The anti-idiotype will have the same conformation as the epitope. It can be made by taking monoclonal abs to the epitope and inoculating them into animals. The anti-idiotype produced can be used as vaccine.
- The anti-idiotype Ab when used as vaccine produced anti-anti-idiotype Abs which is protective because it **binds the original** epitope.

The basis of the interaction is that it was the epitope which induced the antibody idiotype in the first instance and thus provided a complementary site. So, if an antibody is produced against the idiotype, it is designated anti-idiotype. This antibody (anti-idiotype) has the same configuration as the epitope, and therefore, the anti-idiotype can easily be used to produce monoclonal antibodies that will react with the epitope. The anti-idiotype can be used as vaccine easily. Anti-idiotype antibody when used as a vaccine produces anti-anti-idiotype antibodies, which can provide protection against the original epitope (Figure 11.8).

Figure 11.9 demonstrates some new methods of making vaccines. Unfortunately, few of these have been approved for human use. Recombinant vaccines are used against hepatitis B, rabies, and feline leukemia. Synthetic vaccine are generally very expensive.

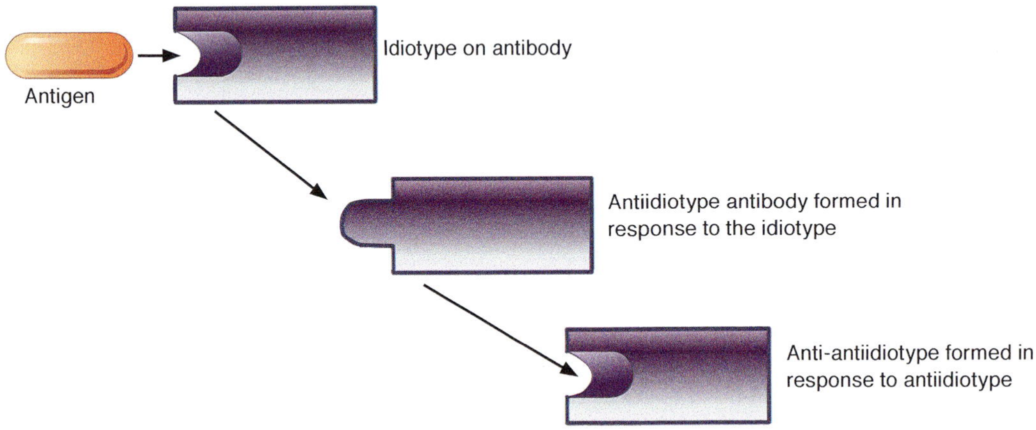

Courtesy of Zainab Ashkanani

Figure 11.8 *A very simple view of the idiotype network.*

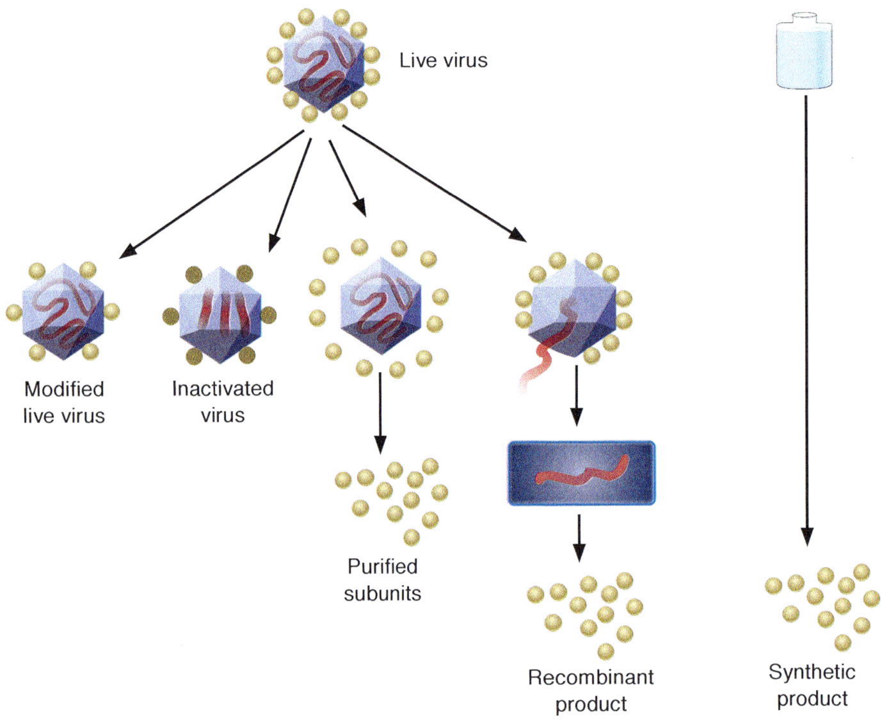

Courtesy of Zainab Ashkanani

Figure 11.9 *Some exciting new methods of making vaccines.*

ADJUVANTS

They are enhancers of immune response. They act by slowing down the release of antigens.

ADJUVANT

- Enhancer of host immune responses.
- Acts by slowing down the release of antigens.
- Adjuvant causes focus formation from which antigens are gradually released.
- Examples are Al(OH)2, Al(PO4)2, Al(K)SO4 (alum) → this will cause macrophage-rich granuloma from which antigens leak to provide sustained antigen stimulation.
- Water-in-oil emulsion is an incomplete adjuvant.
- Water-in-oil emulsion + TB = complete adjuvant, It elicits IL-1 products, enhances phagocytosis, T cell function, and resistance to tumor.

They do this by forming a depot from which antigens are gradually leached into the system. An example is alum such as aluminum phosphate. This will cause a macrophage-rich granuloma, thus delaying the movement of the antigen from the mixture into the host system. Another adjuvant is water-in-oil emulsion, which can be added to the antigen. It is described as an incomplete adjuvant. The oil stimulates local chronic inflammation which is rich in macrophages and fibroblasts, and then antigens are leached from this granuloma. The complete adjuvant is about the same thing except that it is more complex. It consists of agents like killed *Mycobacterium tuberculosis* (TB), as a source of muramyl dipeptide and *Bordetella pertussis* that is added to the antigen system. Therefore, it consists of water-in-oil emulsion, and TB. It elicits a comprehensive response including cytokine release because of the presence of TB, and it enhances phagocytosis, favors T cell function and resistance to tumor (See Tables 11.3–11.6).

TABLE 11.3 SOME COMMON ADJUVANTS

TYPE	ADJUVANT	MODE OF ACTION
Aluminum salts	Aluminum phosphate	Slow-release antigen depot
	Aluminum hydroxide	
	Alum	
Water-in-oil emulsions	Freud's incomplete adjuvant	Slow-release antigen depot
Bacterial fractions	Anaerobic corynebacteria	Macrophage stimulator
	BCG	Macrophage stimulator
	Muramyl dipeptide	Macrophage stimulator
	Bordetella pertussis	Lymphocyte stimulator
	Lipopolysaccharide	Macrophage stimulator
Surface-active agents	Saponin	Stimulates antigen processing
	Lysolecithin	Stimulates antigen processing
Complex carbohydrates	Acemannan	Macrophage stimulator
	Glucans	Macrophage stimulator
	Dextran sulfate	Macrophage stimulator
Mixed adjuvants	Freund's complete adjuvant	Water-in-oil emulsion plus mycobacterium

TABLE 11.4 ACTIVE IMMUNIZING AGENTS (VACCINES) USED AGAINST BACTERIAL DISEASE

DISEASE	ANTIGEN USED	ADJUVANT
Anthrax	Purified proteins	None
Tuberculosis	Modified live (BCG)	None
Cholera	Killed organisms	None
Diphtheria	Toxoid	Aluminum phosphate
Hemophilums	Capsular polysaccharide	None
Meningococcus	Capsular polysaccharide	None
Whooping cough	Killed oraganisms or purified proteins	Aluminum phosphate
Plague	Killed oraganisms	None
Pneumococcus	Capsular polysaccharide	None
Tetanus	Toxid	Aluminum phosphate
Typhoid	Killed or modified live organisms	None

TABLE 11.5 ACTIVE IMMUNIZING AGENTS USED AGAINST VIRAL DISEASE IN HUMANS

DISEASE	ANTIGEN USED	ADJUVANT
Measles	Modified live	None
Mumps	Modified live	None
Rubella	Modified live	None
Poliomyelitis	Inactivated or modified live	None
Influenza	Inactivated	None
Hepatitis B	Recombinant antigen	None
Rabies	Inactivated	None
Yellow fever	Modified live	None

TABLE 11.6 SOME SUBUNIT VACCINES USED IN HUMANS AND OTHER ANIMALS

VACCINE	SUBUNIT
Bacterial	
Tetanus	Toxin
Diphtheria	
S. pheumoniae	Capsular polysaccharide
Meningococci	Capsular polysaccharide
E.Coli	Adherence pili
Viruses	
Rabies	
Foot-and-mouth virus	Capsid proteins
Influenza	
Hepatitis B	Synthetic capsid epitopes
Foot-and-mouth virus	

The depot-causing agent-oil-in water emulsion which also forms granuloma tissue causes the feeling of heaviness on the spot where it has been inoculated. Sometimes, in complete adjuvant, the matrix of lipid micelles containing some viral proteins can also be used as part of the complete adjuvant, so the reaction resembles the complete adjuvant in that there is enhanced macrophage uptake. Also, some macromolecules such as surfactants and detergents may be added to adjuvants to enhance cell membrane permeability to antigens.

SAMPLE QUESTIONS

VACCINES AND VACCINATION

1. The major disadvantage of passive immunization is that it
   a. is ineffective
   b. is expensive
   c. is liable to cause serum sickness
   d. interferes with active immunization
   e. induces short-lived immunity
2. The major disadvantage of active immunization is that it
   a. causes prolonged immunity
   b. induces rapid onset of immunity
   c. induces slow onset of immunity
   d. causes serum sickness
   e. is expensive
3. When given to humans, older forms of rabies vaccines may give rise to
   a. anaphylactoid reactions
   b. disseminated intravascular coagulation
   c. anaphylaxis
   d. serum sickness
   e. allergic encephalitis
4. A rabbit has been immunized with DNP-BSA. Three weeks later you want to induce an anamnestic response to DNP-BGG. This can be accomplished by
   a. boosting with DNP one week before immunization with DNP-BGG.
   b. immunizing with BGG one week after the initial immunization with DNP-BSA.
   c. passively administering anti-BGG antibodies before immunization with BGG.
   d. passively administering anti-DNP antibodies prior to challenging with DNP-BGG.
   e. transfusing purified lymphocytes from a rabbit primed with DNP at least 2 days before challenging with DNP-BGG.

Answer True of False to the following:

Synthetic peptides and naked DNA vaccines

T 5. For synthetic peptide vaccine production, the immunogenic portion of the antigen molecules is chemically synthesized and used for immunization.

F 6. Synthetic peptides are safe and inexpensive.

Anti-idiotype vaccines

T 7. The binding site of the immunoglobulin is the idiotype, induced by an antigenic epitope.

T 8. An antibody to the idiotype is the anti-idiotype, which has the same conformation as the epitope.

Adjuvant

F 9. Adjuvants enhance the immune response ~~by speeding up~~ slowing down the release of antigens from the vaccine site.

T 10. Examples of adjuvants are Al(OH)2, Al(PO4)2, and AL(K)SO4, which cause the formation of a macrophage-rich granuloma.

F 11. Water-in-oil emulsion is ~~complete~~ incomplete adjuvant, which elicits IL-1 products, enhanced phagocytosis, T cell function, and resistance to tumors.

F 12. Water-in-oil emulsion + TB is an ~~incomplete~~ complete adjuvant, which stimulates local chronic inflammation.

SUGGESTED LABORATORY PRACTICALS

- Case Studies on:

1. Criteria for Vaccination
2. Passive and Active Vaccines
3. Methods of Vaccine Production

- Quantification of Antibodies
- Direct and Indirect Antiglobulin Test
- Viral Plaque Assay
- Tuberculin Skin Test
- Embryonated Hen's Egg in Viral Culture

CHAPTER 12

INFLAMMATION

Inflammation is a required process albeit painful due to the production of pain-inducing soluble substances such as IL-1. It is needed for the realization of an effective immune protection. The immune system can also initiate anti-inflammatory responses to ameliorate the effect of inflammation.

Inflammation is the localization of an immune response. The response itself could be acute or chronic. The chronic response occurs over a gradual but longer period. Inflammation, therefore, is the response of tissues to irritation or injury, it is protective, and it initiates the compulsory drafting of protective factors such as immunoglobulins, complements, and phagocytic cells from the blood stream to the site of infection or the site of tissue damage.

INFLAMMATION

- Very important aspect of immune response.
- It is the localization of immune response.
- This enables the immune system maximize its effects.
- It could be acute or chronic—longer period—and usually sustained.

The macrophage is among the earliest cells that play a central role in inflammation. In the illustration given in Figure 12.1, macrophage ingests a gram-negative organism and the lipopolysaccharide (LPS) content of the organism induces the production of soluble substances by the macrophage. The substances elaborated by macrophage include interleukin-1 (IL-1), which activates the vascular endothelium in the area representing the portal of entry of the challenge. The released IL-1 also activates resident lymphocytes that are in the area. This accounts for the observation that the lymph nodes adjacent to the area representing the portal of entry of the organism become inflamed.

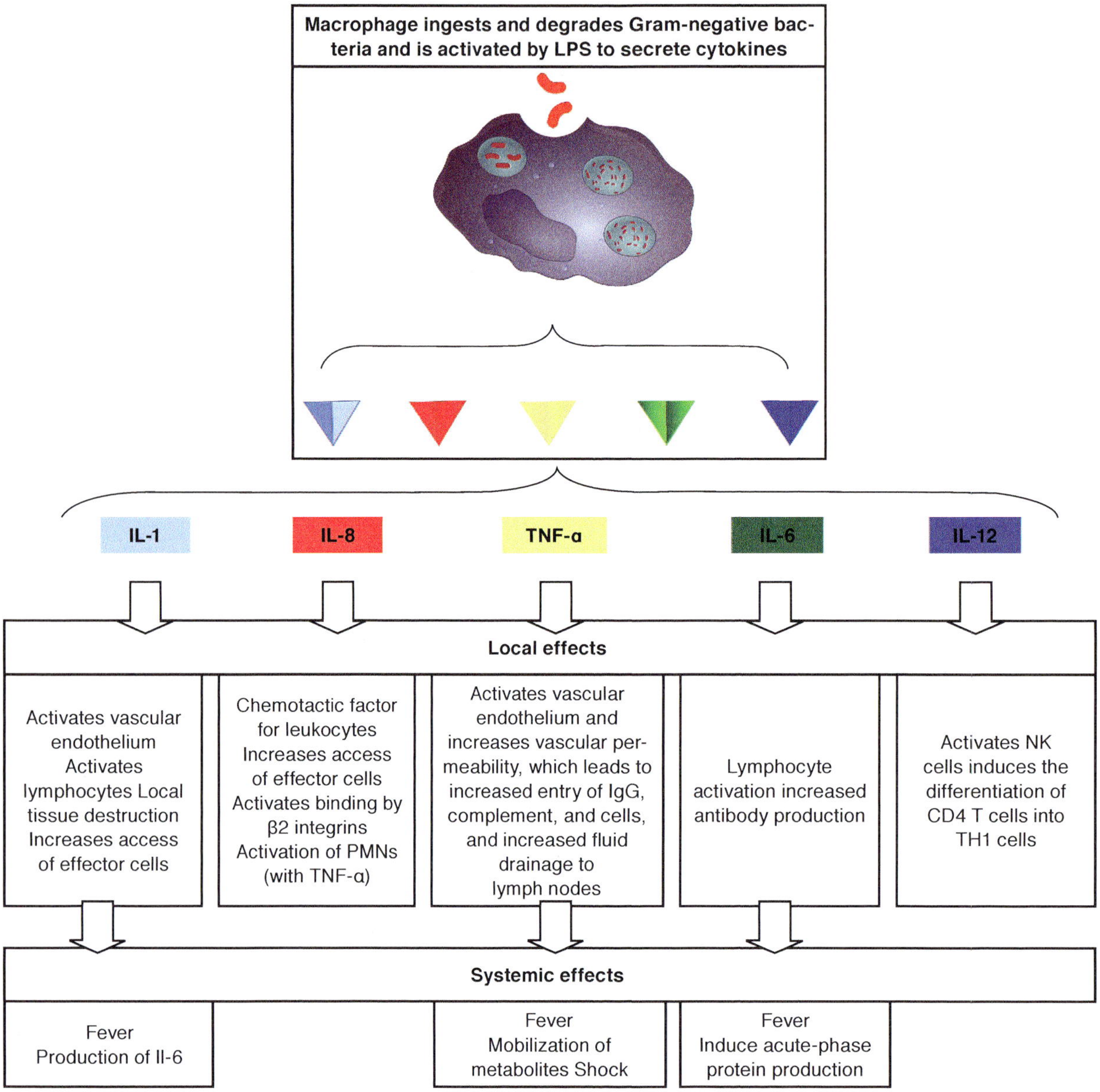

Courtesy of Zainab Ashkanani

Figure 12.1 *Macrophage initiation of the inflammatory response. LPS activation of macrophage results in the macrophage release of cytokines IL-1, IL-8, TNF-a, IL-6, and IL-12.*

Other than IL-1, the body produces IL-8, a chemokine, which causes leukocytes to move to the site. The presence of leukocytes at the site facilitates the impairment of the propagation of the original challenge. This is well illustrated in **Figure 12.2**.

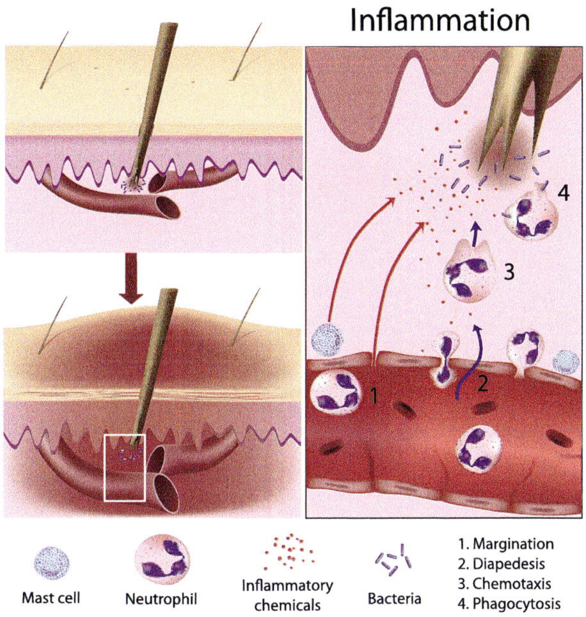

Figure 12.2 *Inflammation is a process by which the effector mechanisms of the immune system, antibodies, complements, and phagocytic cells can escape into tissues and destroy the invading antigen.*

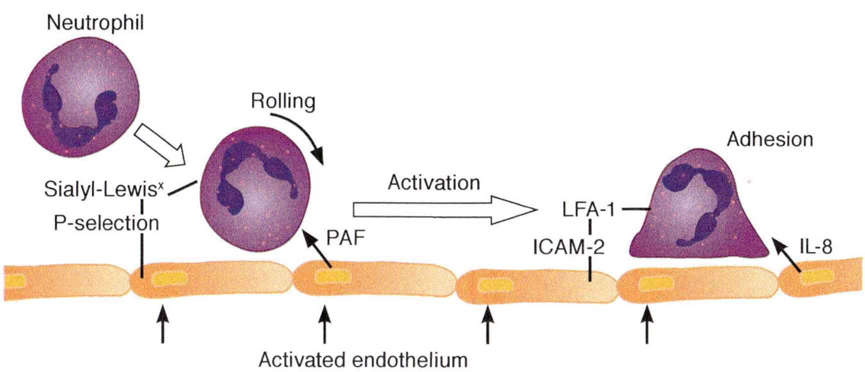

Figure 12.3 *Schematic of rolling process which slows down circulating neutrophils. Prior to emigration from blood vessels, circulating neutrophils must be slowed down and stopped. They are slowed down by a rolling process as their sialyl-Lewis^x binds transiently to P-selectin on endothelial cells. This stimulates local release of PAF, which induces the neutrophil to express LFA-1. The LFA-1 mediates strong binding with endothelial cell ICAM-2 and brings the neutrophil to a complete stop. Local release of IL-8 then ensures that the neutrophil is firmly bound to the endothelium.*

Macrophages will elaborate tumor necrosis factor (TNF), which activates the vascular endothelium and increases vascular permeability, resulting in the efflux of fluid from the blood vessels into the tissue. This fluid influx into tissue causes tenderness and swelling, but also moves soluble substances such as proteins (immunoglobulins, complements, and cytokines) to the site where they are really needed. Through these events, activated lymphocytes produce IL-6 which in turn increases antibody production. Also, cytokines such as IL-12 are elaborated which further enhances the inflammatory process and activates natural killer cells (NK cells) (Figure 12.3).

What are the signs of inflammation? The general signs of inflammation are depicted in Figure 12.4. Inflammation can be acute or chronic. The essential features of acute inflammation include redness, heat, swelling (because of efflux of fluids from vascular space), pain and numbness, and loss of function. These will characterize the early stages of acute inflammation. The progression of these events is marked by a change in vascular permeability, cell emigration, and the release of chemokines from macrophages, mast cells, keratinocytes, hepatocytes, and chemoattractants. Then, coagulation and platelet factors are activated. Because coagulation factors are activated, there is a form of clotting occurring which usually arises from fibrinogen becoming insoluble fibrin. This later process is tightly controlled by the induction of fibrinolytic mechanism; otherwise, there will be thrombosis.

FEATURES OF ACUTE INFLAMMATION

Acute inflammation is marked by following features;

- Changes in vascular permeability: There are two stages involved. First, there is the effect of **vasoactive factors** released from damaged tissue and second, there is **vascular permeability increase**.
- Cellular emigration: This arises from chemo attraction of phagocytic cells and P- selectin-mediated phagocyte adhesion to endothelial cells. P-selectin is secreted in endothelial cells and released in response to histamine or thrombin stimulation.
- Chemokines: These are mediators that have chemotactic activity. IL-8 is an example, it is produced by macrophages, endothelial cells, mast cells, keratinocytes, and hepatocytes in response to bacterial toxin, double-stranded viral RNA, IL-1, and TNF-α. IL-8 is chemotactic for neutrophils, basophils, and some T cells. Its effects include increase of respiratory burst in neutrophils, and leukotrienes synthesis in other cells.
- Coagulatory effects: Inflammation activates platelets, clotting, and fibrinolysis, and causes release of vasoactive agents from platelets.

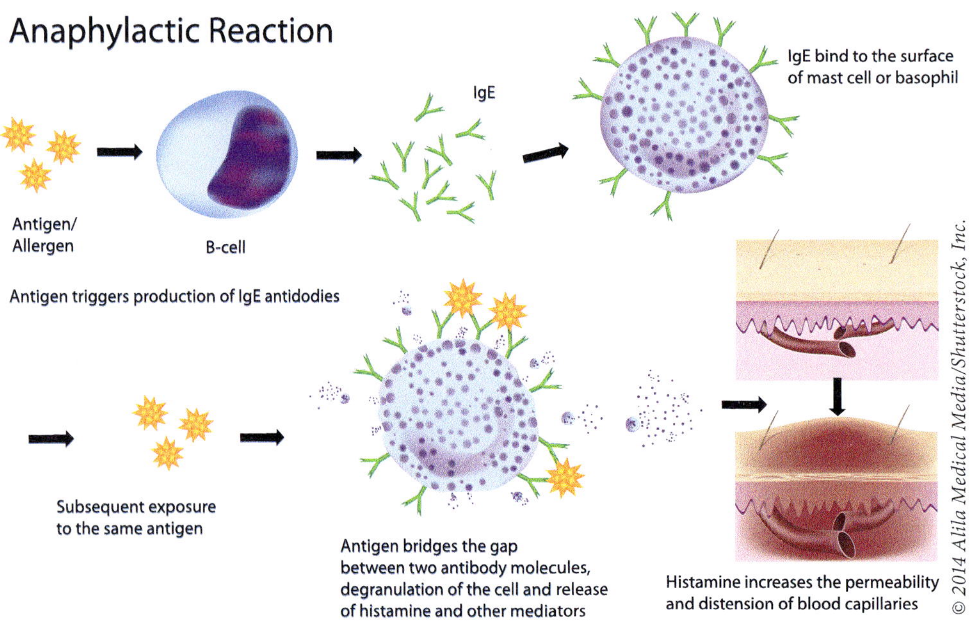

Figure 12.4 *The cardinal signs of inflammation. Redness, heat, pain, and swelling all result from changes in blood vessel properties in the inflamed area.*

The entry of bacteria following a traumatic injury as in the case of the piercing of the skin results in inflammatory response. The tissue compartment in the area interacts with bacteria or some of its products and this elicits responses that draft professional phagocytes to the site. Also, fluid comes into the area in response to enhanced permeability. The fluid brings with it soluble substances such as immunoglobulins, complement, and so on.

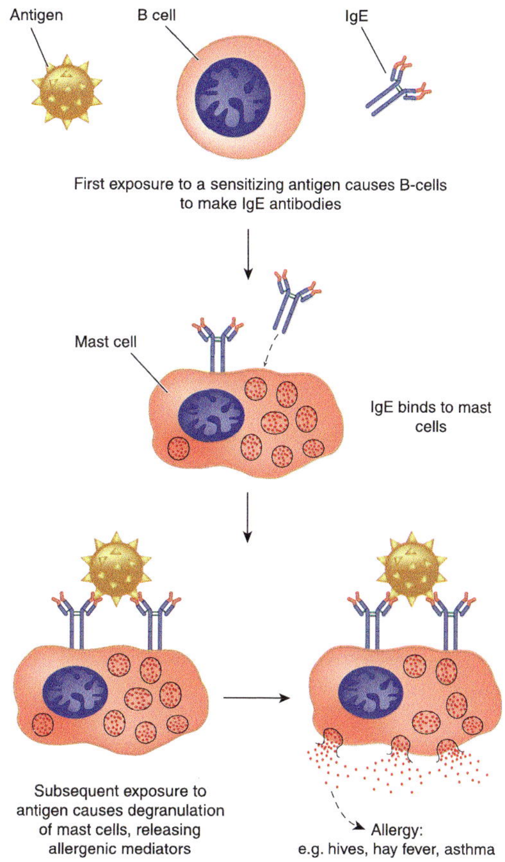

Figure 12.5 *Some of the adhesion molecules that bind neutrophils to capillary endothelial.*

The neutrophils are the earliest cells at the site, they bring about the death of bacteria and in the process they are killed also, resulting in the formation of pus. The movement of neutrophils in intracellular spaces is mediated by adhesion molecules elaborated by endothelial cells. Such molecules include P-selectin that is capable of binding loosely in a noncovalent fashion to sialyl-Lewis receptor (Figure 12.5). The crawling process activates platelet activation factor, which controls the leakage of fluid and regulates excessive edema formation. Other factors produced are intracellular adhesion molecules (ICAM) and leukocyte function associated antigen (LFA). Also, the crawling facilitates the elaboration of a little amount of IL-8, but sufficient to facilitate the drafting of macrophages to this site.

The essential features of inflammation, therefore, include the release of vasoactive factors from damaged tissue; this has the effect of enhancement of vascular permeability. Another feature of inflammation is the enhanced cell migration which arises from the effect of chemoattraction; the migration is effective because of the interaction of cells with selectin and sialyl-Lewis receptor, or ICAM. The P-selectin is secreted by endothelial cells and released in response to histamine or thrombin stimulation.

Interleukin-8 is an example of chemokine. It is produced by macrophage, endothelial cell, mast cell, keratinocytes, and hepatocytes, in response to either whole bacterial infection or bacterial toxin, double-stranded viral RNA, IL-1, TNF. IL-8 is chemotactic for neutrophils, basophils, and some T-cells. Its effect brings about an increase in respiratory burst in neutrophils and it will make the cells start synthesizing some unsaturated fatty acid products that have an immune effect like leukotrienes (Figure 12.6). The cells that are usually activated to secrete these leukotrienes are macrophages and other T cells.

VASOACTIVE FACTORS ASSOCIATED WITH INFLAMMATION

- Histamine: An amine derived from the amino acid histidine and stored in the granules of mast cells and basophils.
- Serotonin (5-hydroxytryptamine): A derivative of the amino acid tryptophan. It is present in nervous tissues, platelets, and mast cells.
- Arachidonic acid derived factors: These are the leukotrienes A4, B4, C4, D4, and E4 derived from lipooxygenase reaction and the prostaglandin, prostacylin, and thromboxanes derived from cyclooxygenase reactions.

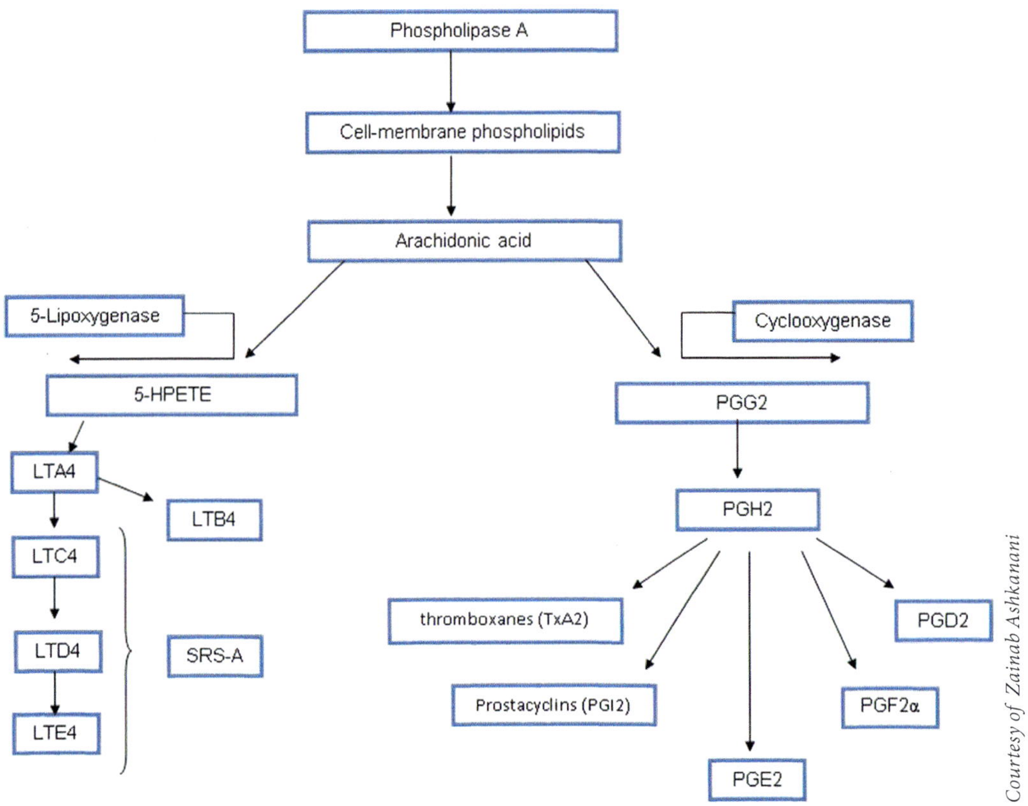

Figure 12.6 *The generation of the leukotrienes, thromboxanes, prostacyclins, and prostaglandins. These compounds, collectively known as prostanoids, are very important mediators of inflammation. Slow-reacting substance of anaphylaxis (SRS-A) is a mixture of leukotrienes.*

The process of inflammation also activates platelets which release proteins associated with the control of the clotting process. This process such as the fibrinolytic step terminates the solid clot of fibrin, thus restoring blood in a fluid form after clotting events.

The vascular factors associated with inflammation include histamine. This is an amine derived from histidine and it is stored in the granules of mast cells and basophils. They are released from mast cells when mast cells are exposed to extracellular fluid as a result of tissue damage. In this circumstance, histamine is released in exchange for sodium ion.

Histamine acts on muscles, blood vessels, and exocrine glands. Another vasoactive factor is serotonin, also described as 5-hydroxytryptamine, it is derived from the amino acid tryptophan. It is present in nervous tissue, in platelets, and in mast cells.

Arachidonic acid, a C20 unsaturated fatty acid, is a very active fatty acid and a vasoactive agent produced during inflammation. The agents that are derived from arachidonic acid are agents like leukotrienes and they are designated A, B, C, D, and E; the reaction that brings about their production is the lipooxygenase reaction. There is another reaction into which arachidonic acid can be fed which brings about prostacyclin, prostaglandins, and thromboxane, this is the cyclooxygenase reaction. Leukotrienes provoke smooth muscle contraction 20 times more than histamine can initiate, while thromboxane is vasoconstrictive. However, prostaglandin and prostacyclin are able to dilate blood vessels. The generation of arachidonic acid is via a phospholipase A reaction. Phospholipase A2 is a membrane-bound enzyme which when activated acts on membrane phosphotidyl choline by cleaving away arachidonic acid. Arachidonic acid is very unstable and very reactive, so it will be fed into either the cyclooxygenase pathway or the lipooxygenase pathway. The 5-HPETE (hydroperoxyeicosatetraenoic acid) is an intermediate between arachidonic acid and leukotrienes.

CLASSIFICATION OF INFLAMMATION

Inflammation is best classified based on the immunotypes. This classification reveals that it is a form of hypersensitivity (Figure 12.7).

CLASSIFICATION OF INFLAMMATION BASED ON IMMUNOLOGIC TYPES

This classification relates them to **hypersensitivity**.

TYPE 1

- Mainly **IgE** mediated.
- IgE interacts with mast cell, and then they react with corresponding antigens.
- Mast cell degranulation occurs.
- Release of vasoactive factors occurs.
- Inflammation results.

TYPE 2

- Mainly IgG, IgM, and complement mediated.
- Target cell interacts with antibodies in the presence of complement.
- Cell destruction occurs.
- Inflammation results.

TYPE 3

- Mainly immune complex mediated.
- Antigen interacts with antibodies in the presence of complement.
- Immune complexes form.
- Neutrophil accumulation occurs.
- Tissue damage and inflammation results.

TYPE 4

- Mainly lymphokines mediated.
- Antigens interact with sensitized T cell.
- Lymphokines are released.
- Mononuclear cell accumulation occurs.
- Tissue damage takes place and inflammation results.

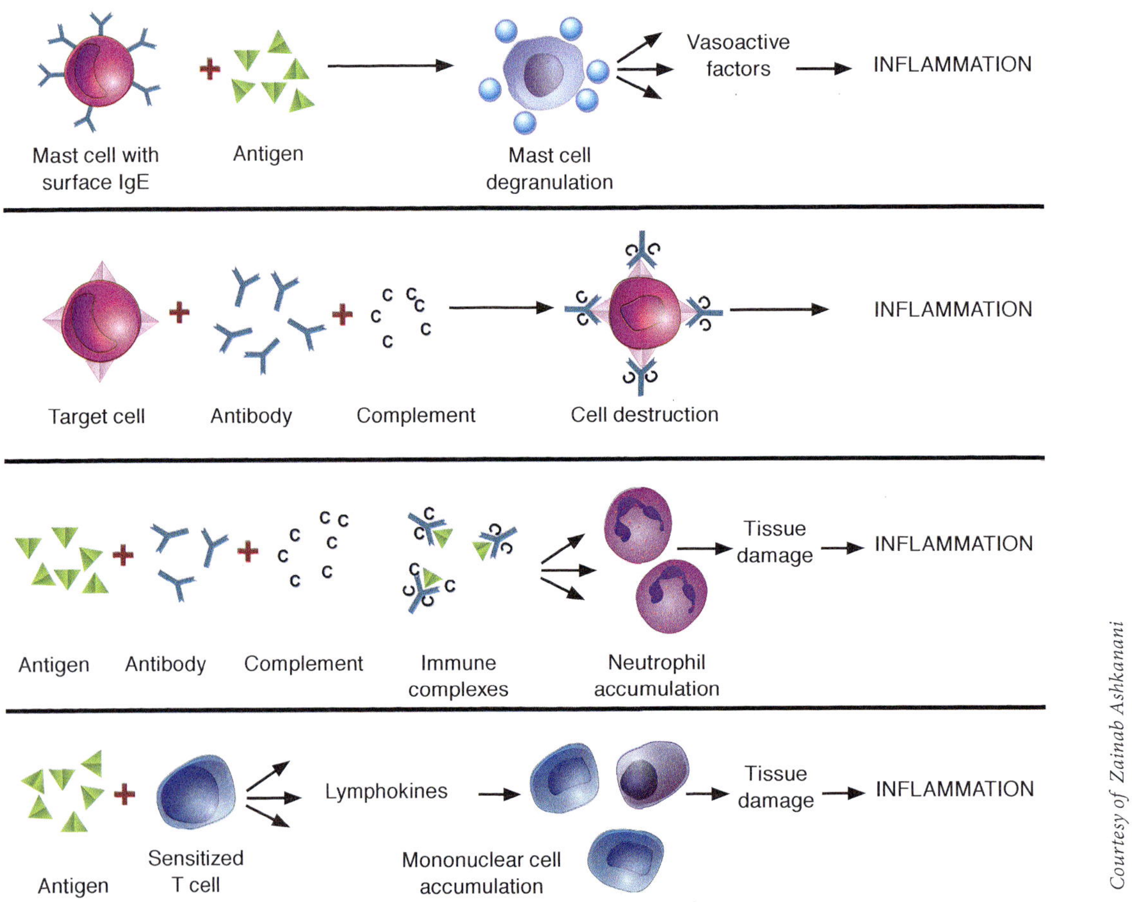

Figure 12.7 *The four types of immunologically mediated inflammation or hypersensitivity as classified by Gell and Coombs.*

Type 1. This is mainly IgE mediated, and IgE interacts with its receptors on mast cells; this results in mast cells degranulation and the release of histamine. The vasoactive effect of histamine is mainly what is observed in type 1 inflammation.

Type 2. It is mainly IgG, IgM, and complement mediated. The target cells interact with these antibodies with subsequent fixing of complement. The activated complement then mediates the destruction of cells and the result of this is inflammation.

Type 3. This is mainly immune complex-mediated. Immune complexes are products of free antigen interaction with antibody. The immune complexes formed fix complement. The difference between type 2 and type 3 is that the antigen is on an organized cell surface for type 2, and in this case the antigen is free. The fixed complement also causes neutrophils to accumulate, tissue damage to occur, and inflammation results.

Type 4. It is lymphokine mediated. It involves the elaboration of cytokines. Antigen interacts with sensitized T cells which have receptors on their surfaces. That makes them release lymphokines. The released lymphokines effect the drafting of mononuclear cells to the site. Mononuclear cells accumulate and initiate tissue destruction. This results in inflammation.

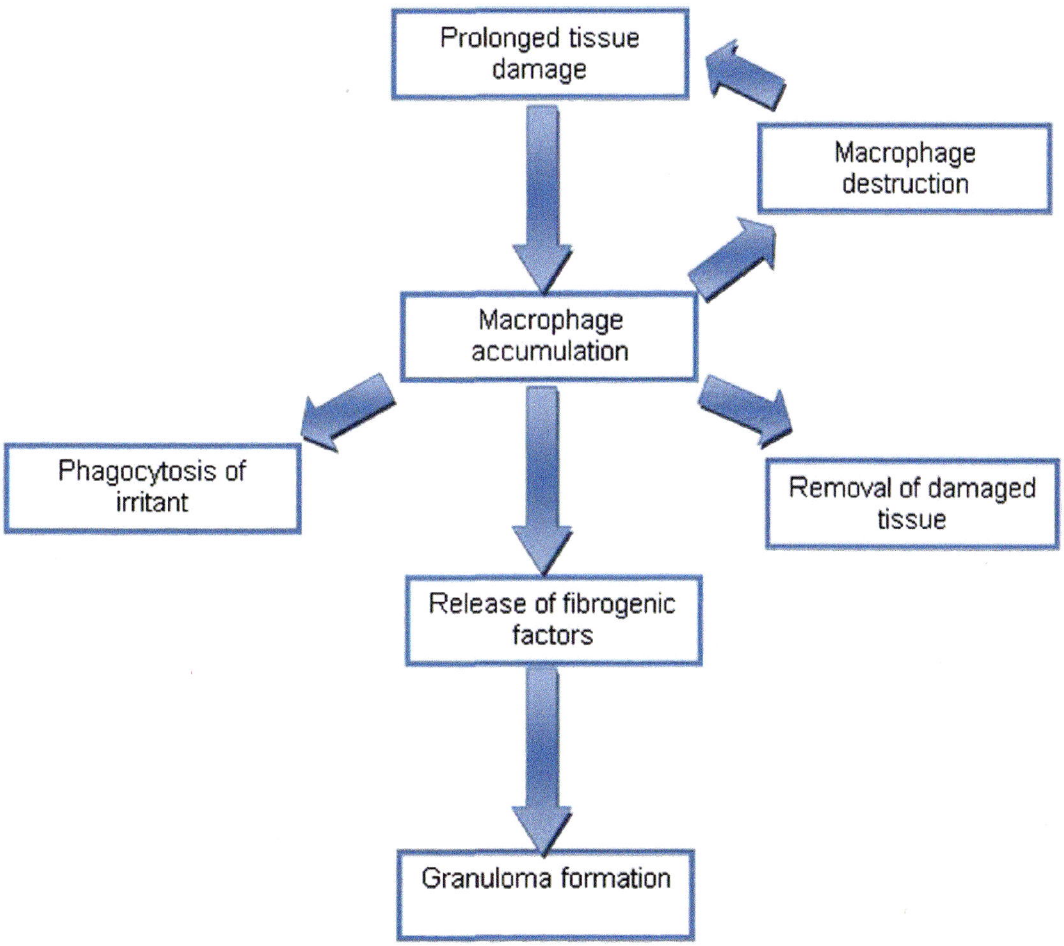

Courtesy of Zainab Ashkanani

Figure 12.8 *The process of chronic inflammation. Prolonged tissue destruction leads to macrophage accumulation and granuloma formation.*

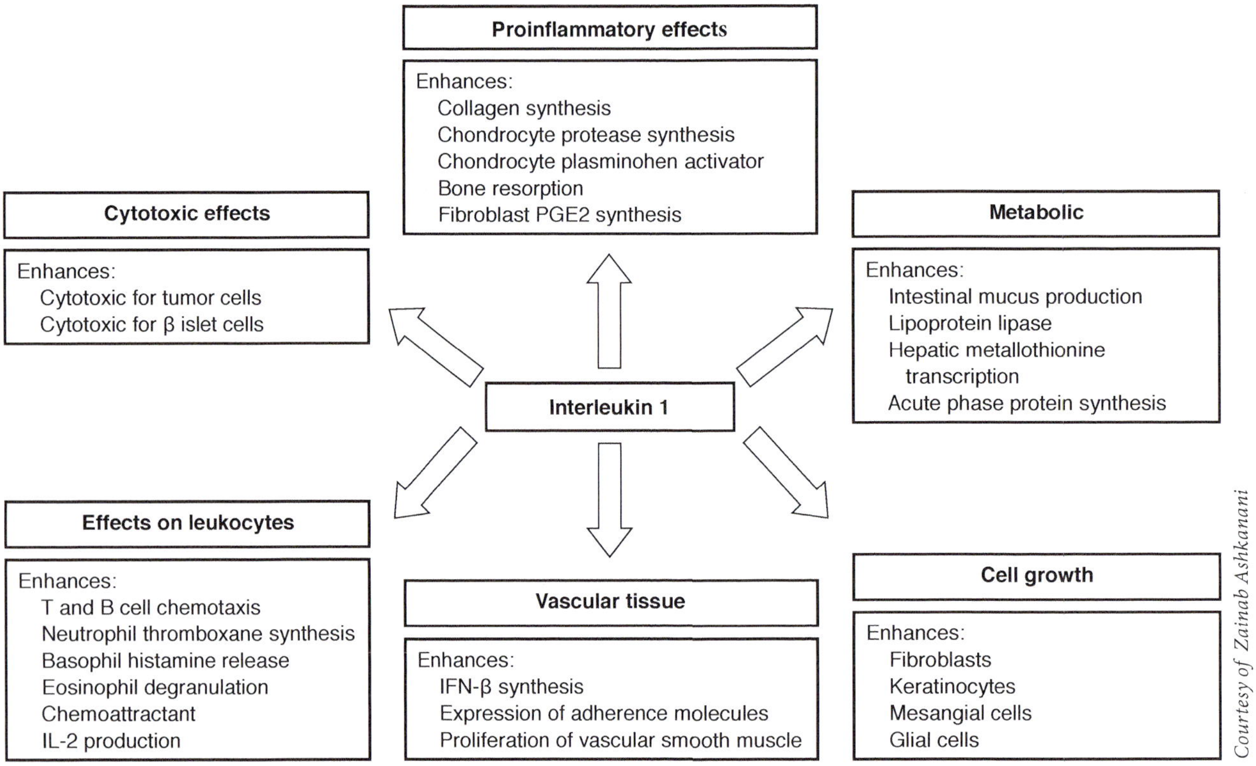

Figure 12.9 *The systemic effects of interleukin-1.*

Inflammation could take a chronic course (Figure 12.8). In chronic inflammation, there is prolonged tissue damage which causes macrophage accumulation. This may cause protracted tissue damage. Chronic inflammation happens for a longer period and is usually sustained. It results from the prolonged presence of infecting agents such as the causative agent of tuberculosis, fungi infections, the presence of ova of parasites, or organic materials such as asbestos. In these cases, the persistence and continuous presence of foreign materials will bring about continuous arrival of new macrophages, fibroblasts, and excessive deposition of collagen around the irritant focus. The lesion that develops is called granuloma because it is granular in appearance. The granules are, in fact, new blood vessels.

CHRONIC INFLAMMATION

- It is for a longer period and usually sustained.
- It results from prolonged presence of bacteria (e.g., TB), fungi, and eggs of parasites or organic materials such as asbestos.
- In these cases, the persistence of foreign materials causes the continuous arrival of new macrophages and fibroblasts and excessive deposition of collagen around the irritant focus.
- The lesion that develops is called granuloma because it is granular in appearance.
- Amyloidosis: Amorphous, waxy, and extracellular substances that infiltrate organs.

The sketch given in Figure 12.9 shows how IL-1 affects the vascular endothelium during chronic inflammation.

SAMPLE QUESTIONS

INFLAMMATION

Answer True or False to the following:

Inflammatory response

1. Following infection vasoconstriction occurs to decrease the velocity of blood flow to the infected site.
2. The inflammatory response includes an increase in cell adhesion molecules, an increase in vessel permeability, and a release of clotting factors.
3. Monocytes differentiate into macrophages in the tissues and migrate to the site of infection.
4. Neutrophils are the first cells to arrive at the site of infection.
5. Chemical mediators of inflammation are released in response to tissue damage or infection.
6. More bacterial cells are attracted to the site of infection by chemotaxis.
7. Localized inflammation will induce fever, increased prostaglandin production, elevated acute phase reactants, and leukocytosis.
8. The hallmarks of inflammation are erythema, elevated temperature, edema, pain, and loss of function.

Major event of inflammatory response

9. Vasoconstriction occurs resulting in engorged vessels causing erythema and increased local temperature.
10. Increased capillary permeability allows for an influx of exudates into extravascular tissue and results in swelling.
11. Macrophages and eosinophils infiltrate infected tissues and engulf invading microorganisms.
12. Plasma proteins and inflammatory mediators infiltrate the infected tissues.

Acute Phase Proteins

13. Acute phase proteins are chemical inflammatory mediators that are produced in response to tissue damage.
14. C-reactive proteins are produced in the bone marrow.
15. C-reactive protein bind to the lipopolysaccharide in the cell walls of bacteria and fungi.
16. Activation of complement results in opsonization and enhanced phagocytosis.

Suggested Laboratory Practicals

- Case Studies on:

1. Hypersensitivity
2. Immune Mediators of Inflammation

- Test for Type II Hypersensitivity
- Test for Type III hypersensitivity
- Test for Delayed Hypersensitivity
- Direct Antiglobulin Test

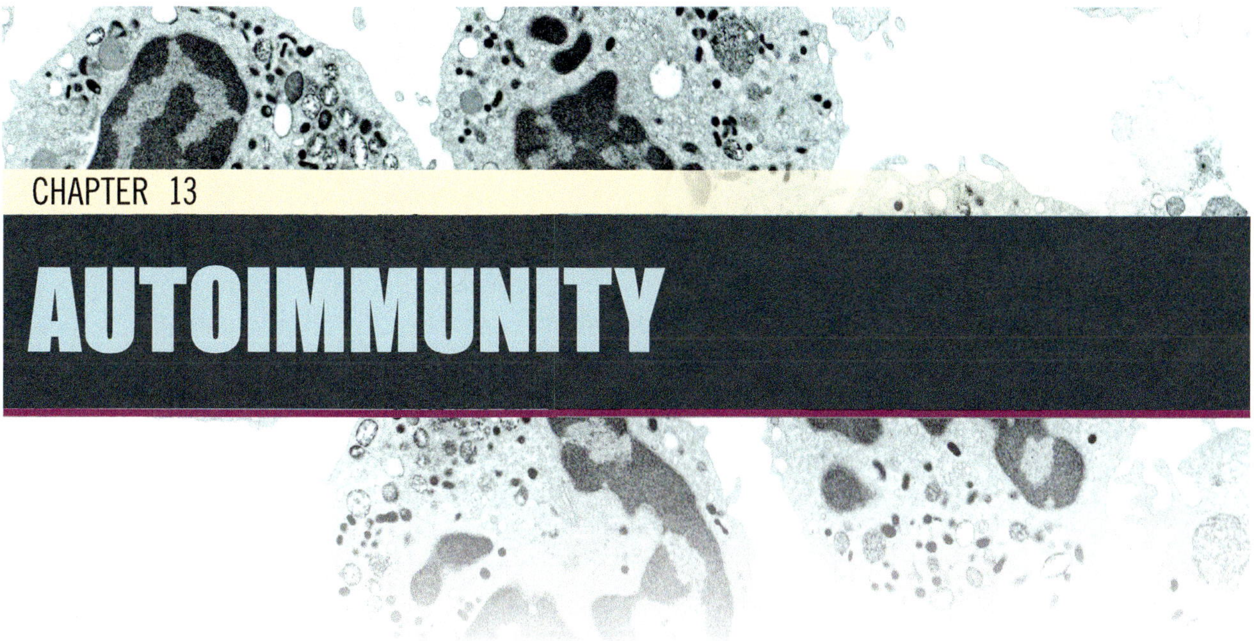

CHAPTER 13

AUTOIMMUNITY

Autoimmune disease is a major threat to health worldwide. At least 10 million Americans suffer from over 80 diseases that have been linked to autoimmune response. Usually, those who are most afflicted are females, constituting up to about 75% of the cases of autoimmune diseases. Although the diseases number up to 80, usually about 10 of them are the most preponderant diseases in the United States.

MAJOR AUTOIMMUNE DISEASES

Some well-known autoimmune diseases are as follows:

1. **Grave's disease:** This is a disease that affects the thyroid gland. It is a serious disease caused by a disorder of antibodies production or a disturbance in the cells of the immune system which become primed in such a way that they begin to react against thyroid secretions. The feedback effect of this is the enlargement of the thyroid gland.
2. **Rheumatoid arthritis:** This is a well-known disorder. It is an affliction in which immune complexes accumulate at the joints resulting in pain and stiffness.
3. **Hashimoto's thyroiditis:** This is another version of autoimmune disease affecting the thyroid gland. In this case, thyroid-stimulating antibodies are elaborated resulting in excessive thyroid stimulation.
4. **Type 1 diabetes:** This arises from a disturbance in glucose metabolism.
5. **Multiple Sclerosis (MS):** This is an affliction in which the myelin sheath covering the neuron is attacked by cytotoxic cells of the immune system. The attacked sheaths are usually coated by autoantibodies. The failure of the desired insulation for adequate transmission of electrical impulses is the cause of the observable symptoms in multiple sclerosis.
6. **Glomerulonephritis:** This is an impairment in renal function which arises from damage to the glomerulus. This is caused by the production of antibodies that attack the cells of the nephron and the glomerulus.

7. **Systemic lupus erythematosus:** It is a syndrome which has a lot of symptoms. It affects the liver, lungs, and kidneys. Antinuclear and antiphospholipid antibodies are produced and they attack the tissues of the whole body system.
8. **Sjorgen's Syndrome:** The lachrymal glands, the gland that secretes tears which help with lubrication of the eye, for some reason, have antibodies produced against them. As the disease progresses, you stop secreting tears and saliva.
9. **Idiopathic thrombocytopenic purpura:** This is a condition of disturbed platelet function which leaves some pinkish patches on the skin. The trigger of the disease is not well known but it is factual that as a result of reduced platelet count, there is the possibility of leaks of blood into the tissues from the blood vessels. The likelihood in idiopathic thrombocytopenic purpura is that there is production of antiplatelet antibodies which attack platelets.
10. **Myasthenia gravis:** In this condition, the neurotransmitter acetylcholine fails to perform its function at the neuromuscular junction, resulting in impaired function at such a junction. The impaired function of acetylcholine is not unconnected with the elaboration of antiacetylcholine antibodies which block acetylcholine receptors in the muscles.

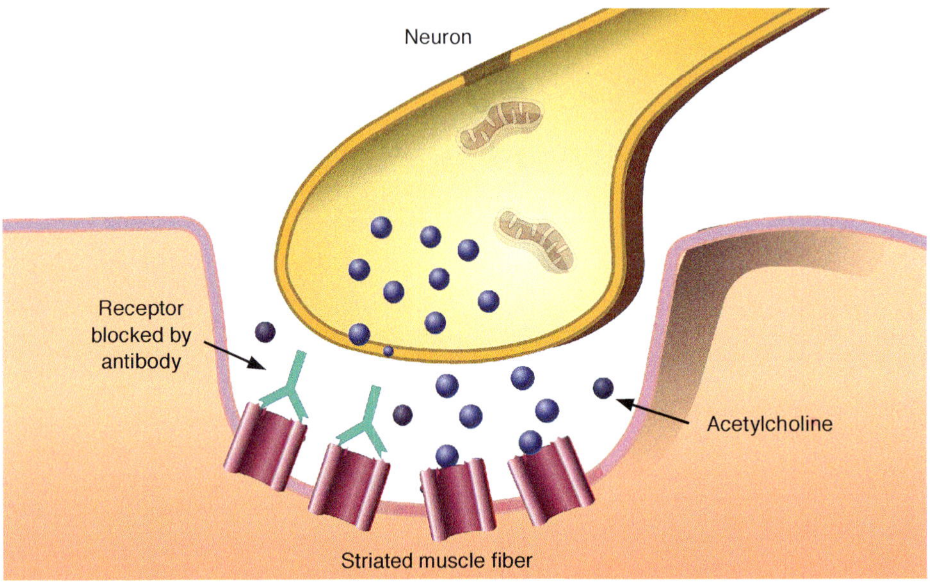

Courtesy of Zainab Ashkanani

Figure 13.1 *The pathogenesis of myasthenia gravis. Blockage of receptors on the motor endplate by autoantibodies reduces the number of receptors that are available to be stimulated by acetylcholine. Anticholinesterase drugs prevent acetylcholine destruction and so ensure that the remaining receptors are stimulated more effectively.*

The transmission of impulses at the neuromuscular junction is impaired in myasthenia gravis (Figure 13.1). In normal function, information is transmitted through this neuromuscular junction and delivered to the muscle in order to elicit a response from the muscle. This is mediated by the neurotransmitter called acetylcholine. In the circumstance of myasthenia gravis, antibodies to acetylcholine block the acetylcholine receptors in muscles resulting in an inadequacy in the acetylcholine availability. The principle of its therapy is to impair the degradation of acetylcholine by impairing the effect of acetylcholinesterase. The antibodies can be transmitted from the mother to the fetus.

AUTOIMMUNITY

GENERAL CONSIDERATIONS

- An immune response against one's own tissue due to breakdown of self-tolerance.
- It is not always bad, because some physiologic functions such as removal of effete (aged) RBCs is thought to take place by an autoimmune process.
- It is predominant in the western hemisphere (Europe and North America).
- It affects 5–7% of adult population worldwide.
- It is associated with diseases such as
  - **insulin-dependent diabetes**,
  - **psoriasis**,
  - **multiple sclerosis**,
  - **systemic lupus erythematosus**,
  - **rheumatoid arthritis**,
  - **thyroiditis**, and
  - **Hashimoto's disease**.

PRESENT UNDERSTANDING

- A small pool of B cells that react with self-antigens is always present in lymphoid tissues. They are extensively stimulated in disease.
- Stimulants are mitogens, for example, bacterial LPS.
- Antibodies produced are directed against autoantigens, for example, DNA, IgG, phospholipids, red cells, and lymphocytes.
  - It is the breakdown in the tightly regulated control mechanism for the activity of autoreactive B cells that results in autoimmunity.

PHYSIOLOGICAL ASPECTS

These aspects affect normal body functions.

- Regulating antibody response via production of anti-idiotypes. These anti-idiotypes produced cause a negative feedback effect, resulting in the termination of antibody production.
- Removal of aged cells: Old red blood cells usually lose their membrane glycoproteins.

Autoimmunity may, therefore, be defined as a condition in which the immune system attacks self-cells. This is by implication an immunological repudiation of a host cell system by the immune system that is supposed to protect it. Autoantibodies and activated T lymphocytes against host cells are the main culprits. The elicitation of autoantibodies is not supposed to be so strange because it is a normal physiological process to be able to destroy a part of self-cell system that is not needed. An immune response against one's own tissue can happen due to a breakdown in self-tolerance. The need to remove one's own cells may be useful. For instance, it is needed for the following;

a. The removal of aged cells. Failure of the removal of red cells may result in polycythemia. Old red blood cells (those that have existed for 90–120 days) usually lose their membrane glycoproteins. When a glycoprotein is worn out to as much as band 3, a new epitope is exposed, and there is elicitation of an immune response and the proliferation of low-grade IgG. The titer is so low, but they do have high affinity for complement component C3. This elaborated antibody reacts with the new epitopes and activates complement. RBC is lysed and cleared from the system via the bilirubin metabolism in the liver.

b. Regulating the antibody response through production of anti-idiotypes. This regulation of antibody response involving the production of anti-idiotypes causes a negative feedback effect, resulting in termination of antibody production. Another physiologic fact is the collection of a small pool of self-reactive B cells that are inactive and which exist normally; they are present in lymphoid tissues, and somehow they have escaped clonal deletion and anergy. They don't cause any problem ordinarily, but they are extensively stimulated during the disease and for such reason, these hitherto quiescent cells begin to expand in population rapidly and bring about autoimmune conditions. The mitogens that stimulate the small pool of B cells are viral proteins, bacterial lipopolysaccharides, and other unique complexes. The antibodies produced are against self-antigens and they can be against self-DNA, immunoglobulins, and phospholipids.

Some important factors such as (i) genetic factors and (ii) environmental factors play a role in autoimmunity. The genetic and the environmental factors may be interrelated in a manner that the environment may select the expression of the genetic factor. In this case, the problem may be expressed only in the appropriate environment.

INDUCTION OF AUTOIMMUNITY

- Exposure of hidden antigen, for example, in the brain or testes.
- Formation of new epitopes, for example, rheumatoid factor, immunoconglutinins (IKs), etc.
- Cross-reactivity with microorganisms (molecular mimicry)
- Loss of control of lymphocyte response.
- Viral-induced autoimmunity.
- Genetic factors.
- Hormonal factors.

EXPOSURE OF HIDDEN EPITOPE OR ANTIGEN

An example of this is when the wearing out of the basement membrane of erythrocyte protein occurs, exposing the band 3. Also, there is a collection of cells that are kept a little outside the regular body structure, for example, the testes are kept away from the body in the scrotal sac, and the brain within the skull is hidden from the immune system; these appear as if they were almost immunologically inert. If for some reason they become exposed to the immune system, antibodies will be produced and they will no longer be hidden. Also, in circumstances of infection, the surfaces of cells are worn out and a new surface is exposed which triggers an immune reaction. The example of the exposure of a new epitope is evident in rheumatoid factor development and immunoconglutinin (IK) formation.

CROSS-REACTIVITY WITH MICROORGANISMS

- Mimicry of host epitopes by parasitic invaders could cause attack of host cells by eliciting an immune response. For example,
  - in *Trypanosoma cruzi*, the antibodies destroy neuronal cells and cardiac muscle cells.
  - in group A streptococci, the antibodies to cell wall proteins, M-proteins, destroy cardiac muscles and glomeruli cells, depending on the strain.

- in case of Epstein-Bar virus, the antibodies to DNA polymerase react with myelin basic protein (multiple sclerosis).
- polio capsid protein antibodies react with acetylcholine receptor—causing myasthenia gravis.

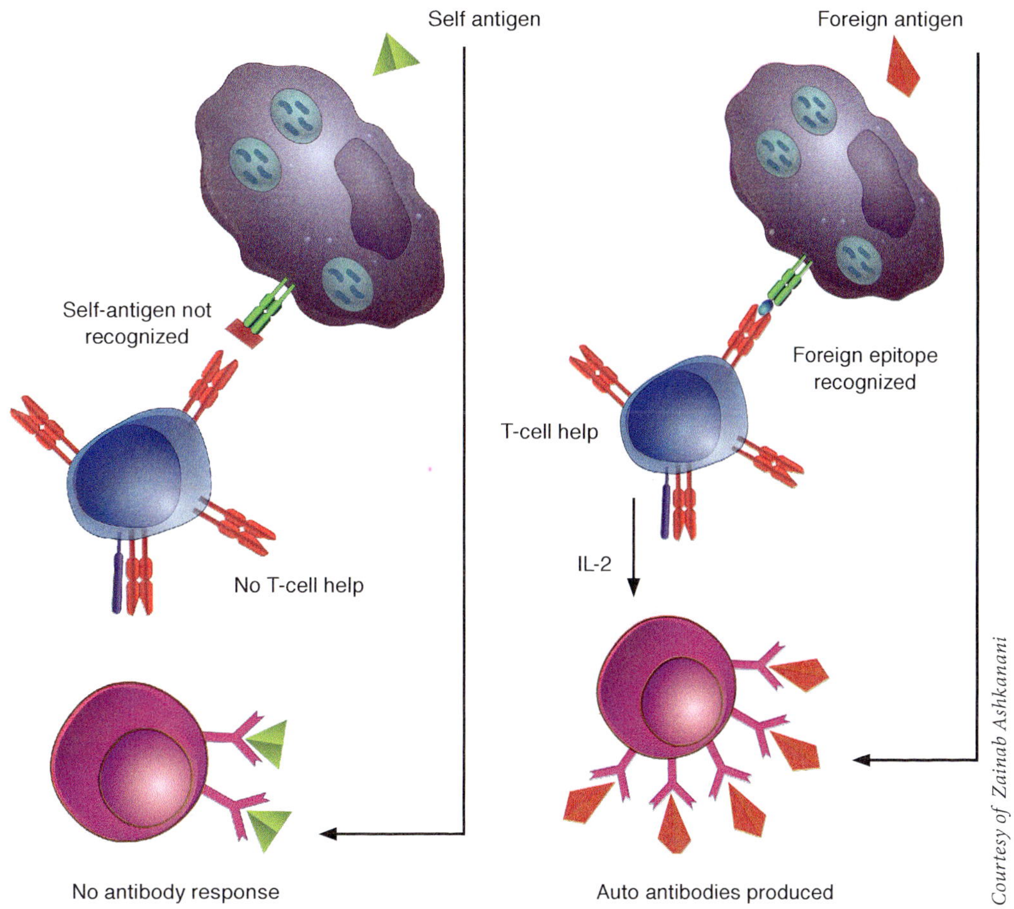

Figure 13.2 *The way in which molecular mimicry antigens may initiate an autoimmune response.*

This is an important factor that will trigger autoimmunity by generating the phenomenon of molecular mimicry (molecular imitation) (Figure 13.2). In this circumstance, the infectious agent acquires a biomolecular component that resembles the one found in the host cells. An immune response against the biomolecular agent is effective against the host cell. Mimicry of host epitopes by parasitic invaders could cause attack of host cells by eliciting an immune response. Some examples include the following;

a. *Trypanosoma cruzi*, a group of trypanosomes that are found in the southern part of North America, including California and Texas, but a lot more in Mexico and South and Central America. This is transmitted by a bug called the reduviid bug. A blood meal by the bug is accompanied by defecation and the fecal material of the bug contains the infective form of the parasite. *T. cruzi* has biomolecular contents that resemble the contents of neuronal and cardiac cells. Therefore, antibodies elaborated against *T. cruzi* will also attack cells of the neuron and heart. That is why they are implicated in cardiovascular disorders and psychiatric ailments.

b. Group A streptococcus. An infection by group A streptococcus results in the elaboration of antibodies to the cell wall protein M which can attack and destroy cardiac muscles and the glomerulus.

c. Epstein-Barr virus. An infection which leads to the elaboration of antibodies to DNA polymerase. These antibodies react with myelin basic protein, an event that has been implicated in the development of multiple sclerosis.

d. Polio capsid protein, to which antibodies could be developed during polio infection. The antibodies react with the acetylcholine receptor and may result in those conditions described in the autoimmune disease called myasthenia gravis. The counterargument is that it is not all cases of polio infection or exposure that leads to myasthenia gravis, thus the mimicry may not be characteristic of all polio strains.

LOSS OF CONTROL OF LYMPHOCYTE RESPONSES

- In responding to antigen stimulation, the host produces some self-antibodies (very few, detected by antiglobulin test) which are rapidly suppressed and cleared. If suppression mechanism fails, destruction results.
- Lymphoid tumor causes autoimmune disease because of control failure
  - Development of forbidden clones of cells
  - Defect in protein responsible for death signal-Fas protein (because of mutation in fas gene). This creates a situation where negative selection of self-reactive cells is impossible.

VIRUSES AS INDUCERS OF AUTOIMMUNITY

- There is interference with immunological control mechanisms due to infection by type C retrovirus or paramyxovirus. Autoantibodies developed are associated with SLE of dog and humans. Also, in cases of polyendocrine disease characterized by diabetes mellitus, retarded growth, etc., antibodies developed are against normal pituitary, growth hormone, pancreas, gastric mucosa, glucagon, and insulin. It is associated with coxsackievirus infection.

There is a tightly in-built control for the response of lymphocytes, so a loss of such control can generate enormous problems. In responding to antigen stimulation, the host produces some self-antibodies, albeit few and they are detectable by antiglobulin test if they coat cells, otherwise they can be detected by indirect antiglobulin test. In the later case, the antibodies are detected by adsorbing them on to appropriate red cells and demonstrating the adhered antibodies with antiglobulin. Simply, it is a situation in which antibodies are used to detect antibodies; the only need is that the antibodies to be detected must be adsorbed on to an organized cell surface (red blood cells) or an organized crystal surface (polyacrylamide beads).

Another way in which a defect in lymphocyte selection can occur is in the protein responsible for death signal (apoptosis process)—the Fas protein. This could arise from the mutation in the Fas gene. So, to clear cells by apoptosis, there is the need for proper Fas protein that is not a variant. If a variant is produced due to mutation, it is ineffective and does not bring about apoptosis. This creates a situation where negative selection of self-reactive cells is impossible, creating room for autoimmunity.

GENETIC FACTORS AND AUTOIMMUNITY

- In Hashimoto's disease, antithyroid antibodies have been described in the blood of relatives.
- Identical twins exhibit a 30% chance of disease developing in the second twin if one has it.
- Genes responsible are associated with MHC classes I and II (they exhibit selective binding). In MHC assembly, transporter genes are defective (causing abnormal protein assembly).

This is a sole defining factor of susceptibility arising from genetic variation. The explicit evidence of the involvement of genetic factor in autoimmune disease is Hashimoto's disease. In this case, it is possible to demonstrate antithyroid antibodies in the blood of relatives, which is the indication of the possible role for a familial factor and therefore it is genetic. In the case of identical twins, where one of them has problems with Hashimoto's disease, data shows that there is a 30% chance that the other twin will develop the disease. Also, the genes responsible for the MHC classes I and II that are associated with this disease have been described, as they exhibit selective binding in the assembly of MHC itself. Also, the transporter genes are defective which will cause abnormal protein assembly in the endoplasmic reticulum. The T-cell receptor genes are also defective, which gives rise to autoreactive T cells. Immunoglobulin genes have been described that are defective. Defect in immunoglobulin genes have been associated with mutation. Complement genes have been described that are defective, and when this happens there is impairment in the clearance of immunoconglutinins; this has to do with antibodies against complement clearance.

HORMONAL FACTORS

- Autoimmune diseases are more in women than in men. They also exhibit a more severe course in women.
- A probable explanation is that estrogen stimulates the enhancer elements for IFN-γ genes.

HOW COMPLEMENT MEDIATION OF IMMUNE REGULATION CAN CONTRIBUTE?

- B-cells have CR1, which binds C3b and blocks B-cell differentiation. A failure results in disease.
- C3a is immunosuppressive; it blocks helper T-cell activity and NK cell activity. When this fails, then there is overactivity of helper T cells and NK cells, which will cause a problem with autoimmunity. Failure results in disease.
- C5a stimulates T- and B-cell responses by enhancing IL-1 production by macrophages. Failure results in failure of T-and B-cell responses, subsequently leading to a disease.

Factors involved in autoimmune diseases are shown in Figure 13.3.

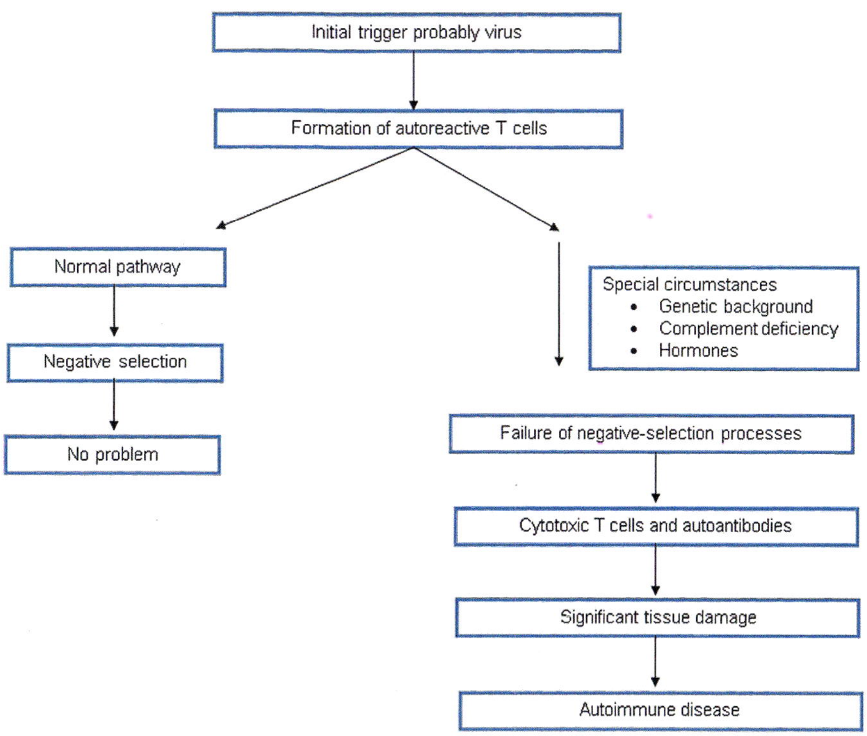

Figure 13.3 *Some of the factors that influence the development of an autoimmune disease.*

Some of the factors that influence the development of an autoimmune disease

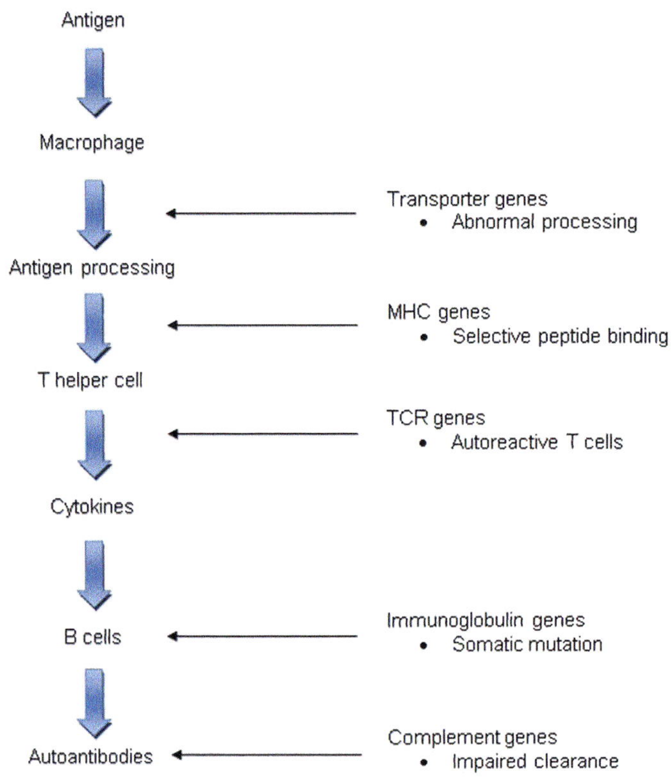

Figure 13.4 *Some of the possible ways in which genes may directly influence the development of autoimmune diseases.*

There is always an initial trigger, such as a virus in the initiation of the process as commonly narrated by the patient. Then, there is the formation of autoreactive T cells.

It is also possible to have a variant pathway in which an antigen is taken up by a macrophage, it is processed, and finally leads to autoantibody production. This generation of autoantibodies may be due to defective transporter genes, such as tapasin, or in antigen processing itself. You can have MHC genes being faulty and exhibiting selective peptide binding. There can also be problems with T cell receptor genes resulting in production of auto-reactive T cells (Figure 13.4).

The mechanism of autoimmune disease development is based on the understanding that it is a chronic inflammatory process which is hypersensitivity itself. So, they are characterized according to hypersensitivity type.

MECHANISMS OF TISSUE DAMAGE IN AUTOIMMUNITY

- Type I hypersensitivity: Development of α-casein IgE autoantibodies in unmilked cow. This becomes an unusual protein at the extra mammary areas. Thus it will cause acute anaphylaxis (binds to mast cells).
- Type II hypersensitivity (IgG, IgM, and complement mediated): This involves autoantibodies directed against cell surface antigens, thus causing lysis with the assistance of complement or cytotoxic cells.

	TYPE I	TYPE II	
Immune reactant	IgE	IgG	
Antigen	Soluble antigen	Cell- or matrix-associated antigen	Cell-surface receptor
Effector mechanism	Mast-cell activation	Complement, FcR$^+$ cells (Phagocytes, NK cells)	Antibody alters signaling
Example of hypersensitivity reaction	Allergic rhinitis, asthma, systemic anaphylaxis	Some drug allergies (e.g. penicillin)	Chronic urticaria (antibody to fce RIα)

	TYPE II	TYPE IV		
Immune reactant	IgG	T_H1 cells	T_H2 cells	CTL
Antigen	Soluble antigen	Soluble antigen	Soluble antigen	Cell-associated antigen
Effector mechanism	Complement phagocytes	Macrophage activation	Eosinophil activation	Cytotoxicity
Example of hypersensitivity reaction	Serum sickness, arthus reaction	Contact dermatitis, tuberculin reaction	Chronic asthma chronic allergic rhinitis	Contact dermatitis

Table 13.1 *There are four types of hypersensitivity reactions, mediated by different types of Abs. Type I is the most common, and the immune reactant is IgE.*

Type I hypersensitivity is IgE mediated. This involves the "hidden epitopes" and some parts of the body are "hidden" away as they are not exposed to regular circulation, such as the brain and the testes. Another example that is suitable here is the mammary gland. The protein of the breast milk is casein. In an event of the blockage of the drains in the mammary gland, casein flows back into the system and anticasein antibodies are developed, which then attack self-cells. This is a feature of common occurrence in unmilked cows. The efflux of α-casein into the system results in an unusual protein in the extramammary area. This itself will cause reactions that will lead to acute anaphylaxis because IgE binds to mast cells, resulting in mast cell degranulation (Figure 13.5). This consequently leads to the release of histamine. It is this histamine release that causes the acute anaphylaxis.

The activation of mast cells and the release of granules will have the following physiological effects:

- One of it is on the gastrointestinal tract, there will be increased fluid secretion, which will consequently increase the movement of the tract (peristalsis). This leads to the expulsion of intestinal tract contents because of intestinal hurrying, thereby causing diarrhea and vomiting.
- If histamine enters the airways, which it will do, it would decrease the diameter of the airways and increase mucus secretion, which leads to expulsion of airway contents.
- In the blood vessels, it increases blood flow and permeability, which leads to edema and inflammation, and increased lymph flow which carries the antigen to the lymph nodes (Figure 13.6).

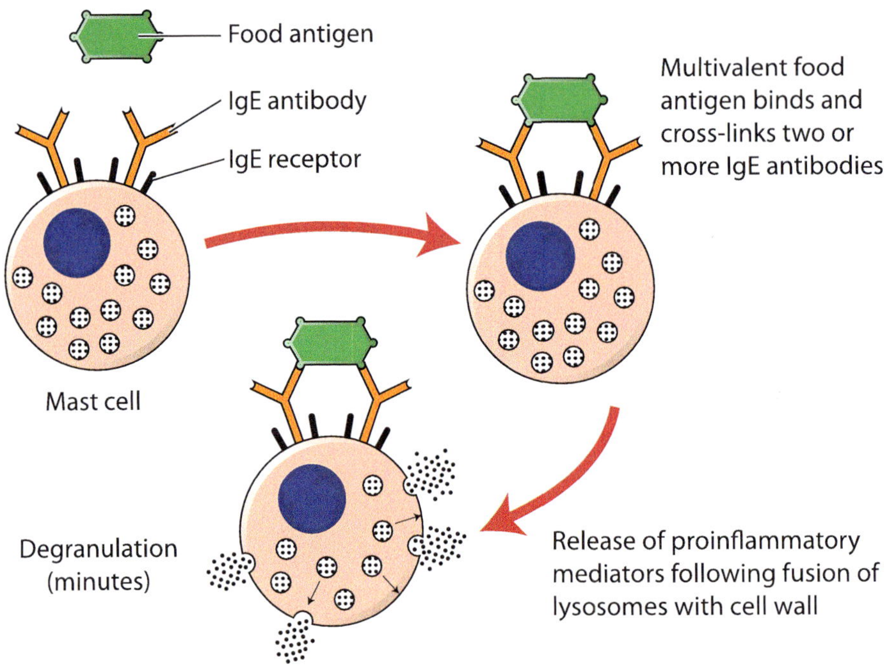

Figure 13.5 *Degranulation of mast cells is the mediator of Type I hypersensitivity reaction, and it occurs by cross-linking of the FcRI receptor on the surface of mast cells by both antigen and IgE.*

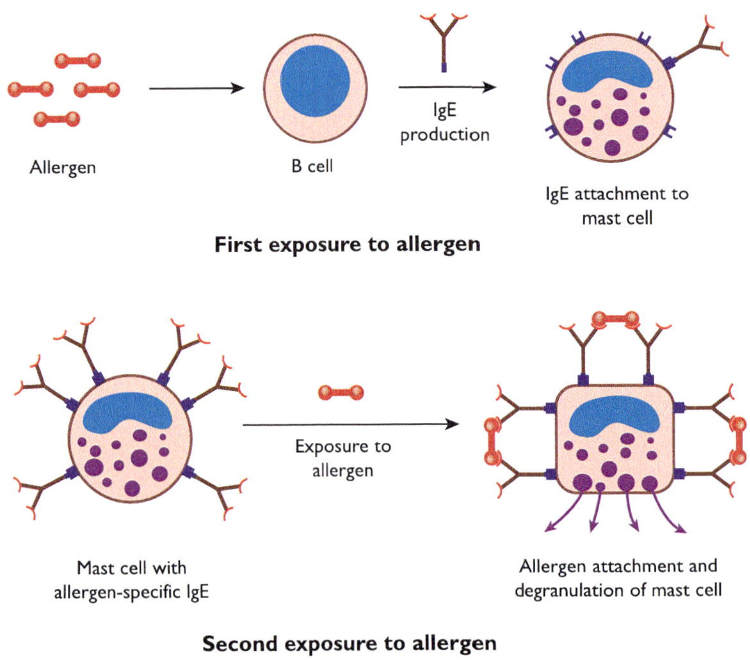

Figure 13.6 *Physical effects of IgE-mediated mast cell degranulation on selected tissues.*

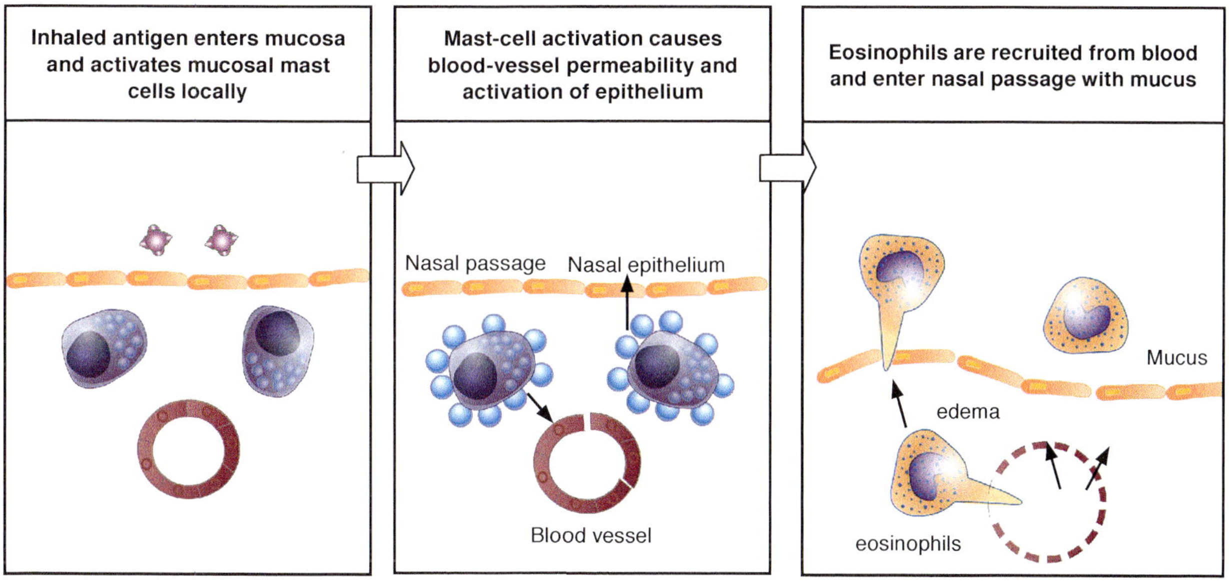

Courtesy of Zainab Ashkanani

Figure 13.7 *Allergic rhinitis is caused by allergens entering the respiratory tract. Histamine and other mediators released by activated mast cells increase the permeability of local capillaries and activate nasal epithelium to produce mucus. Eosinophils attracted into the tissues from the blood become activated and release their inflammatory mediators. Activated eosinophils are shed into the nasal passages.*

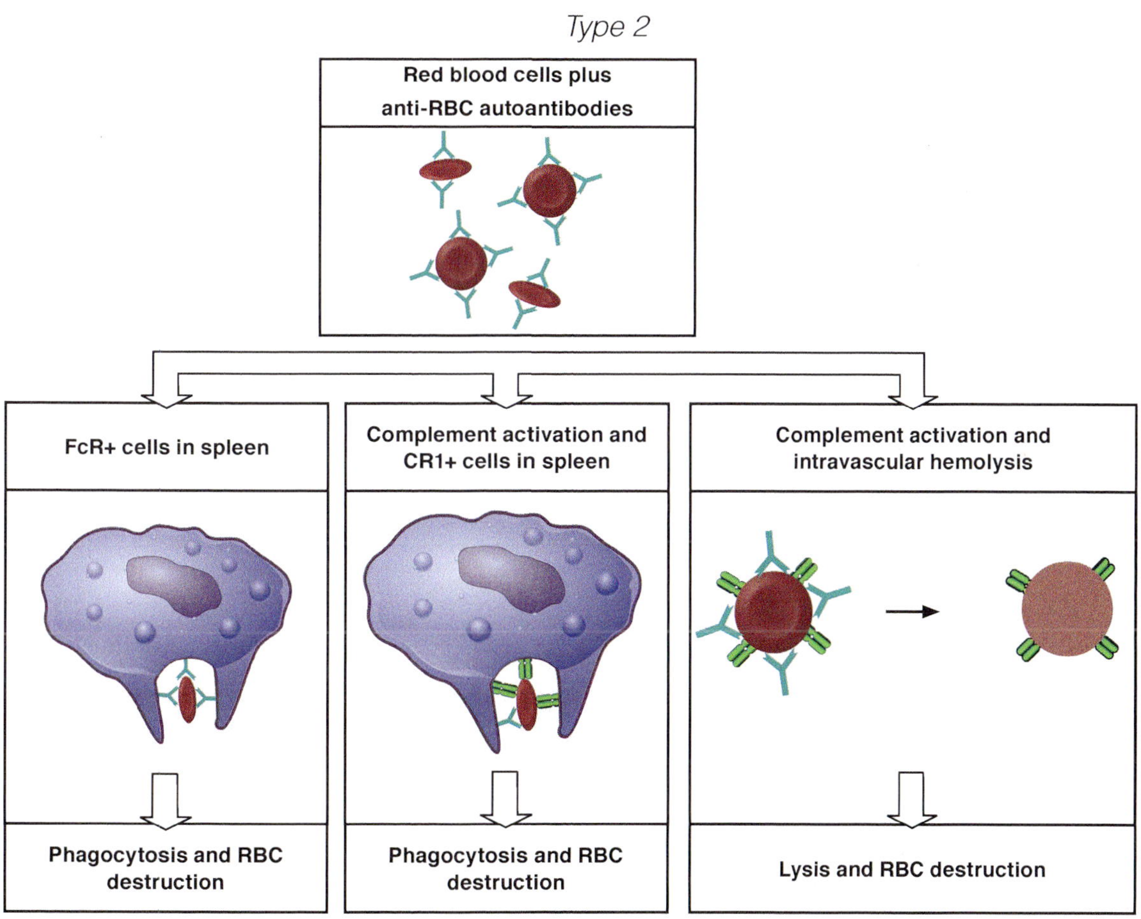

Courtesy of Zainab Ashkanani

Figure 13.8 *Autoimmune hemolytic anemia destroys self red blood cells. Three mechanisms how this occurs are shown.*

Also, an allergic reaction such as allergic rhinitis caused by antigens entering the respiratory tract, cause the release of histamine and other mediators which increase the permeability of local capillaries and activate the nasal epithelium to produce mucus (Figure 13.7). This is one part of the whole reaction, but there is an ameliorating remission follow-up, which has to do with eosinophils, because they also have IgE receptors. Eosinophils are drafted to the site and they bind to IgE too. They then start producing antihistamine agents, such as histaminase which opens up the air passage and reverses the whole process.

Type 2 is IgG, IgM, and complement mediated. It involves autoantibodies directed against cell surface antigens. This results in lysis with the assistance of complement or cytotoxic cells (Figure 13.8).

An example for type 2 is the reaction of red cells with antibodies against red cell proteins; these antibodies against red cell antibodies are autoantibodies. The cells are filtered in the spleen where they are engulfed and destroyed by macrophages. It could also happen that complement is activated and the destruction also takes place in the spleen. But when this occurs, the intravascular hemolysis will produce excessive hemoglobin which will destroy the sieve of the kidney.

- **Type III hypersensitivity**: Autoantibodies bind to free antigens, forming immune complexes which can induce type III hypersensitivity autoimmunity, for example, SLE and rheumatoid arthritis.
- **Type IV hypersensitivity** (lymphokine mediated): This involves mononuclear cells and autosensitized T cells. Examples include autoimmune thyroiditis, ulcerative colitis, and allergic encephalitis.

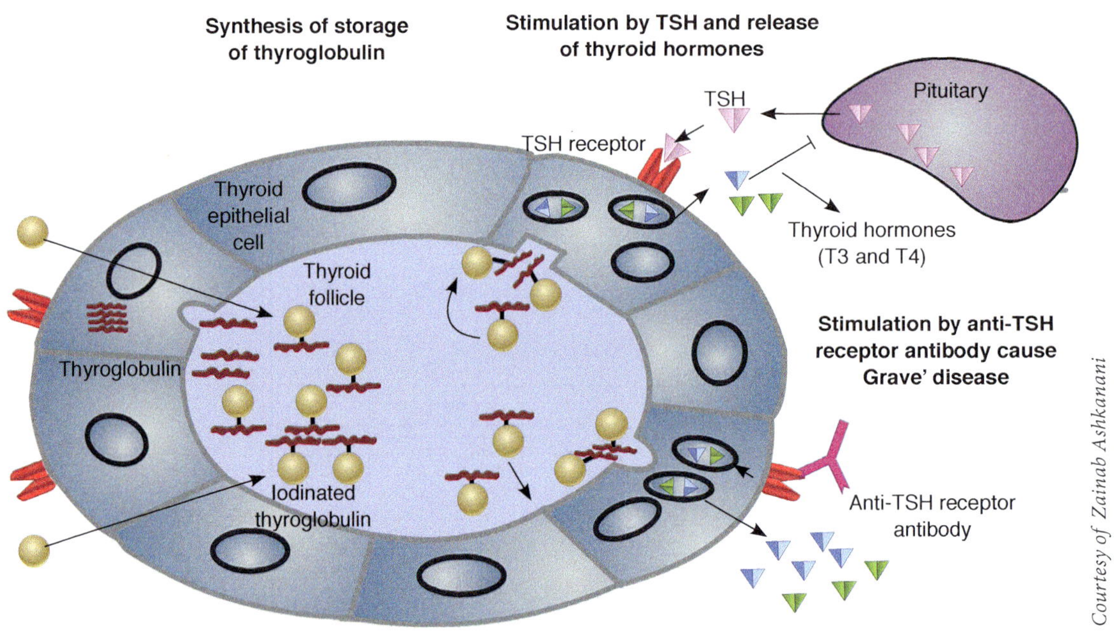

Figure 13.9 *Autoantibodies against TSH receptor cause overproduction of thyroid hormones in Graves' disease.*

In Figure 13.9, the synthesis and storage of thyroglobulin is illustrated. It shows that antibodies against thyroid stimulating hormone (TSH) are excessively produced and it is implicated in Graves's disease. These anti-TSH antibodies cause excessive stimulation of the thyroid gland, making a burst in secretions.

- **In Graves' disease, thyroid stimulating immunoglobulins (TSI)**, a form of IgG, can bind to thyrotropin (TSH) receptors on the thyroid gland. TSIs mimic the action of TSH, causing excess secretion of thyroxine (T4) and triiodothyronine (T3).

- The TSI level is abnormally high in persons with hyperthyroidism due to Graves' disease because its production is not regulated.
- **In Hashimoto's thyroiditis**, there is intense infiltration of the thyroid gland by lymphocytes, macrophages, and plasma cells. The accompanying inflammation causes goiter.
- Also, antibodies to a number of thyroid proteins (thyroglobulin and thyroid peroxidase) involved in the uptake of iodine interfere with the protein activities, thus blocking iodine uptake and leading to a decrease in thyroid hormone production (hypothyroidism). This results in increased TSH production by the pituitary, which causes goiter.

There are three ways in which autoimmune reactions may attack the thyroid gland to produce very dissimilar clinical results (Figure 13.10).

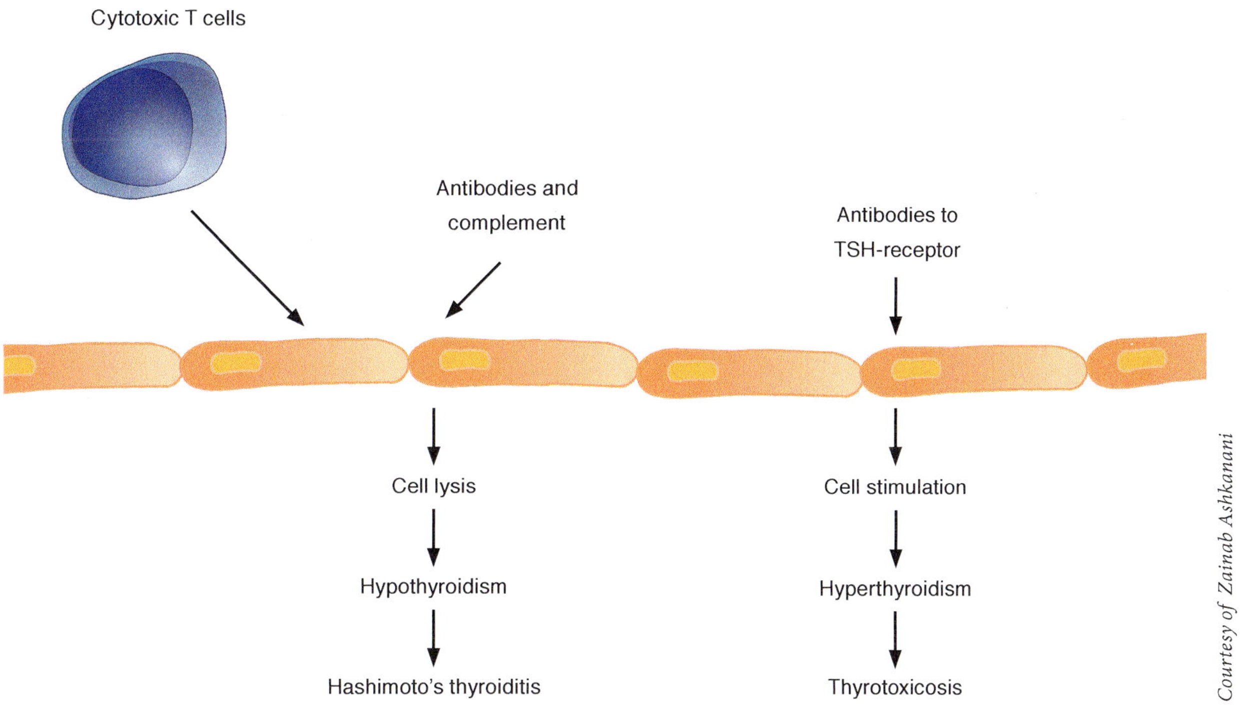

Figure 13.10 *Three ways in which autoimmune reactions may attack the thyroid gland to produce very dissimilar clinical results.*

One way is the cytotoxic T cell attack of the thyroid cells resulting in the destruction of the thyroid and consequent hypoactivity, causing hypothyroidism which is designated as Hashimoto's thyroiditis. This is a type 4 hypersensitivity and there is inflammation of the thyroid. Another way in which the thyroid is affected by autoimmunity is by complement and antibody-mediated activity. This is a type 2 hypersensitivity. An example is the case of TSH receptor antibodies; when these antibodies bind to the TSH receptors, the thyroid gland is stimulated to produce more thyroid hormones causing high hormone levels, which invariably leads to a decrease in TSH levels. Yet the thyroid is still being stimulated by these antibodies that bind the TSH receptor.

MULTIPLE SCLEROSIS

This is an autoimmune disease that afflicts the central nervous system. It is characterized by the destruction of the myelin sheath of neuronal cells of the white matter. This results in the development of neurological symptoms. B and T cells are implicated in this, thus it involves autoantibody activity, cytotoxic T cell activities, and, of course, macrophages.

- An autoimmune disease of the central nervous system.
- Characterized by the destruction of the myelin sheath of neuronal cells in the white matter of the central nervous system.
- Patients develop neurological symptoms.
- B and T cells are implicated, although macrophages are among early infiltrates.
- The resemblance of amino acid sequence in myelin basic protein to the sequence in proteins from adenovirus 2, EBV, hepatitis B virus is also a factor for autoimmunity.
- The disease depends on antigen presentation by MHC molecules.
- T cells recognize an appropriately presented Ag.
- The cytokines activate macrophages, especially microglia, which destroys the myelin on neurons.

In this condition, some viruses are known to have capsid proteins that have resemblance of the amino acid sequence in basic myelin protein; this is the protein of the myelin sheath. The viruses mostly studied in this regard include adenovirus type 2, Epstein-Barr virus, and hepatitis B virus. So, the disease depends on antigen presentation by MHC molecules. Therefore, an individual with HLA-DR2 will be five times more likely to develop the disease than those that lack the receptor. This implies that genetic factor is an additional factor. T cells recognize an appropriately presented antigen, exert a direct cytotoxic effect on the nerve axon, and secrete inflammatory cytokines such as lymphotoxin, TNF-α, and IFN-γ. The cytokines activate macrophages, especially microglia of the CNS, which then mount an attack on neurons.

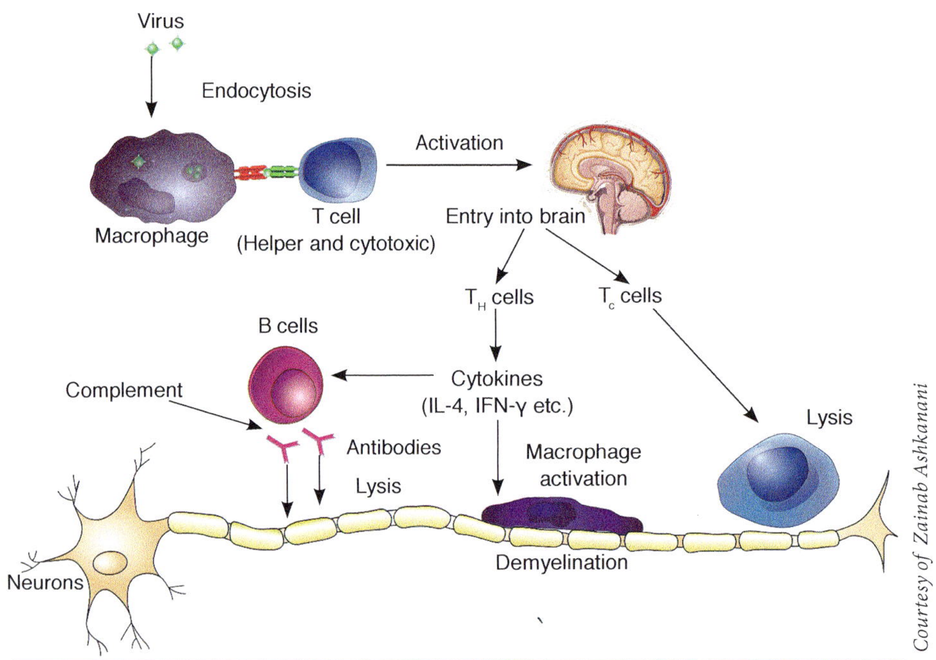

Figure 13.11 *The probable pathogenesis of multiple sclerosis. Infection with a virus of unknown type triggers an immune response against the myelin in an axon sheath. As a result, the myelin is stripped from the axon*

In Figure 13.11, the virus is an important trigger, so microglial cells engulf them and present them to T cells. T cells recognize them and release a profile of cytokines, some of them will make a population of these T cells (that are helper and cytotoxic T cells) to migrate to the site. B cells are drafted to the site, so the activity of macrophage is thought to be a little bit earlier. Activated T cells start exerting their effects on brain cells and then antibodies are produced, which include IgG or IgM antibodies that are complement-activating. These result in the degradation of the neuron covering the myelin sheath. This loss of myelin is termed demyelination. It is thought to be associated with an impairment of the electrical transmission and transductional process which is supposed to be protected by the insulation provided by the myelin sheath. There is leakage of electrical transmission from this insulation.

SYSTEMIC LUPUS ERYTHROMATOSUS

It is erythematosus because of the rash on the skin, or erythema.

- Described in human, mice, dogs, and cats. About 90% of cases found in women.
- Loss of control of B cells resulting in the production of more IL-6.
- Autoantibodies combine with free DNA to form DNA–anti-DNA complexes, deposited in the glomeruli, causing glomerulonephritis.
- Autoantibodies to RBCs are developed in some cases of SLE causing antiglobulin-positive hemolytic anemia
- In primates, immune complexes containing C3b bind to erythrocyte CR1. In nonprimates, platelets bind immune complexes and may thus remove them from the circulation (Figure 13.12).

Women are the most afflicted. There is the loss of control of B cells resulting in production of more IL-6 which activates B cells in an autocrine fashion. This loss of control results in the development of autoantibodies against a wide range of antigens. The evidence so far is that the antibodies are only against housekeeping proteins present in every cell. The autoantibodies combine with free DNA to form DNA–anti-DNA complexes which may be toxic to the glomerulus when deposited there, resulting in glomerulonephritis. Autoantibodies to RBCs are developed in some cases of SLE. The antibodies can be detected by the antiglobulin test. Antiglobulins are antibodies against other antibodies, so we use them to screen for antibodies. If cells *in vivo* are already coated, the antiglobulin will react with the antibodies that are already coating the cell. If they were not coated *in vivo*, then antibodies can be used to coat appropriate cells or polyacrylamide beads *in vitro* and the antibodies are made observable by antiglobulin. In primates, immune complexes containing the complement component C3b bind to erythrocyte CR1, the coated erythrocytes bind to the Kupffer cells of the liver, where they are phagocytosed. The immune complexes may also dissociate from the red cells, permitting the cells to reenter the circulation while the complexes are endocytosed, or swallowed up. In nonprimates, platelets bind immune complexes and may thus remove them from the circulation. The factors that affect systemic lupus erythematosus pathogenesis include infection with herpes virus, failure of B-cell apoptosis, genetic background issue, and estrogen (Figure 13.13).

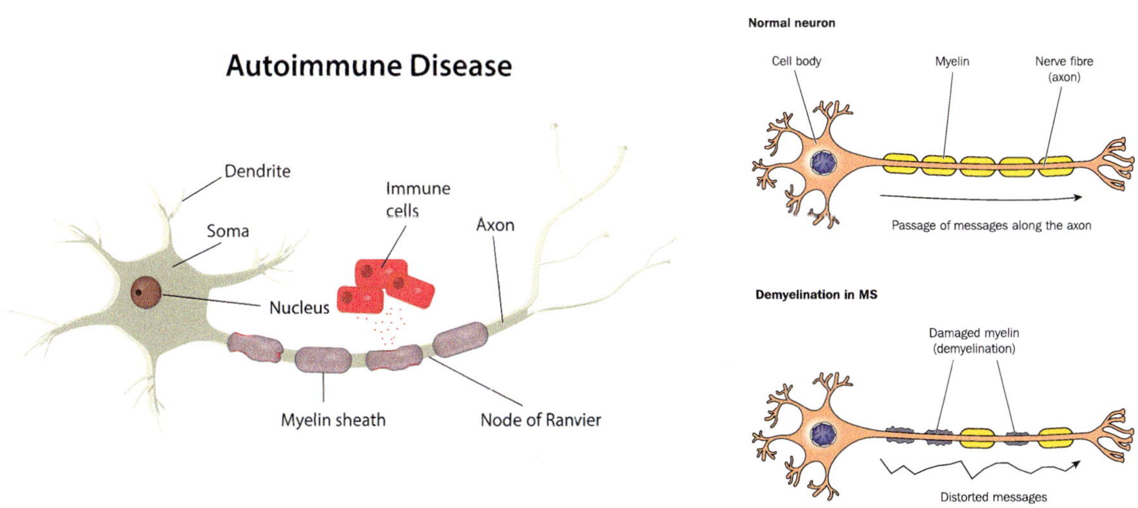

Figure 13.12 *Removal of immune complexes from the circulation.*

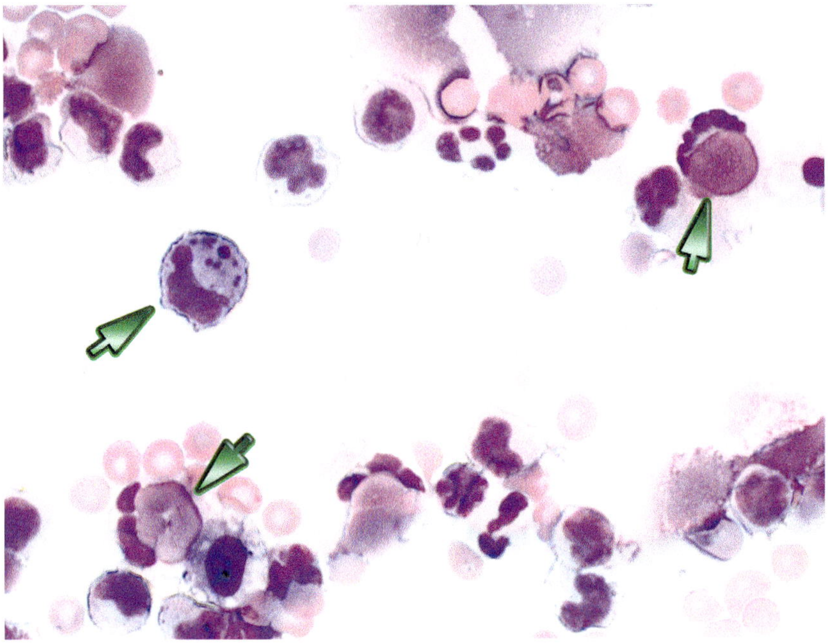

Figure 13.13 *Some of the factors that influence the pathogenesis of SLE.*

The organs, tissues and cells commonly afflicted include thyroid, myocardium, platelets and red cells. The autoantibodies are commonly against the nucleus, or DNA, and phospholipids.

SAMPLE QUESTIONS

AUTOIMMUNITY

Answer True or False to the following:

Induction of autoimmunity

1. A pool of auto reactive T and B cells is present in all individuals.
2. Cross-reactive epitopes from infection agents can lead to activation of autoreactive T and B cells.
3. Molecular mimicry is always antibody mediated.
4. A loss of mechanism responsible for up-regulating immune cell activation can lead to autoimmunity.

Factors affecting autoimmunity

5. Autoimmunity has not been shown to have a genetic component.
6. Women are generally more anti-inflammatory than men.
7. It is believed that estrogen plays a large role in autoimmunity.
8. Autoimmunity usually onsets before puberty.

Autoimmune thyroid disease

9. Hashimoto's thyroiditis is a hyperthyroid condition.
10. Grave's disease involves the formation of antibodies to follicle stimulating hormone.
11. Autoimmune thyroiditis is an example of type IV hypersensitivity.
12. Grave's disease is a hypothyroid condition.

Multiple sclerosis

13. MS is an inflammatory demyelinating disease of the central nervous system.
14. Damage occurs on the nerve soma.
15. Clinical signs and symptoms depend on the location and size of plaques.

Suggested Laboratory Practicals

- Case Studies on:

1. General Mechanisms Involved in the Onset of Autoimmunity
2. Classification of Autoimmunity on the Basis of Immunotypes

- Rheumatoid Factor (RF) Detection and Assay
- Rapid Test for the Detection of Antinucleoproteins found in Systemic Lupus Erythematosus
- Platelets Count for Throbocytopenia

CHAPTER 14

IMMUNITY TO INFECTIONS

This chapter deals with how the body protects itself against infections. Some of the earliest recognized aspects of immunity are based on the observations that those who recovered from infectious diseases did not succumb to subsequent infections. It was for this reason that the concept of "exemption" emerged. The susceptibility to infection is influenced by immunological and nonimmunological factors.

Resistance to infection is influenced by many factors and can be studied under the following classes:

Nonimmunological factors:

- Hormonal: estradiol, affects multiple sclerosis and ↓IL-2 receptor.
- Nutritional status: implicated in TB.
- Genetic background: wiping out of susceptible hosts.

Immunological factors:

- Immunity to bacteria involves
  - antibodies,
  - complements, and
  - activated macrophages.
- Immunity to viruses involves
  - neutralization (neutralizing antibodies),
  - complement,
  - cytolysis (cytotoxic T cells), and
  - ADCC (antibody-dependent cellular cytotoxicity)—cytotoxic process mediated by effector cells which recognize Abs on plasma membrane.
- Immunity to protozoa involves
  - antibody complement in blood and
  - cytotoxic T cell action and macrophage activation in tissue.
- Immunity to helminthes involves
  - IgE, mast cells, and eosinophils degranulation at the site of worm infection.

- Problems involve
  - hypersensitivity
  - evading of immune response by challengers.

NONIMMUNOLOGICAL FORMS OF PROTECTION

- Resistance due to specie insusceptibility: *Neisseria gonorrhea* grows well only in humans, while *Corynebacteriumdiphtheriae* causes disease in humans and guinea pigs, but not in rats.
- Genetic factors: Since infectious diseases tend to wipe out susceptible hosts, a resistant population is left to multiply. Thus, a genetic resistant group prevails.
- Age: The very young and very old are vulnerable to infection. For example, rubella can destroy the fetus during the first trimester of pregnancy without affecting the mother.
- Nutrition: Malnutrition such as protein energy deficiency may impair immunoglobulin production.

Nonimmunological forms of protection are as important as the immunological forms because they serve as backup protection. An important means of protection that may be unrelated to the cells of the immune system is the lack of susceptibility to an infectious agent by a host because of specie barrier. Infectious agents tend to colonize a specie and find it difficult to cross specie barrier. This may be a form of protection for the host out of the vulnerable species. For instance, *N. gonorrhoea* grows well only in humans while *Corynebacterium diptheriae* causes disease in humans and guinea pigs, but not in rats. This is a steep infection barrier and it affords protection for excluded species. Also, in the case of Lassa virus infection, the bush rat, *Rattus fuscipes*, is only a reservoir host in which the virus multiplies without causing any disease, while it causes a very lethal disease in humans. The benefit of specie barrier for the humans is in the fact that bird virus infections such as the lethal Newcastle disease and the Gumboro virus (infectious bursal disease) infections do not infect humans. It is for this important protection based on specie difference that concerns are expressed when infectious agents are able to cross specie barrier through recombination as in the case of avian and swine flu viruses. Such challenges open the immune system to an enormous burden to which it can succumb.

Age. This is a very important factor. The most vulnerable to infections are the very young and the old. Those who are at the prime of their life (25–45 years) have the advantage of being able to mount an adequate immune response to challenges. It is important to note that sometimes such response may be very severe and may produce adverse effects as in the case of severe hemorrhagic fever following response to infection with hemorrhagic fever viruses. The problem in this case is that there is heightened immune reaction which accounts for the symptoms.

Hormonal. One of the prominent nonimmunological factors is hormones. It is now known that the hormone estrogen affects cytokine signaling. It has effect on IL-2 receptors, which are usually found on T and B cells. And since the interaction between IL-2 and its receptor has effect on clonal expansion of T and B cells, it then means that estrogen has effect on the expansion of T and B cells.

Nutritional status. The nutritional status is another example of a factor that affects infection control. The extent to which the affliction with *Mycobacterium tuberculosis* is able to thrive has been found to be closely associated with the nutritional status of an individual. Protein energy malnutrition causes animmunocompromise because immunoglobulin production is impaired. Malnutrition will allow infections of opportunity to establish themselves in the host.

Genetic background. Some individuals are more genetically prone to infections than others. The tendency is that those who are able to survive infections in an infection endemic area are the resistant group and are able to pass on this character to their offspring, thus a genetically resistant group is generated over time. They become more capable of withstanding such familiar challenges. Thus, there emerges the concept of genetic variation and susceptibility.

NONSPECIFIC IMMUNITY TO BACTERIA INFECTIONS

- Lysozyme:
  - These are biomolecular contents of the subcellular organelle called lysosome.
  - They are part and parcel of the innate immune system and are an essential feature of the professional phagocytes. For instance, neuraminidase as a part of the lysozyme is found in tissues and body fluids (except cerebrospinal fluid, sweat, and urine) and is capable of splitting the cell wall of proteoglycans of some grampositive bacteria.
  - It also kills some gram negative organisms in conjunction with complement.
  - Lysozyme is abundant in neutrophils and is released into the body fluid when neutrophils die.
  - It acts best at pH 3 to 6 and sometimes has an opsonin effect.
- Free fatty acids: Inhibit bacteria growth. Unsaturated fatty acids such as oleic acid are bactericidal for gram-positive organisms, while saturated fatty acids are fungicidal.
- Proteins and peptides rich in lysine and arginine: B-lysin (from platelets) is a polypeptide active against *Bacillus anthracis* and the *Clostridium* sp.
- Iron levels in body fluids have effect on *Staphylococcus aureus*, *Escherichia* coli, *Pasteurella multocida*, and *M. tuberculosis* growth. Iron-binding proteins of host system such as transferrin, lactoferrin, and ferritin hinder free iron availability to bacteria for their utilization.

The interaction between complement and lysozyme causes lysis of gram-negative bacteria (Figure 14.1). Although the membrane attack complex of complement origin can create an initial lesion in bacterial cell wall, it is unable to penetrate to the level of the cell membrane. Serum lysozyme, however, can complete the lytic process.

In summary, the innate immune system is very efficient in combating infections and it utilizes antibodies, complement, and lysozyme to kill bacteria. It also effectively utilizes the process of opsonization and phagocytosis of bacteria by neutrophils and macrophages to achieve prompt lethal effect on bacteria. Table 14.1 lists some nonimmunological protective factors. Figure 14.2 illustrates how in many ways the immune system can protect the body against infections and Figure 14.3 depicts evasion of immune response by *Streptococcus pneumoniae*.

TABLE 14. 1 SOME NONIMMUNOLOGICAL PROTECTIVE FACTORS FOUND IN BODY TISSUES AND FLUIDS

GROUP	NAME	MAJOR SOURCES	ACTIVITY AGAINST
Enzymes	Lysozyme	Serum; Leukocytes	Gram-positive and gram-negative bacteria; some viruses
Basic peptides and proteins	β-lysin Phagocytin Leukin Plakin	Platelets Neutrophils Neutrophils Platelets	Gram-positive bacteria
Iron-binding proteins	Transferrin Lactoferrin	Serum Leukocytes; milk	Gram-positive and gram-negative bacteria
Basic amines	Spermine; spermidine	Pancreas; kidney; prostate	Gram-positive bacteria
Complement components	–	Serum	Bacteria; viruses, protozoa
Peroxide-generating mechanisms	Myeloperoxidase; xanthine oxidase	Neutrophils; milk	Bacteria; viruses, protozoa
Interferons	TNF-α-β-γ, and -ω	Most cells but not neutrophils	Viruses; some intracellular protozoa

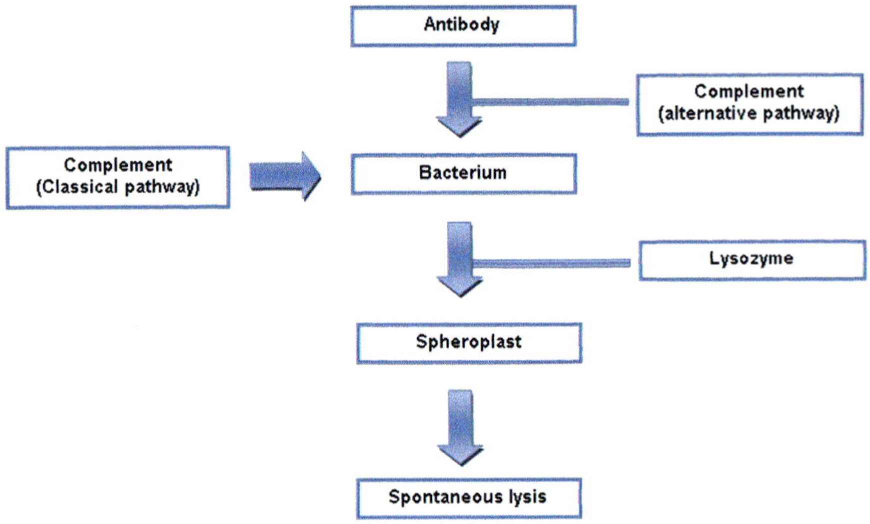

Figure 14.1 *The interaction between complement and lysozyme that causes lysis of gram-negative bacteria. Although it can make an initial lesion in the bacterial cell wall, the membrane attack complex of complement is unable to penetrate the cell membrane. Serum lysozyme, however, can complete the lytic process.*

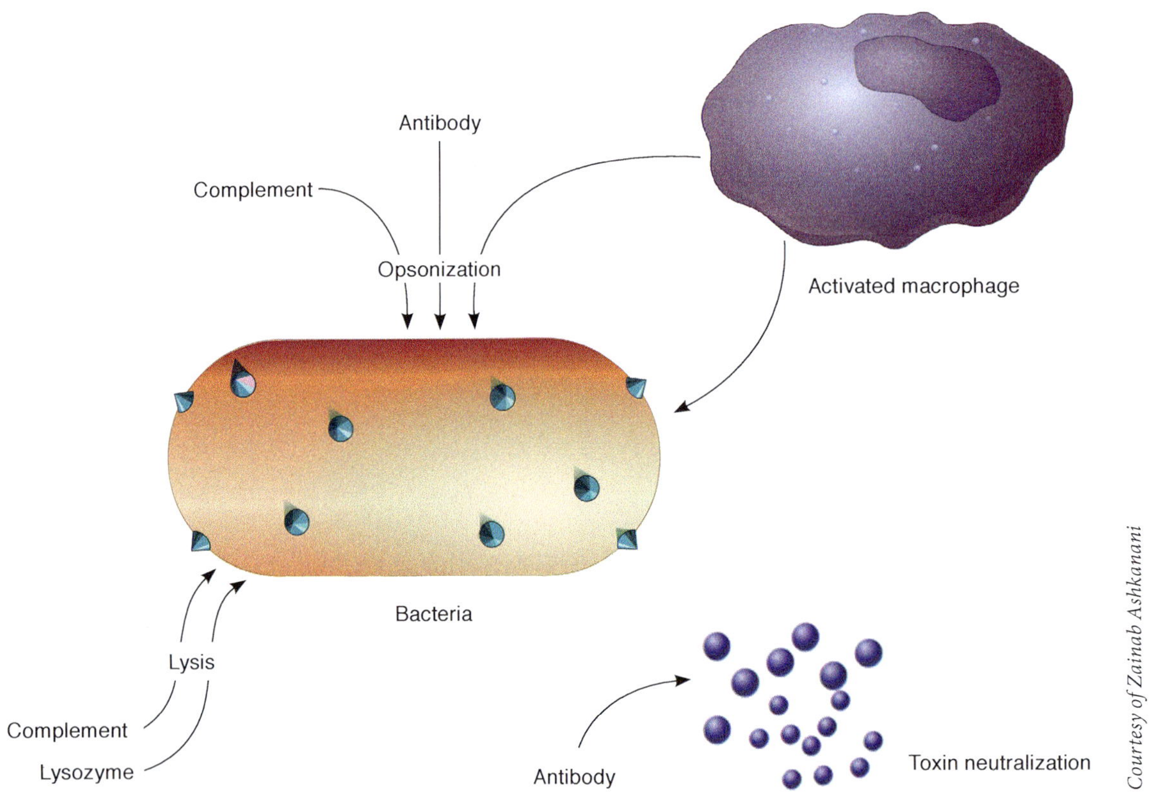

Figure 14.2 *The several ways in which the immune system can protect the body against invasion. These include opsonization, lysis, toxin neutralization, and destruction within activated macrophages.*

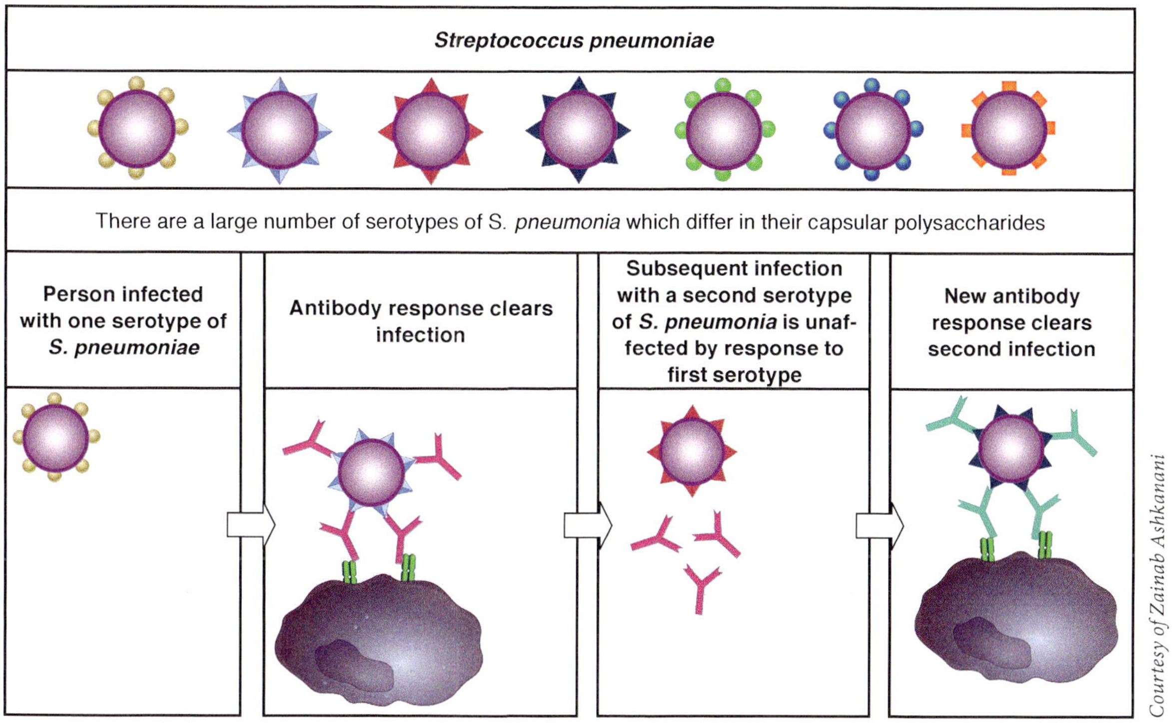

Figure 14.3 *Evasion of immune response by* Streptococcus pneumoniae. *A large number of serotypes of this pathogen exist, and if a secondary infection occurs with a different serotype than the first, it will be unaffected by the initial memory response.*

IMMUNITY TO BACTERIAL INFECTION

This involves antibodies, which serve as opsonins, making the engulfment of opsonized organisms easier for professional phagocytes because antibodies have sites that can bind to receptors on professional phagocytes. If the challenges were just ordinary toxin, then antitoxin is produced which is capable of toxin neutralization. Antibodies do not immediately come into play when the host encounters a new challenge. In that case, the innate immune response is the central player. The engulfment of microorganisms by professional phagocytes can be receptor based or nonreceptor based endocytosis. In the absence of antibodies, nonreceptor-based endocytosis come to play along with some complement component-mediated endocytosis. Macrophages are easily involved in nonreceptor-based endocytosis by producing protuberances that surround the challenge. It is also efficient in the complement component-mediated endocytosis. The complement components commonly involved in such process are C3a, C2a, and C5a. It is important to note that macrophage activation always precedes these processes. The activation of macrophage depends on interferon-gamma.

SPECIFIC IMMUNITY TO BACTERIA INFECTIONS

- Neutralization of toxins or enzymes by antibody.
- Killing of bacteria by antibodies, complement, and lysozyme.
- Opsonization and phagocytosis of bacteria by neutrophils and normal macrophages.
- Phagocytosis and destruction of intracellular bacteria by activated macrophages.
- Immunity to exotoxigenic bacteria:
  - These are exotoxin-producing bacteria, for example, *Clostridium sp.* or *Bacillus anthracis.*
  - Antibodies can readily neutralize exotoxins by competitively blocking the toxin and preventing toxin reaction with its receptor on the host cell.
  - IgG is almost totally responsible for toxin neutralization since IgM does not bind strongly to toxins.
- Immunity to systemic invasive bacteria:
  - Protection against invasive bacteria is directed against their surface antigens.
  - Antibodies directed against capsule may neutralize the antiphagocytic property of the capsule.
  - The class of immunoglobulin produced and the activation of complement are important in determining the fate of bacteria.
  - Antibody and complement may cause the development of membrane attack complexes (MACs) in the outer cell wall.

Immunity to Exotoxigenic Bacteria. Exotoxigenic bacteria are able to express toxins to the outside. The toxins expressed outside that are released into the environment are exotoxins. Examples of such bacteria are *Clostridium* spp. and *B. anthracis.* Antibodies can readily neutralize these toxins; they can also be passively administered. These antibodies act by competitively blocking the toxin and preventing toxin reaction with its receptor on the host cell. It is the efficacy of such ligand–receptor binding that causes the impairment of toxin binding to host receptor when antibodies have bound competitively to the same receptor. Usually, the antibody class of interest here is the IgG, which is responsible for the toxin neutralization since IgM does not bind strongly to toxins. High titer of IgG will be suitable because they are more effective at binding and they are polyclonal at the point of high titer.

Immunity to Systemic Invasive Bacteria. Systemic invasive bacteria are capable of disseminating from the portal of entry and permeating deep into the systemic vital organs. The local portal of entry may be respiratory, oral, or through any other opening to the outside of the body. Protection against invasive bacteria is directed against their surface antigens. Antibodies are directed against surface antigens; however, organisms in their attempt to survive evolve structures such as bacterial capsule that are usually difficult to develop antibodies against, or to attack through various opsonization methods. Capsules are made of such repeated simple structures that antibodies cannot easily be developed to them. The adult humans can, however, develop antibodies against the capsule as opposed to most other animals; antibodies directed against the capsule may neutralize the antiphagocytic properties of the capsule.

The class of immunoglobulin produced and the activation of complement are important in determining the fate of bacteria. For instance, there is a difference between IgG and IgM with regard to neutralizing toxin. The IgM is more effective at precipitating and clumping an antigen, while IgG is more effective as an opsonin in the absence of complement. The IgM is more effective at activating complement than IgG and thus a better opsonin than IgG in the presence of complement. Antibody and complement may cause the development of membrane attack complex (MAC) in the outer cell wall. MAC cannot span the outer and inner cell membrane of gram-negative bacteria, so it requires lysozyme for cell lysis.

Heat Shock Proteins. A common feature of inflammation and infection is the acute phase reactive proteins, including the C-reactive proteins. These proteins are really protective to other proteins and insulate them from the adverse effects of changes that accompany infection and inflammation. These include changes in temperature that could distort proteins. So, the regular configuration, the quaternary and tertiary structure of protein are preserved, even during infection, hence they are described as heat shock proteins. They are non-specific. The infectious agents also make their own heat shock proteins to seek protection from thermolability.

- Heat shock protein (HSP):
  - These are proteins associated with stress such as heat, starvation, ROS, RNI, toxins, protein synthesis inhibitors, and viral infections.
  - HSPs are present in all cells at very low levels at normal temperatures.
  - These proteins control the folding of other proteins so that the cells can function normally at higher temperatures.
  - There are three major HSPs: HSP-90, HSP-70, and HSP-60.
  - HSP-60 is the immunodominant antigen induced by *Mycobacterium, Coxiella, Legionella, Treponema,* and *Borrelia* infections.
  - Antibodies against HSP-70 have been detected in patients with malaria, schistosomiasis, trypanosomiasis, filariasis, and leishmaniasis without any assigned definite role.
  - These HSPs are highly antigenic because they are abundant and rapidly processed by antigen-presenting cells.

MODIFICATION OF BACTERIAL DISEASE BY IMMUNE RESPONSE

- The type of helper T-cell subpopulation that develops during immune response affects the course of the disease.
- Cell-mediated responses are usually required to control diseases caused by intracellular bacteria.
- Only activated macrophages can prevent growth of these organisms and macrophage activation requires that TH1 cells produce IL-2 and IFN-γ.
- When macrophages are activated, they can localize or cure infections. If alternatively only the TH2 cells are stimulated, then cell-mediated immune response fails, macrophages are not activated, and chronic progressive disease results.

MODIFICATION OF BACTERIAL DISEASE BY IMMUNE RESPONSE

Cell-mediated responses are usually required to control infections, especially when such infections concern intracellular bacteria. In such a case, the body's intervention method is to kill the infected cell, an act that is executed by cytotoxic T cell and NK cells, and to some extent macrophages and their secretions that amplify the process. Only activated macrophages can prevent the growth of the organisms, they do so by producing soluble substances, which heighten TH1 responses. Figure 14.4 illustrates three ways in which bacteria can escape destruction by macrophages.

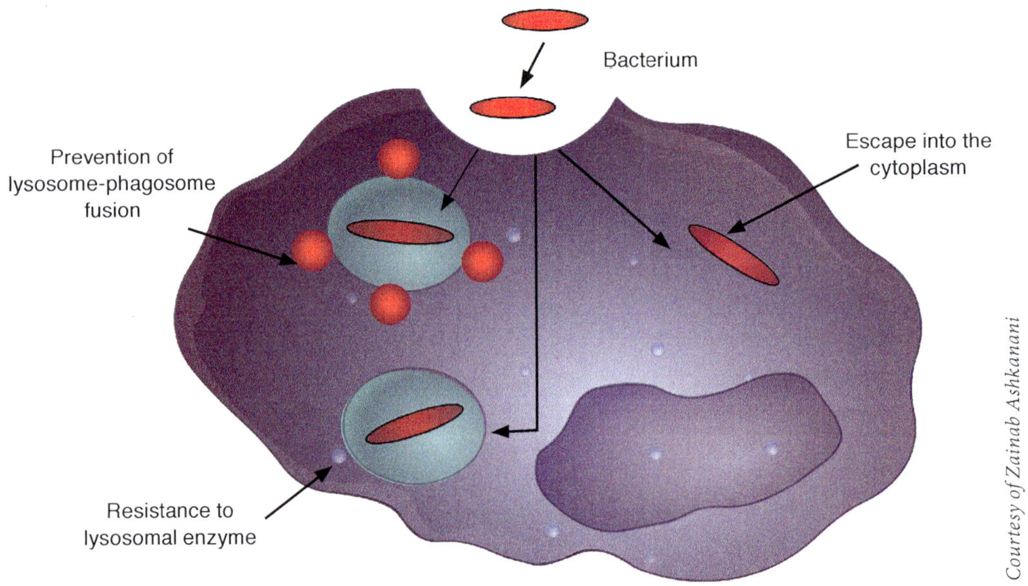

Figure 14.4 *The three major ways by which bacteria and other intracellular parasites can escape destruction within macrophages.*

The type of helper T cell subpopulation that develops during immune response is critical. TH1 response heightens cellular response, while TH2 heightens humoral response, leading to antibodies elaboration. As previously indicated, cell-mediated responses are usually required to control diseases caused by intracellular bacteria. This process mediates macrophage activation which is enhanced by TH1 derived IL-2 and IFN-γ. The role of IL-2 in the activation of macrophages is via the increase in the clones of TH1 cells, which results in increase in total quantity of IFN-gamma production. When macrophages are activated, they can localize or cure infections. The result of localization of infection is inflammation, an event that leads to the maximization of immune response. If alternatively, only TH2 cells are stimulated, then TH1 will be suppressed, cell-mediated immune response will fail, macrophages are not activated, and then the infection takes a chronic course.

EVASION OF IMMUNE RESPONSE BY BACTERIA

- Depression of phagocytosis by microbes such as *E. coli*, *S. aureus*, *M. tuberculosis*, and *Pseudomonas aeruginosa*.
- Induction of apoptosis in infected macrophages can be mediated by *Shigella flexneri*.
- IL-2 destruction by proteases. Some bacteria such as *P. aeruginosa* are capable of producing proteolytic enzymes that degrade IL-2-mediated clonal expansion of lymphocytes.

- Bordetellapertusis induces the secretion of highly active adenylcyclase that raises intracellular cyclic AMP levels and so suppresses cellular activities. It is a reciprocal effect, the greater the AMP levels, the lower the cellular activity.
- Production of free radical scavengers such as SOD, catalase, and some singlet oxygen quenching yellowish pigments by S. aureus.

IMMUNITY TO VIRUSES

- Nonspecific immune responses modify and control the outcome of many viral infections.
  - Lysozyme can destroy several internalized viruses.
  - Bile is a powerful neutralizer of some viruses and helps to protect the intestine against invasion.
  - Interferons are secreted by virus-infected cells within a few hours after viral invasion; cellular elaboration of interferon increases with high concentration achieved in days (see Table 14.2 and Figure 14.5).
    - Four major classes of interferons are recognized. They are IFN-α (from infected leukocytes), IFN-β (from infected fibroblast), IFN-γ (from antigenic stimulated T cells), and IFN-ω (omega) (from embryonic trophoblast).
    - IFNs are produced by viral-mediated activation of target cell genes coding for IFN. All IFNs except IFN-γ are stable at acidic pH.
    - IFN exert their activities by binding to interferon receptors on cells. IFN-α and IFN-β share a common receptor, while IFN-γ uses a different one.

MECHANISMS OF IFN ACTIVITIES

- IFN induces tyrosine phosphorylation and activation of DNA-binding protein. This generates gene activation and new protein production with antiviral activity.
- IFN-γ activates NOS which initiates the degradation of L-arginine to nitric oxide and citrulline. NO has antiviral activity.
- IFN also activates protein kinase which initiates the phosphorylation of an initiation factor eIF2 that prevents the elongation of the double-stranded RNA. This simply means the replication process of RNA contains viruses and protein synthesis is halted.
- IFN activates an Mx protein which inhibits transcription and translation of influenza virus.

TABLE 14.2 THE CLASSIFICATION OF INTERFERONS

SOURCE	NAME	TARGET	EFFECT
Leukocytes	IFN-α	Virus-infected cells	Blocking of viral replication
Fibroblasts	IFN-β		
T, B, or NK cells	IFN-γ	Macrophages, T and NK cells	Activation and enhanced cytotoxicity
Trophoblast cells	IFN-ω	Uterine lymphocytes	Fetal survival

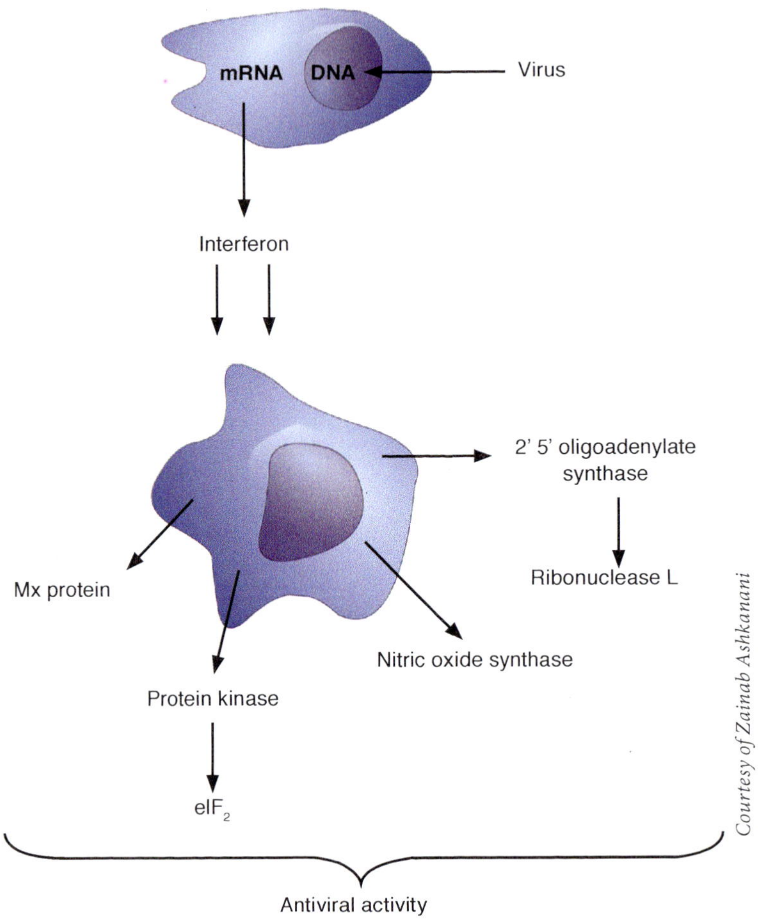

Figure 14.5 *Some of the mechanisms of the antiviral effect of the interferons*

SPECIFIC IMMUNITY

- Cell-mediated immune responses are of great importance in antiviral immunity. Individuals who are deficient in cell-mediated immune response commonly die from uncontrolled viral infections.
- Destruction of antibody is also of enormous importance. Capsids of viruses consist of antigenic glycoproteins to which antiviral antibodies are directed.
  - Since viruses must first bind to receptors on cells in order to infect them, antibodies may prevent viral attachment by blocking these receptors.
  - The combination of antibody with virus is not in itself lethal, but this can have an opsonin effect, promoting the phagocytosis of virons by macrophages.
  - They may also clump virons, so reducing the number of infectious units available for cell invasion.
  - They may initiate complement-mediated virus neutralization, involving alternate or classical pathways.
  - Antibodies and complement are active, not against free virons but against viral antigens expressed on cell surface of infected cells. These infected cells may be destroyed by antibody-mediated opsonization or by complement-mediated lysis.

- An important mechanism by which virus-infected cells are destroyed is the antibody-dependent cellular cytotoxicity (ADCC). In this process, cytotoxic cells with Fc receptors bind and lyse antibody-coated target cells. The cells that are involved in ADCC include macrophages, neutrophils, eosinophils, and NK cells. Antibodies involved in viral neutralization include IgG, IgM, and IgA. IgE may also play a protective role.

Cell-mediated immune responses are of great importance during infection by viruses. This is because viruses are intracellular particles which are not susceptible to immune protection in extracellular fluid except when it involves antibody-mediated viral destruction. Antibody-mediated impairment of viral entry or destruction of viruses is of enormous importance. Viruses are unable to enter cells unless the cells have receptors. Antibodies may prevent viral attachment because of the fact that those antibodies will block the specific site on the virus that is used for attachment, which is just like impairment of receptor–ligand interaction. The binding of antibody with viruses' site is not in itself lethal, but this can have an opsonin effect, making the viruses very susceptible to phagocytosis by professional phagocytes. This is because the phagocytes opsonize the viruses since antibodies have receptor sites that can also bind to professional phagocytes such as macrophages.

In most instances, antibodies are complement activating, so if they do activate complement, then they are capable of initiating the process of complement-mediated viral neutralization, involving alternate or classical complement pathways. Antibodies and complement are active not only against virons but also against viral antigens. This development can result in immune complex formation; such complex is eliminated from the body by scavenger cells such as macrophages. Also, the virus-infected cells usually exhibit markers on their surfaces that antibodies can bind to. These infected cells may be destroyed by antibody-mediated opsonization or complement-mediated lysis.

ANTIBODIES INVOLVED IN VIRAL NEUTRALIZATION

Among antibodies classes, IgM, IgG, and IgA are involved in antibody-mediated protection, while IgE may also play a protective role. The role of IgE in protection may be in the sense that they cause the reduction of histamine effect, thus annulling the effect of soluble substances such as histamine. On binding to eosinophil, histaminase is elaborated by eosinophil and this neutralizes the histamine. When adequate number of IgE is produced, it reduces the effect of those soluble substances that were responsible for compounding the effect of the infection and allergy, bringing about very early recovery.

CELL-MEDIATED IMMUNITY TO VIRAL INFECTIONS

Virus-infected cells commonly develop new antigens on their surface which make them susceptible to destruction. These new antigens include virus proteins exposed when viruses bud from the surfaces of the cell, such markers are characteristic of the infecting virus. Despite the capacity of cell-mediated immune response to combat viral infections, it appears to also allow the host cells to be destroyed in instances of overexpressed immune response. It is this heightened response that may account for severe symptoms reported in some viral infections afflicting the young adults with very healthy immune system. The common examples of this may be found in cases of hemorrhagic episodes accompanying Ebola and Lassa, and the severe symptoms of Dengue viral infection. It is important to note that these symptoms described in such infections are mild in the infected elderly and children with less competent immune response.

Figure 14.6 illustrates how the immune system defends the body against viral infections.

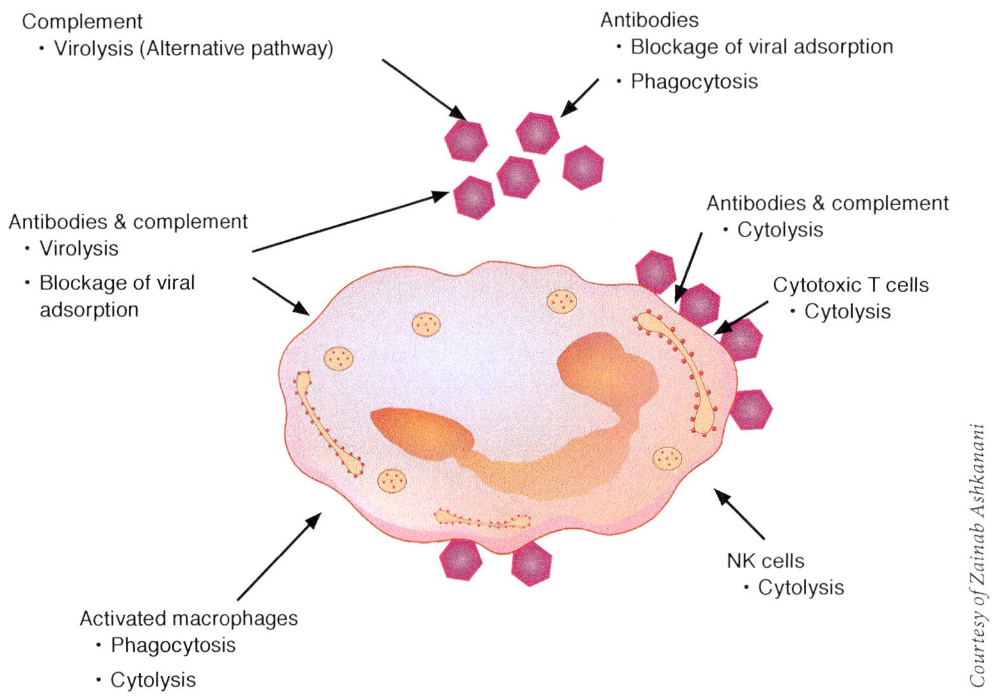

Figure 14.6 *The many ways in which the immune system can defend the body against viral invasion.*

CELL-MEDIATED IMMUNITY

- Virus-infected cells commonly develop new antigens on their surface. These new antigens include
  - Virus proteins exposed when viruses bud from the surfaces of the cell.
  - Other viral antigens expressed on cell surface.
  - Antigens induced by the virus on host cells.
- Immune responses sometimes modify viral diseases; for instance, an enhancement of disease may occur rather than a protection. A good example is lymphocytic choriomeningitis (LCM), a condition in which cytotoxic T cells attack viral infected brain cells.

EVASION OF THE IMMUNE RESPONSE BY VIRUSES

- There are some adaptive mechanisms by which viruses evade the immune system. These include the following:
  - Virus persistence within the cells: In this case they exhibit a slowly replicating or a nonreplicating form as typified by the herpes viruses. The persistent virus may periodically boost the immune response of the infected animal, and in this way generate prolonged immunity. This type of infection can be eliminated by an immune response directed against infected cells, and may even be inefficient if the viral antigens are not presented on the cell surface.

- Viral antigenic variation: The influenza virus has the capacity to change its antigenic structure by mutation affecting their surface hemmagglutinins and neuraminidases gradually, thus altering the antigenicity of each subtype. This antigenic drift permits the virus to persist for many years.
- Presentation of noncritical sites for antibody binding as seen in equine infectious anemia and African swine fever.
- Virus-induced immunosuppression due to virus destruction of lymphoid tissue, for example, herpes virus massive necrosis of the thymic cortex and Gumboro virus destruction of birds bursa of fabricus, T cells destruction by HIV, and EBV infection of B cells which causes cytotoxic T cell attack as in infectious mononucleosis or uncontrolled B-cell growth due to EBV without cytotoxic T cell attack as in Burkitt's lymphoma.
- Suppression of the expression of MHC molecules on infected cells. The viruses involved in this appear to be especially effective in down-regulating the expression of MHC class I molecules.

There are some adaptive mechanisms by which viruses evade the immune system. These include:

1. **Virus persistence within the cells:** During persistence, the virus will exhibit a slow replicating cycle. It is during such period that the virus is able to interact so much with the host, leading to conditions for disease causation. This is especially important in relation to chronic disease processes. The most efficient host response to persistence is cell-mediated attack of viral infected host cells, a process previously stated as dependent on expression of viral-specific marker proteins on cell surface.

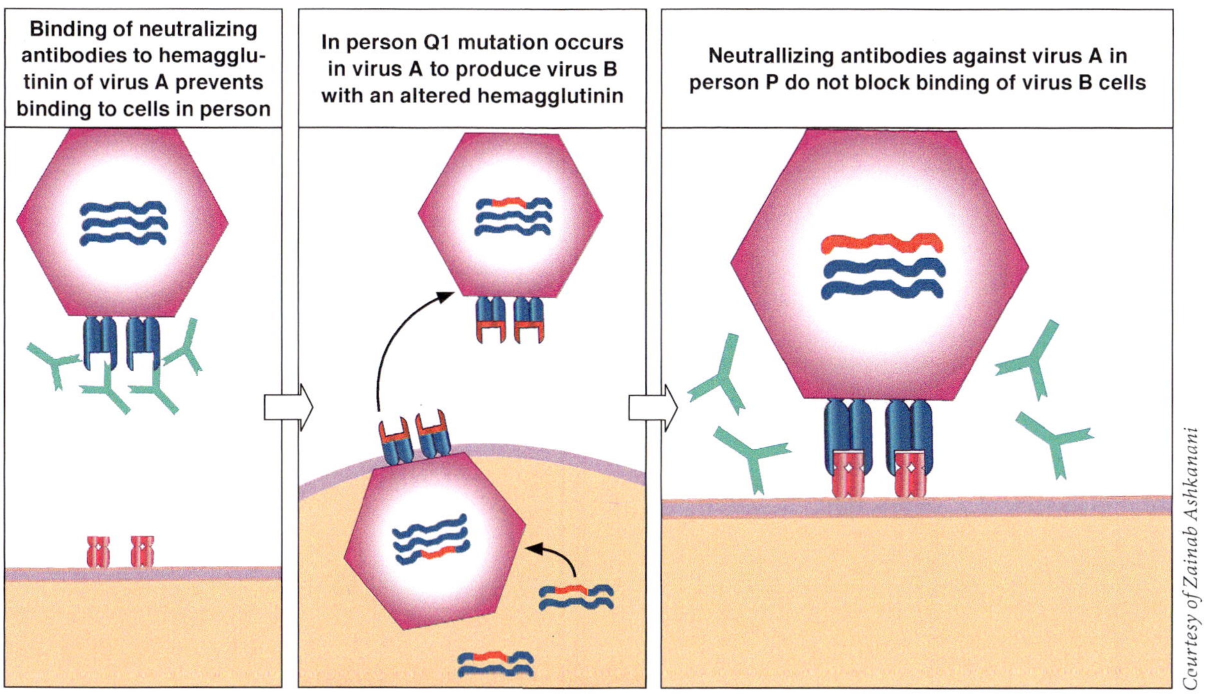

Figure 14.7 *Antigenic drift. The influenza virus contains two glycoproteins in its viral envelope: hemagglutinin and neuraminidase. However, several 'strains' of these glycoproteins exist, and a drift of one of the other protein to a different strain will result in antigenic drift and the evasion of a memory response.*

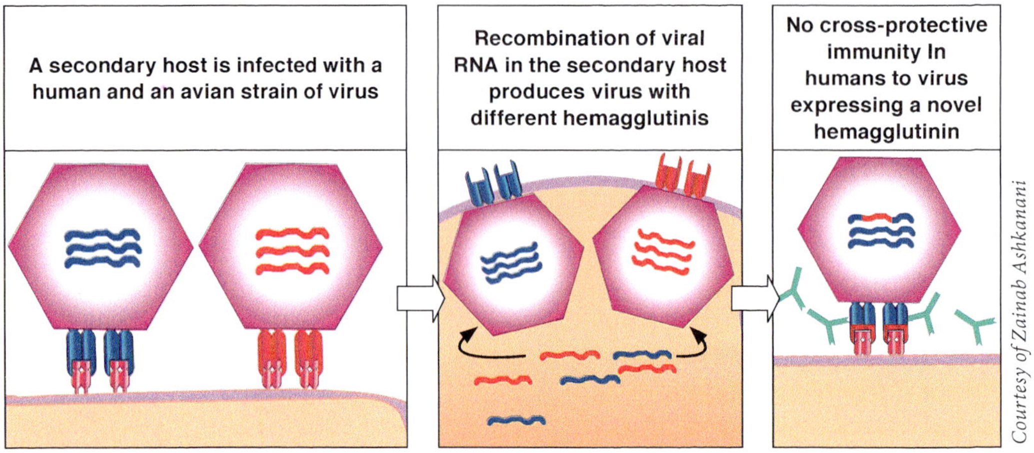

Figure 14.8 *Antigenic shift. Recombination of two different types of the virus (in this case, human and avian) results in a new virus altogether, capable of infection.*

2. **Change in surface protein configuration:** The illustrations given in Figures 14.7–14.8 depict such surface protein manifested in antigenic variations. The first variation is the antigenic drift which represents minor changes in genes determining the surface proteins. When such changes are major genetic changes in the genes determining the surface proteins, the condition is designated antigenic shift. The influenza virus has the capacity to change its antigenic structure by mutating, and the mutation usually affects two types of surface proteins, hemagglutinin and neuraminidase. While antigenic drift may not be serious enough to cause problems of epidemic proportions, antigenic shift is a rare occurrence and when they do occur, they result in apandemia. The changes arising from antigenic drifts from year to year are incorporated into vaccines.
3. **Presentation of noncritical sites:** Since antibodies bind to sites on viruses to neutralize them, viruses have adapted to this problem by adopting a method of producing a protein whose folding can conceal the noncritical sites such that the antibodies raised against such noncritical sites do not count in relation to attachment to cells. Some examples in this regard are the African swine fever virus and equine infectious anemia virus.
4. **Immunosuppression:** The human immunodeficiency virus (HIV) is a typical example in this regard. The HIV infects the pillar of the acquired immune system, the CD4 cells, thereby throwing the immune system into a path that leads to acquired immune deficiency syndrome. In this circumstance, HIV prevails and the host becomes vulnerable to infection by pathogens of opportunity (Figures 14.9 and 14.10). Figures 14.11 depicts opportunistic infections responsible for killing AIDS patients.

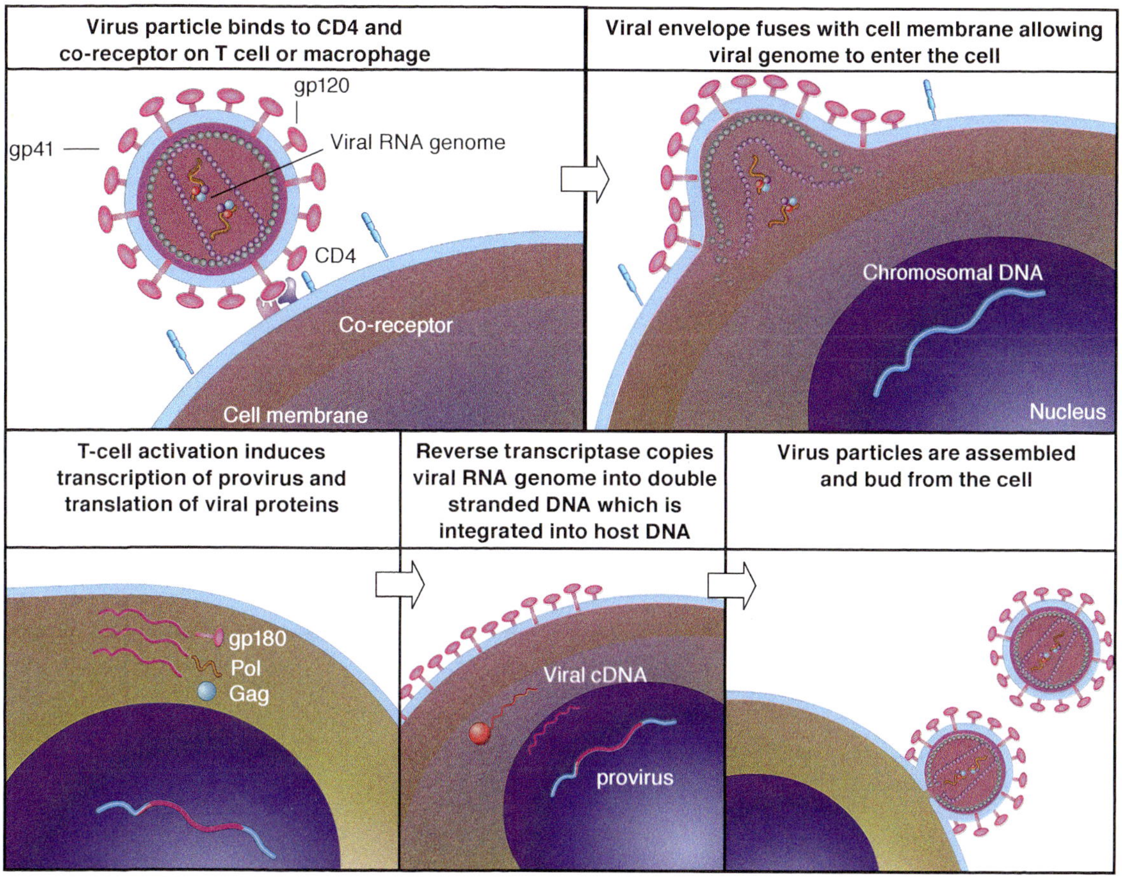

Courtesy of Zainab Ashkanani

Figure 14.9 *Schematic representation of HIV life cycle in human cells. The virus initially binds to CD4 by using gp120, which releases gp41 causing a fusion of the viral envelope to the plasma membrane of the host cell, releasing the viral core into the cytoplasm. Reverse transcriptase copies viral RNA genome into the double-stranded DNA sequence of the host DNA. Assembly and release from the host cell then occurs.*

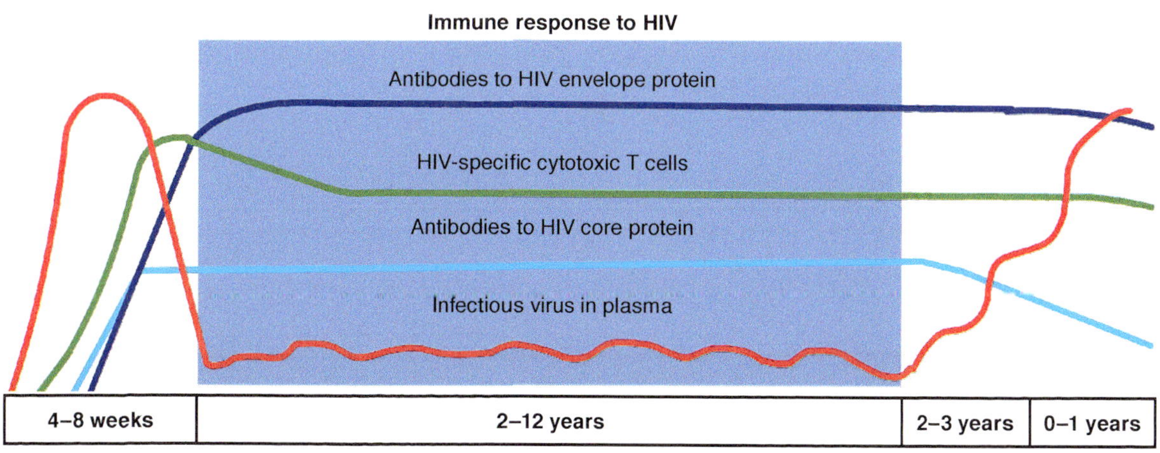

Figure 14.10 *Adaptive immune response limits the effects of HIV infection, which results in low levels of infectious virus in the patient's plasma for many years, and consequently a substantial life span after infection with HIV.*

INFECTIONS	
Parasites	*Toxoplasma* scpecies *Cryptosporidium* species *Leishmania* species *Microsporidium* species
Bacteria	*Mycobacterium tuberculosis* *Mycobacterium avium intracellulare* *Salmonella* species
Fungi	*Pneumocystis carinii* *Cryptococcus neoformans* *Candida* species *Histoplasma capsulatum* *Coccidioides immitis*
Viruses	Herpes simplex Cytomegalovirus Varicella-zoster
Malignancies	Kaposi's sarcoma (associated with herpes virus HHV8) Non-Hodgkin's lymphoma, including EBV-positive Burkitt's lymphoma Primary lymphoma of the brain

Figure 14.11 *Opportunistic infections responsible for killing AIDS patients.*

Another example is the avian infectious bursal disease virus (Gumboro virus) that destroys the repository of the immune system of the bird, which are the bursa cells situated in the bursa of fabricus near the cloaca. The disease is of great economic importance because it could cause the destruction of the poultry industry. Also, the herpes virus is capable of causing massive necrosis of the thymic cortex. Epstein-Barr virus is known to initiate a process that can bring about the destruction of B cells by colonizing them, thereby making them susceptible to cytotoxic T cell attack as seen in infectious mononucleosis. Thus, in this circumstance, the T cells destroy the B cells. In the absence of T cells, the virus will colonize B cells and immortalize them. It is important to note that the destruction of B cells has a positive feedback effect on B cell production. This, together with the capacity of the virus to immortalize B cell accounts for the malignancies, such as Burkitt's lymphoma. Table 14.3 lists some viruses that affect lymphoid tissues and Figure 14.12 depicts various diseases associated with infection by Epstein-Bar virus.

TABLE 14.3 SOME VIRUSES THAT AFFECT LYMPHOID TISSUES

VIRUSES THAT DESTROY LYMPHOID TISSUE
Herpes simplex
Dengue
Measles
Infectious bursal disease
Canine distemper
Bovine virus diarrhea
Simian immunodeficiency virus
Human immunodeficiency virus
VIRUSES THAT STIMULATE LYMPHOID TISSUES
Aleutian disease
Epstein-Barr virus
Visna
VIRUSES THAT CAUSE LYMPHOID CANCERS
Marek's disease
Feline leukemia
Bovine leukemia
Murine leukemias
Human T-cell leukemia virus I

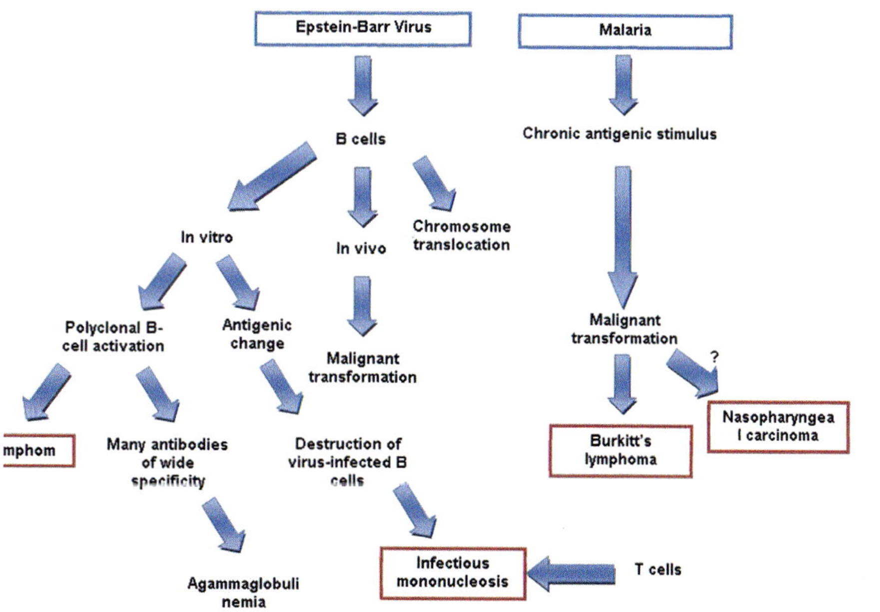

Figure 14.12 *Diseases associated with infection by Epstein-Bar virus.5. Suppression of the expression of major histocompatibility complex (MHC) molecules on infected cells: In this way, antibody production is impaired. The viruses involved in this appear to be especially effective in down-regulating the expression of MHC class I molecules which are involved in viral conserved peptide presentation.*

NONSPECIFIC IMMUNITY TO PROTOZOAN INFECTIONS

Species and genetic influences are very significant in susceptibility consideration. For instance,

- *Trypanosoma lewesi* is found only in rats and *T. musculi* in the mouse, and neither causes disease in animals. Thus, subtle genetic differences prevailing in the species may account for lack of infection.
- A classical case of genetically determined resistance to protozoan infection is the sickle cell anemia in humans. This is a condition in which the 6th amino acid (glutamic acid) of the β-polypeptide linkage of globin moiety of normal adult hemoglobin is replaced by valine. Red cells containing this kind of genetic substitution are not parasitized by *Plasmodium falciparum*.
- Also the lack of Duffy blood group antigens (Fy [a-b-]) confers resistance to malaria. The membrane molecule that carries Fy epitopes is also the receptor for *P. vivax*. Without it, the parasite cannot invade the erythrocyte.

SPECIFIC IMMUNITY TO PROTOZOAN INFECTIONS

- **Specific immunity**.
  - Protozoan also stimulate humoral and cell-mediated immune responses. The level of parasites in blood and tissue fluid is controlled by antibodies, whereas the cell-mediated immune response is directed at intracellular parasites. For instance, the production of reactive nitrogen metabolites stimulated by IFN-α and IFN-γ is effective against Leishmania sp.
  - Opsonization, agglutination, immobilization, and lysis may occur when there is interaction of antibodies with surface antigen, together with complement.
- **Evasion of immune response by protozoa**.
- Parasite-induced immunosuppression may assist parasite survival; for instance, the blood parasite *Babesiabovis* is immunosuppressive for cattle, thus making cattle tick survive easily on infected cattle. Also *T. cruzi* can prevent the expression of IL-2 receptor on T cells and so induce immunosuppression.
- Hypoantigenicity and alteration of surface antigens. An example of hypoantigenicity is found in *Toxoplasma gondii*, which does not stimulate a significant host response. Also *Trypanosoma theileri* in cattle and *T. lewesi* in rats can become functionally nonantigenic by masking themselves with host antigen (see Figures 14.13 and 14.14).

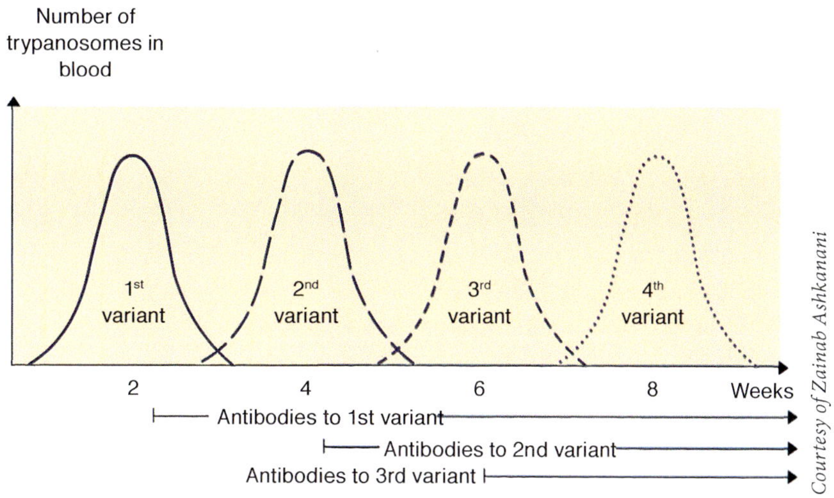

Figure 14.13 *Antigenic variation in cell membrane variant-specific glycoprotein results in the cyclic parasitaemia observed in trypanosomiasis. Each peak represents the growth of a population of parasites expressing new cell surface antigens.*

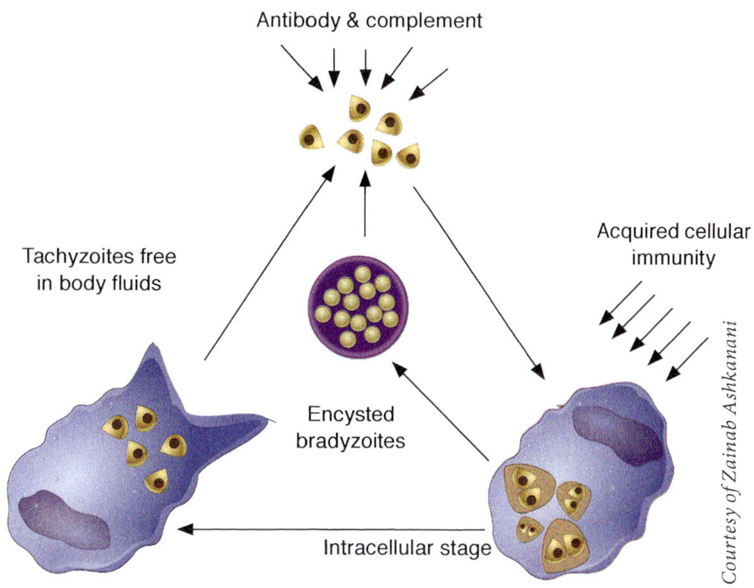

Figure 14.14 *The ways in which both humoral and cell-mediated immune responses act together to destroy the protozoan parasite Toxoplasma gondii. (Tachyzoites are the replicating forms found in the body. Bradyzoites are the forms found within cyst.)*

Immunity to Helminthes

- Parasitic worms are highly prevalent in animals and humans in developing countries, thus more than one species may coexist in an individual resulting in intraspecies and interspecies competition.
- Age and sex play important role in nonspecific immunity. Young children tend to acquire parasitic worm infection more than adults do because of their behavior.
- In animals with seasonal sexual cycle, parasites tend to synchronize their reproductive cycle with that of the host.

SPECIFIC IMMUNITY TO PARASITIC WORMS

- The most important Ig class produced is IgE, others include IgG, IgM, and IgA.
- Many worm infections are associated with the characteristic signs of type 1 hypersensitivity, including eosinophilia, edema, asthma, skin rashes, and positive passive cutaneous anaphylaxis reaction (urticaria) to worm antigens.
- Helminthes antigens preferentially stimulate TH2 and depress TH1 cells, so IL-4 and 5 production is stimulated, while IL-2 and IFN-γ production is low.
- IL-4 stimulates IgE production, while IL-5 stimulates eosinophil differentiation.
- When worm antigens bind to mast cells, they cause mast cell degranulation and secretion of vasoactive molecules.
- By causing mast cell degranulation, IgE stimulates secretion of eosinophil chemotactic factors. These peptides and also IL-5 mobilize bone marrow eosinophils and cause their release into circulation.
- Other Ig play protective roles by
  - Complement-mediated cuticular damage.
  - Antibody-mediated neutralization of proteolytic enzyme used by larva to penetrate tissue.
  - Blockage of the pores of the larva by immune complexes, thus preventing excretion and secretion in the larva.
- Sensitized T cells and macrophages may successfully attack worms that are deeply embedded in the intestinal wall or migrating through tissue (Figure 14.15).

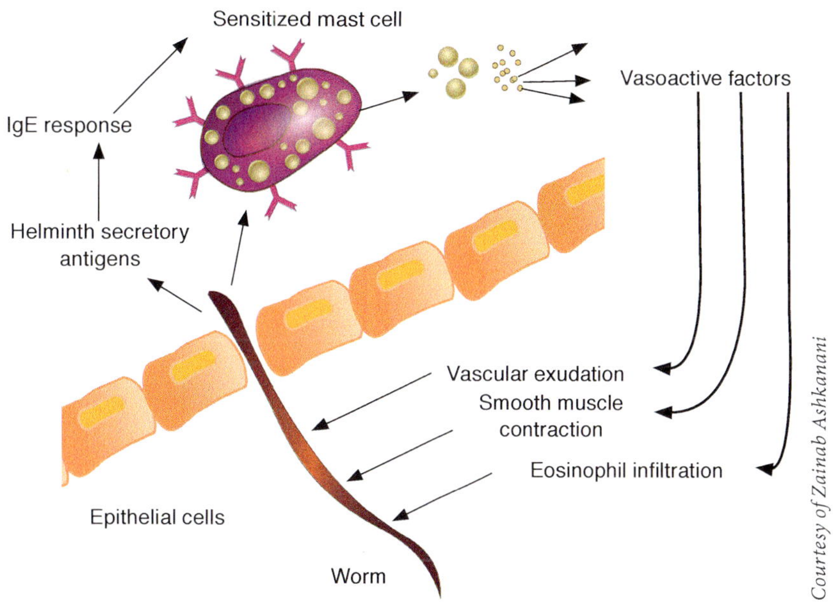

Figure 14.15 *The way in which a local type I hypersensitivity reaction in the intestinal wall can discourage helminthes infestation.*

EVASION OF THE IMMUNE RESPONSE BY HELMINTHES

- Molecular mimicry: This involves the synthesis of histocompatibility or blood group antigens to match those of the host.
- Adsorption of host antigen on to the surface of migrating larval worm for example, *Schistosoma mansoni*, a worm that lives in the mesenteric blood vessels of humans, can also evade alternative complement pathway by adsorbing host CD55 (DAF) on to its surfaces.
- Interfering with antigen presentation: Macrophages from schistosome-infected mice are poor antigen presenters. They may act by secreting molecules that block the actions of lysosomal proteases. Teaniastatin is a protease inhibitor from tape worm larva that inhibits neutrophil chemotaxis as well as T-cell proliferation and production of IL-2.

SAMPLE QUESTIONS

IMMUNITY TO INFECTIONS

1. Cells obtained from the tissues of an animal infected with *Leishmania major*, an intracellular parasite, show increased transcription of mRNA for IL-4 and IL-10. The synthesis of these two cytokines can be interpreted as meaning that
   a. antibody levels to *L. major* are likely to be elevated.
   b. IL-12 mRNA is also likely to be overexpressed in the same tissues.
   c. TH1 cells are actively engaged in the immune response against the parasite.
   d. the ability of infected macrophages to eliminate *L. major* is enhanced.
   e. the mice carry an expanded population of cytotoxic T cells able to destroy.

2. Which of the following would be a major problem for the therapeutic administration of IgA antibodies to individuals congenitally unable to synthesize them?
   a. Affinity to mucosal cells
   b. Lack of complement fixing capacity
   c. Low concentration in serum
   d. Molecular heterogeneity
   e. Short half-life

3. The protective effect of preformed antiviral antibodies is related to their ability to
   a. agglutinate circulating viral particles.
   b. form soluble immune complexes with viral antigens.
   c. induce phagocytosis of the virus.
   d. lyse the virus.
   e. prevent the virus from infecting its target cell(s).

Answer True of False to the Following:

Physical and chemical barriers

4. Epithelial surfaces are the first line of defense against infection.
5. Lysozyme and defensins are specific to bacterial cell walls.
6. Defensins cleave specific linkages in peptidoglycan.
7. Lysozyme creates pores in the plasma membrane of bacterial cells.

Evasion of immune response by bacteria

8. *M. tuberculosis* and *S. flexneri* can induce apoptosis in infected macrophages.
9. *B. pertussis* produces proteases that destroy IL-2.
10. *E. coli* secretes highly active adenylcyclase that raises intracellular cyclic AMP levels and so suppresses cellular activities.
11. *E. coli, S. aureus, M. tuberculosis*, and *P. aeruginosa* can cause a depression of phagocytosis.

Non-Specific Immunity to Viruses

12. Lysozyme is only effective against bacteria and plays no role in immunity to viruses.
13. Bile is a powerful neutralizer of some viruses and helps to protect the intestine against invasion.
14. Interferons (IFN) are secreted by virally infected cells within a few seconds after viral invasion, with high concentration achieved in hours.
15. IFN-α and IFN-β share a common receptor, while IFN-γ uses a different one

Mechanisms of IFN activities

16. IFN induces tyrosine de-phosphorylation and inactivation of DNA binding proteins, which switches off gene transcription and protein production.
17. IFN-γ activates iNOS which initiates the degradation of L-arginine to nitric oxide and citrulline; NO has antiviral activity.
18. IFN activates a protein kinase which initiates the phosphorylation of an initiation factor, preventing the elongation of double-stranded RNA.
19. IFN inactivates an Mx protein (GTPase), which inhibits the transcription and translation of influenza virus.

Specific immunity to viruses

20. Specific immunity to viruses is mainly antibody-mediated, not cell-mediated.
21. Antibodies may block viral attachment by blocking receptors on cells that antibodies would bind to, and they also enhance the phagocytosis of viral particles by macrophages.
22. Antibodies may also clump virions, reducing the number of infectious units available.
23. Antibody-dependent cellular cytotoxicity plays no role in the destruction of virus-infected cells.

Suggested Laboratory Practicals

- Case Studies on:

1. Strategies for the Evasion of Immune Response by Infectious Organisms
2. Strategies for the Killing of Intracellular Microbes by the Immune System

- Serologic Test for the Detection of Streptococci Infection
- Rapid Plasma Reagin Test for Syphilis
- Paul-Bunnel Test
- Detection of Heterophile Antibodies of Infectious Mononucleosis
- Enumeration of CD4 T Cell
- Serologic Assay for Protozoan Diseases
- Serologic Assay for Mycotic Diseases

GLOSSARY

Acquired immune deficiency syndrome (AIDS) The disease caused by infection with the human immunodeficiency virus (HIV). It involves a gradual destruction of the CD4 T-cell population and increasing susceptibility to infection. **Acquired immunity** *see* **adaptive immunity**

Acute Rejection of transplanted cells, tissues, or organs that is due to a T-cell response stimulated by the transplant.

Acute phase proteins Plasma proteins made by the liver, their synthesis is rapidly increased in response to infection. They include mannose-binding lectin (MBL), C-reactive protein (CRP), and fibrinogen.

Acute phase response A response of innate immunity that occurs soon after the start of an infection and involves the synthesis of acute phase proteins by the liver and their secretion into the blood.

Adaptive immune response The response of antigen-specific B and T lymphocytes to antigen, including the development of immunological memory.

Adaptive immunity The state of resistance to infection that is produced by the adaptive immune response.

Adenoids mucosa-associated secondary lymphoid tissues located in the nasal cavity.

Adenosine deaminase (ADA) Enzyme involved in purine breakdown. Its absence leads to the accumulation of toxic purine nucleosides and nucleotides, resulting in the death of most developing lymphocytes within the thymus. The disease that results from a genetically determined lack of adenosine deaminase is called **adenosine deaminase deficiency**. Its symptoms are severe combined immunodeficiency.

Adjuvant Substance used to enhance the adaptive immune response to any antigen. To exert its effect an adjuvant must be mixed with the antigen before injection or vaccination.

Afferent lymphatic vessels The several vessels that bring lymph draining from connective tissue into a lymph node en route to the blood.

Affinity A measure of the strength with which one molecule binds to another via a single binding site.

Agglutination The clumping together of particles, usually caused by antibody or some other multivalent binding molecule interacting with antigens on the surfaces of adjacent particles. Such particles are said to be agglutinated. When the particles are red blood cells, the phenomenon is called hemagglutination. When they are white blood cells, it is called leukoagglutination.

Agonist Any molecule that binds to a receptor and causes it to function.

Alleles The natural variants of a single gene.

Allelic exclusion In reference to antibody production, the case that, in a heterozygous individual, only one of the two C-region alleles at the immunoglobulin heavy-chain or light-chain loci is expressed in each B cell. In the B-cell population, for each locus roughly half the cells express one allele and the remaining cells express the other.

Allergen An antigen that elicits hypersensitivity or allergic reactions. Allergens are usually innocuous proteins that do not inherently threaten the integrity of the body.

Allergic asthma Disease caused by an allergic reaction to inhaled antigen, in which the bronchi constrict and the patient has difficulty breathing.

Allergic conjunctivitis Allergic reactions in the conjunctiva of the eye, usually caused by airborne antigens.

Allergic reaction The result of a secondary immune response to an otherwise innocuous environmental antigen, or allergen. Allergic reactions can involve either antibodies or effector T cells.

Allergic rhinitis An allergic reaction in the nasal mucosa that causes runny nose, sneezing, and tears. It is also known as hay fever.

Allergy A state of hypersensitivity to a normally innocuous environmental antigen. It results from the interaction between the antigen and the antibodies or T cells produced by earlier exposure to the same antigen.

Alloantibody Antibody that is made by immunization of one member of a species with antigen derived from another member of the same species. Alloantibodies recognize antigens that are the result of allelic variation at polymorphic genes. Common types of alloantibody are those recognizing blood group antigens and HLA class I and class II molecules.

Alloantigen An antigen that differs between members of the same species, such as HLA molecules and blood group antigens. Alloantigens are determined by the different alleles of polymorphic genes.

Allogeneic Describes two members of the same species who are genetically different.

Allograft A tissue graft made between genetically nonidentical members of the same species.

Alloreaction An adaptive immune response made by one member of a species against an allogeneic antigen from another member of the same species.

Alloreactive T cell T cell in one member of a species that responds to an allogeneic antigen from another member of the same species.

Allotypes Natural protein variants that are encoded by the alleles of a gene.

Alternative C3 convertase The **C3 convertase** of the alternative pathway of complement activation. It is composed of C3 bound to proteolytically active Bb (C3Bb) and cleaves C3 into C3a and C3b.

Alternative C5 convertase The **C5 convertase** of the alternative pathway of complement activation. It is composed of two molecules of C3h bound to Bb (C3b2Bb) and cleaves C5 into C5a and C5b.

Alternative pathway of complement activation One of the three pathways of complement activation. It is triggered by the presence of infection but does not involve antibody.

Anaphylactic shock IgE-mediated allergic reaction to systemically administered antigen that causes circulatory collapse and suffocation due to tracheal swelling. Also called systemic anaphylaxis.

Anaphylactoid reactions Reactions that are clinically similar to anaphylactic shock but do not involve IgE.

Anaphylatoxins Complement fragments C5a, C4a, and C3a, which are produced during complement activation. They recruit fluid and inflammatory cells to sites of antigen deposition.

Anergy A state of nonresponsiveness to antigen. People are said to be anergic when they cannot mount delayed-type hypersensitivity reactions on challenge with an antigen. T and B cells are said to be anergic when they cannot respond to their specific antigen.

Angioedema Swelling of the skin as a result of IgE-mediated allergic reactions, which cause increased permeability of subcutaneous blood vessels with consequent leakage of fluid into the skin.

Antagonist Any molecule that binds to a receptor and prevents its function.

Antibody The secreted form of the immunoglobulin made by a B cell.

Antibody repertoire The total variety of antibodies that a person can make.

Antibody-dependent cell-mediated cytotoxicity (ADCC) The killing of antibody-coated target cells by NK cells having the FcγRIII receptor (CD16) that recognizes the Fc region of the bound antibody.

Antigen Originally defined as any molecule that binds specifically to an antibody, the term now also refers to any molecule that can produce peptides that bind specifically to a T-cell receptor.

Antigen-binding site The site on an immunoglobulin or T-cell receptor molecule that binds specific antigen.

Antigen presentation The display of antigen as peptide fragments bound to MHC molecules on the surface of cells. This is the form in which antigen is recognized by most T cells.

Antigen-presenting cells Cells that express either MHC class I and/or MHC class II molecules and thus display complexes of MHC molecule and peptide antigen on their surfaces.

Antigen processing The intracellular degradation of proteins into peptides that binds to MHC molecules for presentation to T cells.

Antigen receptor for a B cell, the antigen receptor is its cell-surface immunoglobulin; for a T cell the antigen receptor is a rather similar molecule called the T-cell receptor. Each individual lymphocyte bears receptors of a single-antigen specificity.

Antigenic drift A process by which point mutations in influenza virus genes cause differences in the structure of viral surface antigens. This causes year-to-year antigenic differences in strains of influenza virus.

Antigenic shift A process by which influenza viruses reassort their segmented genomes and change their surface antigens radically. New viruses arising by antigenic shift are the usual cause of influenza pandemics.

Antilymphocyte globulin (ALG) A preparation of antibodies made by immunizing animals with human lymphocytes. It is used clinically to prevent rejection in organ transplantation.

Antiserum (plural antisera) The fluid component of clotted blood from an immune individual that contains antibodies against an antigen. An antiserum contains a heterogeneous collection of antibodies that bind the antigen.

Antithymocyte globulin (ATG) A preparation of antibodies made by immunizing animals with human thymocytes. It is used clinically to prevent rejection in organ transplantation.

AP-1 A family of transcription factors, some of which participate in lymphocyte activation.

Apoptosis A mechanism of cell death in which the cells to be killed are induced to degrade themselves from within, in a tidy manner. Also called programmed cell death.

Appendix A gut-associated secondary lymphoid tissue located at the beginning of the colon.

Arthus reaction An immune reaction in the skin caused by the injection of antigen into the dermis. The antigen reacts with specific IgG antibodies in the extracellular spaces, activating complement and phagocytic cells to produce a local inflammatory response.

Atopic allergy (atopy) The genetically determined tendency of some people to produce IgE-mediated hypersensitivity reactions against innocuous substances.

Autoantibody An antibody produced by an individual against an antigen produced by their own body.

Autoantigen A self-antigen, an antigenic component of the body that provokes an immune response by the individual's own immune system.

Autocrine Describes a cytokine or other secreted molecule that acts on the same type of cell as the one that secreted it.

Autograft a graft of tissue made from one anatomical site to another on the same individual.

Autoimmune disease Disease in which the pathology is caused by an immune response to normal components of healthy tissue.

Autoimmune hemolytic anemia A disease characterized by reduced numbers of red blood cells (anemia). The reduction is caused by autoantibodies that bind to surface antigens of red blood cells and destroy them.

Autoimmune polyendocrinopathy-candidiasis ectodermal dystrophy (APECED) An autoimmune disease caused by a lack of a protein called **autoimmune regulator (AIRE)**, which results in the production of T cells reactive against a number of tissues in the body. Also known as **autoimmune polyglandular disease (APD)**.

Autoimmune response An adaptive immune response directed at an antigenic component of the individual's own body.

Autoimmunity Adaptive immunity specific for an antigenic component of the individual's own body.

Autologous Describes cells, HLA molecules, and so on that derives from the individual in question.

Autologous bone marrow transplant A bone marrow transplant in which the donor and recipient are the same person.

Azathioprine An immunosuppressive drug that kills dividing cells. It is used in transplantation.

B cells Lymphocytes that are dedicated to making immunoglobulins and antibodies.

B-cell receptor The antigen receptor on B cells. Each B cell is programmed to make a single type of immunoglobulin. The cell surface form of this immunoglobulin serves as the B-cell receptor for specific antigen. Associated in the membrane with the immunoglobulin are the signal transduction molecules Igα and Igβ.

B-cell coreceptor A complex of the CD19, TAPA-1, and CR2 polypeptides that associates with the B-cell receptor and augments its response to specific antigen.

B-1 cells The minority population of B cells. They express the CD5 glycoprotein and make antibodies of broad specificities. They are also known as CD5 B cells.

B-2 cells The majority population of B cells. They do not express the CD5 glycoprotein and make antibodies of narrow specificities.

B7 molecules The B7.1 and B7.2 proteins, which are costimulatory molecules present on the surface of professional antigen-presenting cells.

Bare lymphocyte syndromes Genetically determined diseases in which MHC class I or II molecules are not expressed on cells. They can be caused by various different regulatory gene defects, and their effect is severe immunodeficiency.

Basophil White blood cell present in small numbers in the blood; it is one of the three types of granulocyte. Basophils contain granules that stain with basic dyes.

Benign tumor A growth due to abnormal proliferation of cells that is localized and contained by epithelial barriers.

Bone marrow The tissue in the center of certain bones that is the major site of generation of all the cellular elements of blood (hematopoiesis).

Bronchial-associated lymphoid tissues (BALT) The lymphoid cells and organized lymphoid tissues in the respiratory tract.

C-reactive protein (CRP) An acute phase protein that binds to phosphocholine, a surface constituent of various bacteria. CRP binds bacteria, opsonizing them for uptake by phagocytes.

C1 inhibitor (C1INH) A regulatory protein in plasma that inhibits the activity of activated complement component C1. C1INH deficiency causes the disease hereditary angioneurotic edema, in which spontaneous complement activation causes episodes of epiglottal swelling and suffocation.

C3 convertases Proteolytic enzymes that are formed during complement activation and cleave complement component C3 to C3b and C3a, thereby enabling C3b to bond covalently to antigens.

C4-binding protein (C4BP) A regulatory protein in plasma that activates the classical C3 convertase by binding to C4b and displacing C2b.

C5 convertases Proteolytic enzymes that are formed during complement activation and cleave complement component C5 to form C5a and C5b.

Calcineurin A cytosolic serine/threonine phosphatase that contributes to T-cell activation. The immunosuppressive drugs cyclosporin A and tacrolimus act by inhibiting calcineurin.

Calnexin A membrane protein in the endoplasmic reticulum that facilitates the folding of MHC molecules and other glycoproteins.

Calreticulin A soluble protein in the endoplasmic reticulum that is structurally related to calnexin and helps MHC molecules and other glycoproteins to fold properly.

Cancer Diseases caused by abnormal and invasive cell proliferation.

Carcinogen Chemical or physical agent that increases the risk of cancer.

Carcinoma Cancer of epithelial cells.

Carrier Foreign protein to which small nonimmunogenic antigens, or haptens, can be coupled to render the hapten immunogenic. *In vivo*, self proteins can also serve as carriers if they are suitably modified by the hapten; this is important in allergy to drugs.

Caseation necrosis A form of necrosis seen in the center of some large granulomas. The term comes from the white cheesy appearance of the central necrotic area.

Catalytic antibody An antibody that binds an antigen, chemically changes it, and then releases it.

CCL2 A chemokine produced by activated T cells that attracts macrophages into a site of infection. Formerly known as macrophage chemotactic protein (MCP).

CCL2l A chemokine made by vascular endothelial cells and which is involved in extravasation of leukocytes. Formerly known as SLC.

CD2 An adhesion molecule of T cells that binds to the LFA-3 adhesion molecule of antigen-presenting cells. Also called LFA-2.

CD3 complex A complex of signaling molecules that associates with T-cell receptors. It consists of CD3y, 5, and E chains, and chains.

CD4 a cell-surface glycoprotein on some T cells that recognize antigens presented by MHC class II molecules. CD4 binds to MHC class II molecules on the antigen-presenting cell and acts as a coreceptor to augment the T cell's response to antigen.

CD4 T cells The subset of T cells that express the CD4 coreceptor and recognize peptide antigens presented by MHC class II molecules.

CD8 A cell-surface glycoprotein on some T cells that recognize antigens presented by MHC class I molecules. CD8 binds to MHC classl molecules on the antigen-presenting cell and acts as a coreceptor to augment the T cell's response to antigen.

CD8 T cells The subset of T cells that express the CD8 coreceptor and recognize peptide antigens presented by MHC class I molecules.

CD19 A component of the B-cell coreceptor.

CD21 Another name for complement receptor 2 (CR2). It is a component of the B-cell receptor.

CD28 the low-affinity receptor on T cells that interacts with B7 costimulatory molecules to promote T-cell activation.

CD34 A vascular addressin expressed on high endothelial venules in lymph nodes, and which is involved in extravasation of white blood cells.

CD40 Cell-surface glycoprotein on B cells whose interaction with **CD40 ligand** on T cells triggers B-cell proliferation.

CD81 A component of the B-cell receptor that is also a cellular receptor for hepatitis C virus. Also called TAPA-1.

Celiac disease Inflammatory autoimmune disease of the gut mucosa caused by an immune response to the gluten proteins present in some cereals such as wheat.

Cell adhesion molecules (CAMs) Cell-surface proteins that enable cells to bind to each other.

Cell-mediated immunity (cellular immunity) Any adaptive immune response in which antigen-specific effector T cells dominate. It is defined operationally as all adaptive immunity that cannot be transferred to a naive recipient with serum antibody.

Central lymphoid tissues The anatomical sites of lymphocyte development. In humans, B lymphocytes develop in bone marrow, whereas T lymphocytes develop in the thymus.

Central MHC The class III region of the MHC, located between the class I and II regions.

Centroblast Large dividing B cell present in germinal centers. Somatic hypermutation occurs in centroblasts, and antibody-secreting and memory B cells derive from them.

Centrocyte Nondividing B cell in germinal centers. Centrocytes have undergone isotype switching and somatic hypermutation.

Chediak-Higashi syndrome A genetic disease in which phagocytes malfunction. Their lysosomes fail to fuse properly with phagosomes, and killing of ingested bacteria is impaired.

Chemokines Large group of small proteins involved in guiding white blood cells to sites where their functions are needed. They have a central role, in inflammatory responses.

Chronic asthma A disease characterized by chronic inflammation of the airways and difficulty in breathing. Although probably initiated by exposure to an allergen, chronic asthma can be perpetuated in its absence.

Chronic granulomatous disease An immunodeficiency disease in which multiple granulomas form as a result of defective elimination of bacteria by phagocytic cells. It is caused by a defect in the NADPH oxidase system of enzymes, which generates the superoxide radical involved in bacterial killing.

Chronic rejection Rejection of organ grafts that occurs years after transplantation and is characterized by degeneration and occlusion of the blood vessels in the graft. It is caused by an antibody response to the HLA class I alloantigens of the graft.

Chronic thyroiditis an autoimmune disease that causes progressive destruction of the thyroid gland. Also called Hashimoto's thyroiditis or Hashimoto's disease.

Class I region The part of the major histocompatibility complex that contains the MHC class I heavy-chain genes.

Class II region The part of the major histocompatibility complex that contains the MHC class II a- and 3-chain genes.

Class II-associated invariant chain peptide (CLIP) A peptide of variable length cleaved from the class II invariant chain by proteases in the endosomal pathway. It remains associated with the MHC class II molecule in an unstable form until it is removed by the HLA-DM protein.

Class III region A region of the major histocompatibility complex between the class I and II regions. Also known as the **central MHC**, it contains no genes for class I or II MHC molecules.

Classical C3 convertase A surface-associated serine protease of the classical pathway of complement activation. It is composed of the complement components C4b2a and cleaves C3 into C3a and C3b.

Classical C5 convertase C5-cleaving enzyme consisting of the complement fragments C4b, C2b, and C3b.

Classical pathway of complement activation One of three pathways of complement activation. It is activated by antibody bound to antigen, and involves complement components Cl, C4, and C2 in the generation of the C3 and C5 convertases. *See also* **alternative pathway of complement activation; lectin pathway of complement activation.**

Clonal deletion The elimination of immature lymphocytes that bind to self antigens. Clonal deletion is the main mechanism that produces self-tolerance.

Clonal selection The central principle of adaptive immunity It is the mechanism by which adaptive immune responses derive only from individual antigen-specific lymphocytes, which are stimulated by the antigen to proliferate and differentiate into antigen-specific effector cells.

Co-receptor A cell-surface protein that increases the sensitivity of an antigen receptor to its antigen. A coreceptor can accomplish this by increasing adhesive interactions between the interacting cells, and/or by enhancing signal transduction from the main receptor.

Costimulator molecule A molecule on an antigen-presenting cell that delivers signals to an interacting naive lymphocyte that are required in addition to the antigen-binding signal for the lymphocyte to respond. Costimulator molecules include the B7.1 and B7.2 proteins on professional antigen-presenting cells, which engage molecules CD28 and CTLA-4 on T cells. **CD40 ligand** serves a costimulatory role when it binds to CD40 on B cells.

Cognate interactions Cell–cell interactions between B and T lymphocytes specific for the same antigen.

Collectins A family of calcium-dependent sugar-binding proteins or lectins containing collagen-like sequences. An example is mannose-binding lectin.

Combination therapy Antiviral therapy (for HIV, for example) in which several antiviral drugs are used together to try and avoid the rapid generation of mutant viruses resistant to one of the drugs alone

Combination vaccine Vaccine that contains antigens derived from more than one pathogen and is designed to provide protection against more than one disease.

Common lymphoid progenitor Stem cell that gives rise to all lymphocytes and is derived from a pluripotent hematopoietic stem cell.

Complement A set of plasma proteins that act in a cascade of reactions to attack extracellular forms of pathogens. As a result of complement activation, pathogens become coated with complement components, which can either kill the pathogen directly or cause its engulfment and destruction by phagocytes.

Complement activation The initiation by pathogens of a series of reactions involving the complement components of plasma, leading to the death and elimination of the pathogen. *See also* **alternative pathway of complement activation; classical pathway of complement activation; and lectin pathway of complement activation.**

Complement control protein (CCP) modules Family of structurally similar protein modules found in many of the proteins that regulate complement activity.

Complement receptors (CR) Cell-surface proteins on various cell types that recognize and bind complement proteins bound to antigens. Complement receptors on phagocytes facilitate the phagocytic engulfment of pathogens coated with complement. Complement receptors include CR1, CR2, CR3, CR4, and the receptor for Clq.

Complementarity-determining regions (CDRs) The localized regions of immunoglobulin and T-cell receptor chains that determine the antigenic specificity and bind to the antigen. The CDRs are the most variable parts of the variable domains and are also called hypervariable regions.

Conformational epitopes Epitopes on a protein antigen that are formed from several separate regions in the primary sequence of a protein brought together by protein folding. Antibodies that bind conformational epitopes bind only to native folded proteins. Also called **discontinuous epitopes.**

Conjugate vaccine A vaccine made from capsular polysaccharides bound to an immunogenic protein such as tetanus toxoid. The protein provides peptide epitopes that stimulate CD4 T cells to help B cells specific for the polysaccharide.

Constant domains (C domains) The constituent domains of the constant regions of immunoglobulin and T-cell receptor polypeptides.

Constant region (C region) The part of an immunoglobulin or T-cell receptor (or of its constituent polypeptide chains) that is of identical amino acid sequence in molecules of the same isotype but different antigen-binding specificities.

Contact sensitivity A form of delayed-type hypersensitivity in which T cells respond to antigens that are introduced into the body by contact with the skin.

Corticosteroids Compounds related to the steroid hormones produced in the adrenal cortex, such as cortisone. They suppress immune responses and are widely used as anti-inflammatory and immunosuppressive agents in medicine.

Cross-match testing A test used in blood typing and histocompatibility testing to determine whether donor and recipient have antibodies against each other's cells that might interfere with successful transfusion or transplantation.

Cryptic epitope Antigenic determinant on a molecule that is normally hidden from the immune system but becomes revealed under conditions of infection or inflammation.

CTLA-4 A high-affinity inhibitory receptor on T cells that interacts with B7 costimulatory molecules.

Cutaneous T-cell lymphoma A malignant growth of T cells that home to the skin. Also known as mycosis fungoides.

CXCL8 A chemokine involved in the extravasation of neutrophils. Formerly known as IL-8.

Cyclophilins Family of cytoplasmic proteins that bind to the immunosuppressive drugs cyclosporin A and tacrolimus. The complex of drug and cyclophilin binds calcineurin and this prevents T-cell activation.

Cyclophosphamide An allcylating agent used as an immunosuppressive drug. It acts by killing rapidly dividing cells, including lymphocytes proliferating in response to antigen.

Cyclosporin A An immunosuppressive drug that specifically prevents T-cell activation and effector function. Also called cyclosporine.

Cytokines Proteins made by cells that affect the behavior of other cells. Cytokines made by lymphocytes are often called lympholcines or interleukins (abbreviated IL). Cytokines bind to specific receptors on their target cells.

Cytotoxic CD8 T cells The subset of T cells that express the CD8 coreceptor and recognize peptide antigen presented by MHC class I molecules.

Cytotoxic T cells T cells that can kill other cells. Almost all cytotoxic T cells are CD8 T cells. Cytotoxic T cells are important in host defense against viruses and other cytosolic pathogens, because they recognize and kill the infected cells. Cytotoxins proteins made by cytotoxic T cells that participate in the destruction of target cells. Perforins, granzymes or fragmentins, and granulysin are examples of cytotoxins.

Dark zone The part of a germinal center in secondary lymphoid tissue that contains dividing centroblasts.

Decay-accelerating factor (DAF) A cell-surface protein that prevents complement activation on human cells. DAF binds to C3 convertases of both the alternative and classical pathways of complement activation and, by displacing Bb and C2b respectively, prevents their action.

Degenerate binding specificity The type of antigen-binding specificity exhibited by MHC class I and II molecules, in which each MHC allotype can bind numerous peptides of different amino acid sequences.

Delayed-type hypersensitivity (DTH) A form of cell-mediated immunity elicited by antigen in the skin and mediated by CD4 TH1 cells. It is called delayed-type hypersensitivity because the reaction appears hours to days after antigen is injected.

Dendritic cells Professional antigen-presenting cells with a branched, dendritic morphology. They are the most potent stimulators of T-cell responses. Also known as interdigitating reticular cells, they are derived from the bone marrow and are distinct from the follicular dendritic cell that presents antigen to B cells.

Immature dendritic cells Take up and process antigens but cannot yet stimulate T cells. Mature or activated **dendritic cells** are present in secondary lymphoid tissues and are able to stimulate T cells.

Dendritic epidermal T cells (dETC) A specialized class of y.6 T cells found in the skin of mice and some other species, but not humans. All dETCs have the same y:8 T-cell receptor; their function is unknown.

Desensitization A therapeutic procedure in which an allergic individual is exposed to increasing doses of allergen with the goal of inhibiting their allergic reactions. It probably works by shifting the balance between CD4 TH 1 and TH2 cells and thus changing the antibody produced from IgE to IgG.

Diapedesis The movement of white blood cells from the blood across blood vessel walls into tissues.

DiGeorge syndrome A recessive genetic immunodeficiency disease in which thymic epithelium fails to develop.

Diphtheria toxin The toxin secreted by the bacterium *Corynebac terium diphtheriae*, the cause of diphtheria, which causes the disease symptoms. The diphtheria vaccine consists of an inactive form of the toxin called diphtheria toxoid.

Direct pathway of allorecognition Type of alloreactive response in which T cells of the recipient of a transplant are stimulated by direct interaction of their receptors with the allogeneic HLA molecules expressed by dendritic cells from the donor, present in the transplant.

Directional selection Type of natural selection that replaces older alleles with newer variants (for example in the MHC). Its characteristic outcome is change.

Diversity (D) gene segments Short DNA sequences present in immunoglobulin heavy-chain loci and in T-cell receptor 13- and 6-chain loci. In the rearranged functional genes at these loci, a D region connects the V and J regions.

Double-negative thymocyte Immature T cell within the thymus that expresses neither CD4 nor CD8.

Double-positive thymocyte T cell at an intermediate stage of development in the thymus. It expresses both CD4 and CD8.

Draining lymph node The lymph node to which extracellular fluid collected at a site of infection first travels.

Eczema A common skin disease of children, appearing as scaly, reddened and itchy patches on the skin. Its etiology is poorly understood. Also called atopic dermatitis.

Edema Abnormal accumulation of fluid in connective tissue, leading to swelling.

Effector cells Lymphocytes that can mediate the removal of pathogens from the body without the need for further differentiation.

Effector mechanisms The physiological and cellular processes used by the immune system to destroy pathogens and remove them from the body.

Efferent lymphatic vessel The single vessel in which lymph and lymphocytes leave a lymph node en route to the blood.

Encapsulated bacteria Bacteria that possess thick carbohydrate coats that protect them from phagocytosis. Encapsulated bacteria cause extracellular infections and can be dealt with by phagocytes only if the bacteria are first coated with antibody and complement.

Endocytic vesicle Membrane vesicle that is pinched off from the plasma membrane and takes extracellular material into cells.

Endocytosis The uptake of extracellular material into cells by endocytic vesicles that form by pinching off pieces of plasma membrane.

Engraftment The time at which a bone marrow transplant is making new blood cells.

Eosinophil White blood cell that is one of the three types of granulocyte. It contains granules that stain with eosin and whose contents are secreted when the cell is stimulated. Eosinophils contribute chiefly to defense against parasitic infections.

Eotaxin-1 and eotaxin-2 Chemokines that act specifically on eosinophils. Now called CXCLI I and CXCL24, respectively.

Epidemic An outbreak of infectious disease that affects many individuals within a population.

Epitope The portion of an antigenic molecule that is bound by an antibody or gives rise to the MHC-binding peptide that is recognized by a T-cell receptor. Also called an antigenic determinant.

Extravasation The movement of cells or fluid from within blood vessels to the surrounding tissues.

F(a13')2 A proteolytic fragment of IgG that consists of the two Fab arms held together by a disulfide bond. It is produced by digesting IgG with pepsin.

Fab fragment A proteolytic fragment of IgG that consists of the light chain and the amino-terminal half of the heavy chain held together by an interchain disulfide bond. It is called Fab because it is the Fragment with antigen binding specificity. In the intact IgG molecule the parts corresponding to the Fab fragment are often called Fab or Fab arms.

Factor B Plasma protein that binds to C3(OH) or C3b and is cleaved to form part of the C3 convertases (C3(OH),Bb and C3b,Bb) in the alternative pathway of complement activation.

Factor D Plasma protease that cleaves factor B to Bb and Ba in the alternative pathway of complement activation.

Factor H A complement regulatory protein of plasma that inactivates the C3 convertase of the alternative pathway and C5 convertases by binding to C3b and rendering it susceptible to cleavage by factor I to produce inactive iC3b.

Factor I A regulatory protease of complement that can cleave C3b and C4b into inactive forms.

Farmer's lung A hypersensitivity disease caused by the interaction of IgG antibodies with large particles of inhaled allergen in the alveolar wall of the lung. The resulting inflammation compromises gas exchange by the lungs. The disease is caused by chronic exposure to large quantities of the allergen.

Fas A member of the TNF receptor family that is expressed on certain cells and makes them susceptible to killing by cells expressing Fas ligand, a cell-surface member of the TNF family of proteins. Binding of Fas ligand to Fas triggers apoptosis in the Fas-bearing cell.

Fc fragment A fragment of an antibody, resulting from proteolytic cleavage, that consists of the carboxy-terminal halves of the two heavy chains disulfide-bonded to each other by the residual hinge region. It is called Fc because it was the fragment that was most readily crystallized in early studies of IgG antibody structure. In an intact antibody the part corresponding to the Fc fragment is called **Fc, Fc region,** or **Fc piece**.

Fc receptors Cell-surface receptors for the Fc portion of some immunoglobulin isotypes. They include the Fey and Fcs receptors.

FCE receptor (FceRI) A receptor present on the surface of mast cells, basophils and activated eosinophils that binds free IgE with very high affinity. When antigen binds to IgE and cross-links FccRI it causes cellular activation and degranulation.

Fcyreceptors Receptors present on various cell types that are specific for the Fc regions of IgG antibodies. There are different receptors for different subclasses of IgG.

Fever A rise of body temperature above the normal. It is caused by cytokines produced in response to infection.

FK-binding proteins Another name for the cyclophilins that bind tacrolimus (FK506). *See also* **cyclophilins.**

Follicular center cell lymphoma A malignancy of mature B cells.

Follicular dendritic cells (FDCs) Characteristic nonlymphoid cells of follicles in secondary lymphoid tissues. They have long branching processes that make intimate contact with B cells and have Fc and complement receptors that hold antigen:antibody:complement complexes on their surfaces for long periods. These cells are crucial in selecting antigen-binding B cells during antibody responses.

Framework regions Relatively invariant regions within the variable domains of immunoglobulins and T-cell receptors that provide a protein scaffold for the hypervariable regions.

Freund's complete adjuvant An adjuvant consisting of an emulsion of mineral oil and water containing killed mycobacteria.

Fungi Single-celled and multicellular eukaryotic organisms, including the yeasts and molds, that can cause a variety of diseases. Immunity to fungi involves both humoral and cell-mediated responses.

Gene family A set of genes encoding proteins of similar structure, and often of similar function, such as the MHC class I genes.

Gene segments Multiple short DNA sequences in the immunoglobulin and T-cell receptor genes. These can be rearranged in many different combinations to produce the vast diversity of immunoglobulin or T- cell receptor polypeptide chains. *See also* **D gene segments; J gene segments; V gene segments.**

Genetic polymorphism Variation in a population due to the existence of two or more alleles of a gene.

Germinal center Area in secondary lymphoid tissue that is a site of intense B-cell proliferation, selection, maturation, and death. Germinal centers form around follicular dendritic cell networks when activated B cells migrate into lymphoid follicles.

Germline configuration The organization of the immunoglobulin and T-cell receptor genes in the DNA of germ cells and in the vast majority of somatic cells that do not undergo somatic recombination.

GlyCAM-1 A vascular addressin found on the high endothelial venules of lymphoid tissues. It is an important ligand for the L-selectin molecule on naive lymphocytes and directs these cells to leave the blood and enter the lymphoid tissues.

Granulocyte Colony-stimulating factor (G-CSF) A glycoprotein of 20 kDa produced by macrophages, endothelial cells, and fibroblasts. It regulates the maturation of granulocyte progenitors into mature neutrophils. The term *colony-stimulating factor* refers to its ability to promote the growth of bone marrow stem cell "colonies" in tissue culture.

Granulocyte-macrophage colony-stimulating factor (GM-CSF) A protein of 14 kDa produced by T cells, macrophages, fibroblasts, and endothelial cells. It is the major regulator of granulocyte and macrophage stem cells. It induces phagocytosis, superoxide production, and ADCC by neutrophils.

Goodpasture's syndrome An autoimmune disease in which autoantibodies against type IV collagen of the basement membrane of blood vessel endothelium cause extensive vasculitis.

Graft-versus-host disease (GVHD) Pathological condition caused by the **graft-versus-host reaction (GVHR),** which is the response of mature donor-derived T cells in transplanted bone marrow against the alloantigens of the recipient's tissues.

Graft-versus-leukemia (GVL) effect An effect in bone marrow transplantation as therapy for leukemia where some degree of genetic incompatibility between donor and recipient is thought to help T cells or NK cells from the transplant to eliminate residual leukemia cells in the recipient. Also known as a **graft-versus-tumor effect.**

Granulocyte-macrophage colony-stimulating factor (GM-CSF) A cytokine involved in the growth and differentiation of cells in the granulocyte and monocyte lineages.

Granulocytes White blood cells with irregularly shaped, multilobed nuclei and cytoplasmic granules. There are three types of granulocyte: neutrophils, eosinophils, and basophils. They are also known as polymorphonuclear leukocytes.

Granuloma A site of chronic inflammation usually triggered by persistent infectious agents such as mycobacteria, or by a nondegradable foreign body. Granulomas have a central area of macrophages, often fused into multinucleate giant cells, surrounded by T lymphocytes.

Granulysin A membrane-perturbing protein present in the granules of cytotoxic T cells. With perforin it is thought to make pores in the target cell's membrane.

Granzymes Serine esterases present in the granules of cytotoxic T cells and NK cells. On entering the cytosol of a target cell, granzymes induce apoptosis of the target. Also called fragmentins.

Graves' disease An autoimmune disease in which antibodies against the thyroid-stimulating hormone receptor cause the overproduction of thyroid hormone and the symptoms of hyperthyroidism.

Gut-associated lymphoid tissues (GAIT) Lymphoid tissues closely associated with the gastrointestinal tract, including the palatine tonsils, Payer's patches in the intestine, and layers of intraepithelial lymphocytes.

HAART *see* **highly active anti-retroviral therapy** HANE *see* **hereditary angioneurotic edema**

Haploidentical transplant A transplant from a donor who shares one HLA haplotype with the patient but differs in the second.

Haplotype In respect of a linked cluster of polymorphic genes, the set of alleles carried on a single chromosome is called a haplotype. Every person inherits two haplotypes, one from each parent. The term was first used in connection with the genes of the major histocompatibility complex.

Hashimoto's thyroiditis An autoimmune disease characterized by persistent high levels of antibodies against thyroid-specific antigens. These antibodies recruit NK cells to the thyroid, leading to damage and inflammation.

Heavy chain (H chain) The larger of the two component polypeptides of an immunoglobulin molecule. Heavy chains come in a variety of heavy-chain classes or isotypes, each of which confers a distinctive effector function on the antibody molecule.

Helper CD4 T cells CD4 T cells are sometimes generally known as helper cells because their function is to help other cell types to perform their functions. The term helper T cell sometimes refers to TH2 cells only, the cells that help B cells to produce antibody.

Hematopoiesis The generation of the cellular elements of blood, including the red blood cells, white blood cells, and platelets. These cells all originate from pluripotent **hematopoietic stem cells** whose differentiated progeny divide under the influence of various **hematopoietic growth factors.**

Hematopoietic stem cell transplantation Any transplantation in which the role of the graft is to replace the hematopoietic system. Sources of hematopoietic stem cells include bone marrow and umbilical cord blood.

Hemolytic anemia of the newborn A potentially fatal disease caused by maternal IgG antibodies directed towards paternal antigens expressed on fetal red blood cells. The usual target of this response is the Rh blood group antigen. Maternal anti-Rh IgG antibodies cross the placenta to attack the fetal red blood cells. Also called erythroblastosis fetalis.

Herd immunity The phenomenon whereby those people in a population who have no protective immunity against a pathogen are largely protected from infection when the majority of the population is resistant to the pathogen.

Hereditary angioneurotic edema (HANE) A genetic disease due to deficiency of the Cl inhibitor of the complement system. In the absence of Cl inhibitor, spontaneous activation of the complement system causes diffuse fluid leakage from blood vessels, the most serious consequence of which is epiglottal swelling leading to suffocation.

Heterozygous Describes an individual who has inherited different forms (alleles) of a given gene from their two parents.

Highly active anti-retroviral therapy (HAART) Combination therapy for HIV infection, in which several antiviral drugs are used together to try and avoid the rapid generation of drug-resistant mutant viruses that occurs when one of the drugs is used alone.

Highly polymorphic Genes that have many alleles and for which most individuals in a population are heterozygotes.

Histamine A vasoactive amine stored in mast cell granules. Histamine is released when antigen binds to IgE molecules on mast cells and causes dilation of local blood vessels and contraction of smooth muscle, producing some of the symptoms of immediate hypersensitivity reactions. Antihistamines are drugs that counter histamine action.

Histocompatibility Literally, the ability of tissues (Greek *histo*) to get along with each other. The term is used in immunology to describe the genetic systems that determine the rejection of tissue and organ grafts as a result of the immunological recognition of alloantigens (known in this context as **histocompatibility antigens).**

Hives Itchy red swellings in the skirt caused by IgE-mediated reactions. Also called urticaria or nettle rash.

HLA The acronym for Human Leukocyte Antigen. It is the genetic designation for the human MHC. Individual loci are designated by capital letters, as in HLA-A, and alleles are designated by numbers, as in HLA-A*0201.

HLA class I molecules The name for the human version of the **MHC class I molecules.**

HLA class II molecules The name for the human version of the **MHC class II molecules.**

HLA-A, HLA-B, and HLA-C The highly polymorphic human MHC class I genes.

HLA-DM An invariant MHC class II molecule in humans that is involved in the intracellular loading of MHC class II molecules with peptides.

HLA-DO A relatively invariant human MHC class II molecule. Although not precisely defined, the function of HLA-DO is thought to modify that of HLA-DM.

HLA-DP, HLA-DQ, and HLA-DR The highly polymorphic human MHC class II molecules. Each class II molecule is made from a and 13 chains encoded by A and B genes respectively. For example, the HLA-DPa and HLA-DP13 chains are encoded by the HLA-DPA and HLA-DPB genes respectively. All the genes are in the MHC.

HLA-E, HLA-G Relatively invariant human MHC class I molecules that form ligands for NK-cell receptors.

HLA-F A monomorphic human MHC class I molecule of unknown function.

HLA type the combination of HLA class I and class II allotypes that a person expresses.

Hodgkin's disease A malignant disease caused by transformed germinal center B cells.

Homing The movement of naive T cells into secondary lymphoid tissues, or of effector T cells to an effector site.

Homozygous Describes an individual who has inherited the same form (allele) of a given gene from both parents.

Human immunodeficiency virus (HIV) The causative agent of the acquired immune deficiency syndrome (AIDS). HIV is a retrovirus of the lentivirus family that infects CD4 T cells, leading to their slow depletion, which eventually results in immunodeficiency.

Human leukocyte antigen (HLA) complex The human major histocompatibility complex (MHC).

Humanize To replace, by means of genetic engineering, the CDR loops in a human antibody with the corresponding CDR sequences of a desired specificity from a mouse antibody.

Humoral immunity Immunity that is mediated by antibodies and can therefore be transferred to a nonimmune recipient by serum.

Hybridomas Hybrid cell lines that make monoclonal antibodies of defined specificity They are formed by fusing a specific antibody-producing B lymphocyte with a myeloma cell that grows in tissue culture and does not make any immunoglobulin chains of its own.

Hygiene hypothesis Hypothesis advanced to explain the increasing incidence of hypersensitivity and autoimmune diseases in developed countries, in which the increase is proposed to be due to widespread hygiene, vaccination, and antibiotic therapy, preventing children's immune systems from becoming used to dealing correctly with infections.

Hyperacute rejection Rejection of an allogeneic tissue graft as a result of preformed antibodies that react against A,B4O blood group antigens or HLA class I antigens on the graft. The antibodies bind to endothelium and trigger the blood clotting cascade, leading to ischemia and death of the transplanted organ or tissue.

Hyper-IgM syndrome A genetically determined X-linked immunodeficiency disease in which B cells cannot switch their immunoglobulin heavy-chain isotype. It arises from the absence of CD40 ligand.

Hypereosinophilia Abnormally high numbers of eosinophils in the blood.

Hypersensitivity reactions Immune responses to innocuous antigens that lead to symptomatic reactions on re-exposure. These can cause **hypersensitivity diseases** If they occur repetitively. This state of heightened reactivity to an antigen is called hypersensitivity. Hypersensitivity reactions are classified by mechanism: type I hypersensitivity reactions involve the triggering of mast cells by IgE antibodies; type II hypersensitivity reactions involve IgG antibodies against cell-surface or matrix antigens; type III hypersensitivity reactions involve antigen: antibody complexes; and type IV hypersensitivity reactions are mediated by effector T cells.

Hyperthyroid Refers to an abnormally high production of thyroid hormones by the thyroid gland.

Hypervariable regions (HV regions) Small regions of high amino acid sequence diversity within the variable regions of immunoglobulin and T-cell receptors. They correspond to the complementarity-determining regions.

ICAM-1, ICAM-2, and ICAM-3 The three different types of ICAM. *See also* **intercellular adhesion molecules**.

Iccosomes Immune-complex coated bodies. Small fragments of membrane coated with immune complexes that bud off from the processes of follicular dendritic cells in lymphoid follicles.

IDDM *see* **insulin-dependent diabetes mellitus**

IFN-a, IFN-f3, IFN-y *see* **interferons**

Ig domain *see* **immunoglobulin domains Iga, Ig13** *see* **B-cell antigen receptor**

IgA The class of immunoglobulin having a heavy chains. IgA antibodies in dimeric form are the antibodies present in mucosa] secretions. IgA in monomeric form is present in the blood.

IgD The class of immunoglobulin having ö heavy chains. It appears as surface immunoglobulin on mature naive B cells but its function is unknown.

IgE The class of immunoglobulin having e heavy chains. It is involved in allergic reactions.

IgG The class of immunoglobulin having y heavy chains. It is the most abundant class of immunoglobulin in plasma.

IgM The class of immunoglobulin having u heavy chains. It is the first immunoglobulin to appear on the surface of B cells and the first antibody secreted during an immune response. It is secreted in pentameric form.

Interferon-a (IFN-a) Produced in at least 23 different variants, with molecular masses ranging from 19 to 26 kDa. It has a common conserved sequence region but highly variable amino terminus. It is produced in large quantities by plasmacytic dendritic cells and in much smaller amounts by lymphocytes, monocytes, and macrophages. It activates NK cell mediated cytotoxic activity, and it stimulates the differentiation of monocytes into dendritic cells, as well as the maturation and activity of dendritic cells. IFN-a also drives certain -y/6 T cell responses. It has, of course, potent antiviral activities.

Interferon-I3 (IFN-I3) A 20-kDa protein produced by fibro-blasts and is coded for by a single gene in most mammals. Produced in response to viral infections, it has similar properties to IFN-a.

Interferon-y (IFN-y) The only type II interferon, it is a 17-kDa glycoprotein produced mainly by CD4+ THl cells, by some CD8 T cells, and by NK cells. IFN-7 acts on B cells, T cells, NK cells, and macrophages and is the key mediator of cell-mediated immune responses.

Interferon-a (IFN-co) A protein of 20 kDa produced by lymphocytes and monocytes and human, horse, pig, rabbit,and dog trophoblast cells. It has significant antiviral activity.

Interferon-T (IFN-c) A protein of 20 kDa produced by ruminant trophoblast cells during early pregnancy. It regulates immune responses in the placenta.

Interferon-8 (IFN-43) A protein of 19 kDa produced by pig trophoblast cells. It probably controls the maternal immune response to the fetus.

Interferon -? (IFN-X) A collective name for IL-28A, IL-28B, and IL-29. All are 20-kDa proteins distantly related to the 1L-10 family. All three use a distinct receptor system to trigger antiviral defense.

Interleukin-1 (IL-1) A family of at least 11 proteins produced by macrophages, dendritic cells, T cells, B cells, NK cells, vascular endothelium, fibroblasts, and keratinocytes. They originate as 31-1(Da procytokines but are cleaved by caspase-1 to 17-1(Da active peptides. The two most important forms of IL-1 act on TH2 cells, B cells, NK cells, neutrophils, eosinophils, dendritic cells, fibroblasts, endothelial cells, and hepatocytes. It is a proinflammatory mediator and a TH2 cell stimulator.

Interleukin-2 (IL-2) A 15.4-kDa glycoprotein produced by THl and NK cells. Its targets include other T cells, B cells, and NK cells. IL-2 activates helper and cytotoxic T cells and NK cells. 1L-2 stimulates T cell proliferation and cytotoxicity.

Interleukin-3 (IL-3) A 15-kDa protein produced by activated T cells, NK cells, eosinophils, and mast cells. It is a hematopoietic growth factor that stimulates the growth and maturation of bone marrow stem cells for eosinophils, neutrophils, and monocytes.

Interleukin-4 (IL-4) A 15-kDa protein produced by activated TH2 cells, mast cells, and activated basophils. It acts on B cells, T cells, macrophages, endothelial cells, fibroblasts, and mast cells. IL-4 stimulates the growth and differentiation of B cells.

Interleukin-5 (IL-5) A 26-kDa disulfide-linked homodimeric glycoprotein produced by activated TH2 cells, mast cells, and eosinophils. In humans its main activity is the control of eosinophil production.

Interleukin-6 (IL-6) A 20- to 30-kDa glycoprotein that occurs in at least 5 isoforms. It is produced by activated macro-phages, T and B cells, mast cells, vascular endothelial cells, fibroblasts, keratinocytes, and mesangial cells. It is also produced by muscle cells during exercise. It acts on T cells, B cells, hepatocytes, and bone marrow stromal cells as well as the brain.

Interleukin-7 (IL-7) A 17-kDa glycoprotein produced by bone marrow and thymic stromal cells. It regulates the activity of lymphoid stem cells. Its major role, however, is to control lymphocyte function by regulating V(D).1 recombination in both B and T cells.

Interleukin-8 (IL-8) The prototypical chemokine (CXCL8). Like other chemokines, it is a relatively small (8.4-kDa) protein produced by macrophages and endothelial cells. IL-8 attracts and activates neutrophils.

Interleukin-9 (IL-9) A 14-kDa stem cell growth factor produced by TH2 cells. It promotes the growth of helper T cells and mast cells. It also potentiates the effects of IL-4 on IgE production.

Interleukin-10 (IL-10) An 18.6-kDa nonglycosylated homodimeric protein that acts as an immunosuppressive and anti-inflammatory cytokine that suppresses inflammation as well as T cell, NK cell, and macrophage function. It is mainly produced by TH2 cells but also from M2 cells, NK cells, and some dendritic cells. Its targets are THl cells, B cells, macrophages, NK cells, and mast cells.

Interleukin-11 (IL-11) A 19-kDa nonglycosylated protein produced by bone marrow stromal cells, epithelial cells, and fibroblasts. It stimulates B cell growth in association with IL-6. IL-11 also stimulates megakaryocyte formation in association with IL-3 and promotes the production of acute phase proteins.

Interleukin-12 (IL-12) A 75-kDa heterodimer consisting of disulfide-linked 35- and 40-kDa subunits (p35 and p40). It is produced by monocytes and macrophages, dendritic cells, B cells, and keratinocytes. It is the major activator of TH1 cells and NK cells.

Interleukin-13 (IL-13) A 12.5-kDa glycoprotein produced by TH2 cells, cytotoxic T cells, mast cells, and dendritic cells. It has biological activities similar to those of IL-4, because it acts through a receptor (CD213) that shares a common a chain with the IL-4R.

Interleukin-14 (IL-14) A 53-kDa glycoprotein produced by T cells and some malignant B cells. It is a B cell growth factor that inhibits immunoglobulin secretion and selectively expands some B cell subpopulations.

Interleukin-15 (IL-15) A 14-kDa glycoprotein produced by activated macrophages, dendritic cells, endothelial cells, and fibroblasts. It shares many biological activities with IL-2. IL-15 acts as a T cell, B cell, and NK cell growth factor. IL-15 is essential for the prolonged survival of memory T cells.

Interleukin-16 (IL-16) A 13-kDa protein produced by CDS' T cells, eosinophils, dendritic cells, and mast cells. Its receptor is CD4 through which IL-16 regulates CD4 T cell recruitment and activation, it also acts on eosinophils and macrophages.

Interleukin-17 (IL-17) A mixture of at least 6 proteins produced mainly by TH17 helper cells. They exist as 31- to 40-kDa disulfide-linked homodimers. IL-17 molecules stimulate macrophages and endothelial cells to secrete proinflammatory cytokines and chemokines leading to the recruitment and activation of neutrophils. IL-17 thus appears to play a key role in the development of acute inflammation.

Interleukin-18 (IL-18) A member of the IL-1 family that is produced, like IL-1, by antigen-presenting cells. It originates as a 24-kDa pro-protein that is cleaved by caspase-1 to an 18-kDa active molecule. It activates THl cells to promote the production of IFN-7, TNF-a, IL-1, CD95L, and several chemokines. This can lead to positive feedback where the IL-18 and IFN-y reinforce each other's activities.

Interleukin-19 (1L-19) An 18-kDa protein and a member of the IL-10 family produced by B cells and activated monocytes. It is a proinflammatory cytokine that acts on monocytes to stimulate production of IL-1, IL-6, and TNF-a.

Interleukin-20 (IL-20) A 35.2-kDa homodimeric protein and a member of the IL-10 family. It is produced by monocytes and keratinocytes and acts as a hematopoietic growth factor.

Interleukin-21 (IL-21) A protein of 15-kDa produced by activated TH2 cells and structurally related to IL-2 and IL-15. It regulates NK, B, and T cell function. It up-regulates production of IL-18R and IFNI/.

Interleukin-22 (IL-22) A 33.6-kDa homodimeric protein and a member of the IL-10 family produced by activated TH17 cells and mast cells. It induces acute-phase protein production in the liver. IL-22 acts on cells of the skin and digestive and respiratory systems to increase expression of several P-defensins and presumably promotes innate immunity in these tissues.

Interleukin-23 (IL-23) A heterodimer consisting of a 19kDa peptide chain (IL-23p19) paired with the IL-12p40 chain. IL-23 is produced by macrophages, dendritic cells, and activated 7/6 T cells. It is a major cytokine produced by activated M1 cells. It stimulates TH17 cells to secrete IL-17 and IL-22, and these T cells in turn promote acute neutrophil-mediated inflammation.

Interleukin-24 (IL-24) A 37-kDa dimeric protein is a member of the IL-10 family produced by activated monocytes and TH2 cells. It is involved in antitumor activity since it stimulates apoptosis in many tumor cell lines and stimulates acute phase responses in hepatocytes. It may play a role in wound healing.

Interleukin-25 (IL-25) Unassigned.

Interleukin-26 (IL-26) A 37-kDa protein is a member of the IL-10 family produced by virus-transformed CD4±T cells, activated memory cells, and activated T and NK cells. It induces the proliferation of keratinocytes and T cells. It signals through a novel receptor composed of IL-20 receptor 1 and IL-10 receptor 2.

Interleukin-27 (IL-27) A heterodimer with one chain (p28) also called 1L-30 and the other called EB-13 related to IL-12p40. It is expressed by activated monocytes and dendritic cells. 1L-27 suppresses the activation of all three helper T cell subsets and prevents neutrophil activation. It thus serves a major regulatory role.

Interleukin-28 (IL-28) Two protein isoforms of 22 kDa produced by virus-infected cells. 1FN-2 (1L-28A) and IFN-3 (IL-28B) share a common three-dimensional structure with IL-ID but have limited sequence similarity.

Interleukin-29 (IL-29) (IFN-A,1) A 20-kDa member of the IL-10 family produced by virus-infected cells. It is an interferon closely related to IL-28A and IL-28B.

Interleukin-30 (IL-30) A 2841 protein secreted by antigen-presenting cells. It forms one chain of heterodimeric IL-27. It acts on naive CD4 T cells. It synergizes strongly with IL-12 to promote IFN-y production by THl cells.

Interleukin-31 (IL-31) A 15.5-kDa protein related to 1L-6. It is produced by stimulated TH2 cells. Its receptor is expressed on keratinocytes and induced on monocytes by IFN-y. It may be involved in the pathogenesis of allergic skin diseases.

Interleukin-32 (IL-32) A protein of 15 kDa that exists in four isoforms. It is produced by activated human lymphocytes, NK cells, and endothelial cells. It acts on macrophages to enhance the production of TNF-a, IL-113, IL-6, and IL-8.

Interleukin-33 (IL-33) An 18-kDa member of the IL-1 family that serves as a matched counterpart to IL-18. Like IL-1, it is derived from cleavage of a 31-kDa precursor by caspase-1. IL-33 is expressed by endothelial and smooth muscle cells. It is a chromatin-associated nuclear factor. It acts through an IL-1 receptor to drive production of IL-4, IL-5, and IL-13 by TH2 cells. IL-33 may play a key role in TH2 diseases.

Immature dendritic cells Dendritic cells present in tissues, which take up antigen but do not express co-stimulatory molecules and cannot yet act as professional antigen-presenting cells to naive T cells.

Immediate reactions Reactions occurring within minutes of exposure to antigen. They are mediated by preexisting antibodies in the circulation. Also called immediate hypersensitivity reactions.

Immune Resistant to infection.

Immune complex The protein complex formed from the binding of antibodies to soluble antigens. The size of the immune complexes formed depends on the relative concentrations of antigen and antibody. Large immune complexes are cleared by phagocytes bearing Fc and complement receptors. Small soluble immune complexes tend to be deposited on the walls of small blood vessels, where they can activate complement and cause damage.

Immune-complex **coated bodies** *see* **iccosomes**

Immune stimulatory complexes (ISCOMs) Lipid carriers that act as adjuvants.

Immune system The tissues, cells, and molecules involved in host defense mechanisms, primarily against infectious agents.

Immunity The ability to resist infection.

Immunization The deliberate provocation of an adaptive immune response by introducing antigen into the body.

Immunodeficiency diseases A group of inherited or acquired disorders in which some part or parts of host defense are either absent or defective.

Immunogenetics A subfield of immunology that was originally concerned with the analysis of genetic traits by means of antibodies against genetically polymorphic molecules such as blood group antigens and NIHC proteins. Immunogenetics now encompasses the genetic analysis, by any technique, of molecules that are of specific importance to the immune system.

Immunoglobulin A *see* **IgA Immunoglobulin D** *see* **IgD**

Immunoglobulin domains (Ig domains) Components of protein structure consisting of about 100 amino acids that fold into a sandwich of two 13 sheets held together by a disulfide bond. **Immunoglobulin** heavy and light chains are made up of a series of immunoglobulin domains. Similar domains are present in many other proteins.

Immunoglobulin E *see* **IgE Irnmunoglobulin G** *see* **IgG Immunoglobulin M** *see* **IgM**

Immunoglobulin superfamily (Ig superfarnily) The name given to all the proteins that contain one or more immunoglobulin or immuno glob ulin - like domains.

Immunoglobulin-like domains Protein domains that resemble the immunoglobulin domain in structure but are present in a variety of other proteins.

Immunoglobulins (Ig) The antigen-binding molecules of B cells.

Immunological memory The capacity of the immune system to make quicker and stronger adaptive immune responses to successive encounters with an antigen. Immunological memory is specific for a particular antigen and is long-lived.

Immunoph ilins Intracellular proteins with peptidyl-prolyl *cis-trans* isomerase activity that bind the immunosuppressive drugs cyclosporin A, tacrolimus, and sirolimus (rapamycin).

Immunoreceptor tyrosine-based Activation motifs (ITAMs) sequences in the cytoplasmic domains of membrane receptors that are sites of tyrosine phosphorylation and of association with tyrosine ldnases and phosphotyrosine-binding proteins involved in signal transduction . Related motifs with opposing effects are **immunoreceptor tyrosine-based inhibitory motifs (ITIMs),** which recruit phosphatases that remove the phosphate groups added by tyrosine kinases.

Immunosuppressive drugs Compounds that inhibit adaptive immune responses.

Inactivated virus vaccines *see* **killed virus vaccines**

Indirect pathway of allorecognition One means by which alloreactive T cells in a transplant recipient can be stimulated to react against the transplant. The alloreactive T cells do not directly recognize the transplanted cells but recognize subcellular material that has been processed and presented by autologous antigen-presenting cells.

Inflarrunation A general term for the local accumulation of fluid, plasma proteins, and white blood cells that is initiated by physical injury, infection, or a local immune response. This is also known as an **inflammatory response.** The cells that invade tissues undergoing inflammatory responses are often called **inflammatory cells** or an inflammatory **infiltrate.**

Inflammatory mediators A variety of substances released by various cell types that contribute to the production of inflammation at a site of infection or trauma.

Influenza hemagglutinin A glycoprotein of the influenza virus coat that binds to certain carbohydrates on human cells, the first step in viral infection. Changes in the hemagglutinin are the major source of antigenic shift.

Innate immunity The host defense mechanisms that act from the start of an infection and do not adapt to a particular pathogen. Also called the **innate immune response.**

Insulin-dependent diabetes mellitus (IDDM) An autoimmune disease in which insulin-secreting 13 cells of the pancreatic islets of Langerhans are gradually destroyed.

Insulitis An infiltration of the pancreatic islets of Langerhans with lymphocytes and other leukocytes. This is a symptom of incipient diabetes.

Integrins A class of cell-surface glycoproteins that mediate adhesive interactions between cells and the extracellular matrix.

Interallelic conversion A mechanism of genetic recombination between two alleles of a locus in which a segment of one allele is replaced with the homologous segment from the other. This mechanism is used to generate new HLA class I and II alleles.

Intercellular adhesion molecules (ICAMs) Ligands for the leukocyte integrins that enable lymphocytes and other leukocytes to bind to other cells, including antigen-presenting cells and endothelial cells.

Interdigitating reticular cells *see* **dendritic cells**

Interferons Cytolcines that help cells to resist viral infection. **Interferon-a (IFN-a)** and **interferon-0 (IFN-0)** are produced by leukocytes and fibroblasts respectively, as well as by other cells, whereas **interferon-y (IFN-y)** is a product of CD4 TH1 cells, CDB T cells, and NK cells. IFN-y acts principally to activate macrophages.

Interferon response Changes in the expression of a variety of genes in cells exposed to interferon.

Interferon-producing cells (IPCs) Specialized lymphocyte-like cells in the blood that secrete up to 1000-fold more type I interferon than other cells. *See also* plasmacytoid **dendritic cells**.

Interleuldn (IL) A generic term used for many of the cytokines produced by leukocytes. *See also* **IL-1, IL-2, IL-3,** etc.

Intermolecular epitope spreading The process by which the immune response initially reacts against an epitope of one antigenic molecule and then progresses to epitopes on different proteins.

Intramolecular epitope spreading The process by which the immune response initially reacts against epitopes in one part of an antigenic molecule and then progresses to other, noncross-reactive, epitopes of the same molecule.

Invariant chain (Ii) Polypeptide that associates with major histocompatibility complex (IVIHC) class II proteins in the endoplasmic reticulum and prevents them from binding peptides there. It guides the MHC class II molecules to endosomes where Ii is degraded, enabling MHC class II molecules to bind peptides present in the endosomes.

Ischemia Deficient blood supply due to obstructed blood vessels. **ISCOMs** *see* **immune stimulatory complexes**

Islets of Langerhans The endocrine hormone-producing tissue of the pancreas, which includes the p. cells that produce insulin.

Isoforms The different forms of a protein that are encoded by the alleles of a gene or by different but closely related genes.

Isograft A tissue or organ graft from one genetically identical individual to another.

Isotype switching The process by which a B cell changes the class of immunoglobulin made while preserving the antigenic specificity of the immunoglobulin. Isotype switching involves somatic recombination that attaches a different heavy-chain constant-region gene to the variable-region exon.

Isotypes Classes of immunoglobulin IgM, IgG, IgD, IgA, and IgE each of which has a distinct heavy-chain constant region encoded by a different constant-region gene. The heavy-chain constant region determines the effector properties of each antibody class.

J gene segments *see* **joining (J) gene segments**

Janus kinases (JAKs) A family of tyrosine kinases that transduce activating signals from cytokine receptors.

Joining (J) gene segments One of the types of gene segment in immunoglobulin and T-cell receptor genes that is rearranged to make functional variable-region exons.

Junctional diversity Diversity present in immunoglobulin and T-cell receptor polypeptides that is created during the process of gene rearrangement by the addition of nucleotides into the junctions between gene segments.

kappa (Ic) One of the two types of immunoglobulin light chain.

Killed virus vaccines Vaccincs that contain viral particles that have been deliberately killed by heat, chemicals, or radiation.

Killer cell immunoglobulin-like receptors (Mils) Receptors on NK cells that bind to MHC class I molecules and can send either activating or inhibitory signals to the NK cell.

Kupffer cells Phagocytic cells of the liver that line the hepatic sinusoids. X5 *see* **pre-B-cell receptor**

L chain *see* **light chain**

L-selectin An adhesion molecule of the selectin family found on lymphocytes. It binds to CD34 and GlyCAM-1 on high endothelial venules to initiate the migration of naive lymphocytes into secondary lymphoid tissue.

lambda(k) One of the two types of immunoglobulin light chain.

Langerhans' cells Phagocytic dendritic cells found in the epidermis. They can migrate in lymph from the epidermis to lymph nodes, where they differentiate into dendritic cells.

Large granular lymphocytes *see* **natural killer cells**

Large pre-B cells Immature B cells that have a cell-surface pre-B-cell receptor.

Late pro-B cell *see* **pro-B cell**

Late-phase reaction That part of a type 1 immediate hypersensitivity reaction that occurs 7-12 hours after contact with antigen and is resistant to treatment with antihistamine.

Latency A state adopted by some viruses in which they have entered cells but do not replicate.

Lectin pathway of complement activation One of the three pathways of complement activation. It is activated by the binding of a mannose-binding lectin present in blood plasma to mannose-containing peptidoglycans on bacterial surfaces. *See also* **alternative pathway of complement activation; classical** pathway of **complement activation**.

Lentiviruses Group of slow retroviruses that includes the human immunodeficiency virus (HIV). They have a long incubation period and disease can take years to become apparent.

Leukemia The unrestrained proliferation of a malignant white blood cell characterized by abnormally high numbers of white cells in the blood. A leukemia can be lymphocytic, myelocytic, or monocytic depending on the type of white blood cell that became malignant.

Leukocyte A general term for a white blood cell. Lymphocytes, granulocytes, and monocytes are all leukocytes.

Leukocyte adhesion deficiency An immunodeficiency disease in which the common 13 chain of the leukocyte integrins is absent. This mainly affects the ability of leukocytes to enter sites infected with extracellular pathogens, so such infections cannot be effectively eradicated.

Leukocytosis Increased numbers of leukocytes in the blood. It is commonly seen in acute infection.

LFA-1 *see* **lymphocyte function-associated antigen-1 LFA-3** *see* **lymphocyte function-associated antigen-3**.

Light chain (L chain) The smaller of the two types of polypeptide chain that make up immunoglobulins. It consists of one variable and one constant domain, and in the immunoglobulin molecule it is disulfide-bonded to a heavy chain.

Light zone The part of a germinal center in secondary lymphoid tissue that contains nondividing centrocytes interacting with follicular dendritic cells.

Linear epitope Epitope of a protein recognized by antibody that consists of a linear sequence of amino acids within the protein's primary structure.

Linkage disequilibrium (LD) The situation when particular alleles of two or more polymorphic genes (for example those comprising an

Live-attenuated viral vaccines Vaccines composed of live viruses that have an accumulation of mutations that impedes their growth in human cells and their capacity to cause disease.

LPS-binding protein Plasma protein that binds bacterial lipopolysaccharide (LPS) and delivers it to LPS receptors on neutrophils and macrophages.

Lymph Mixture of extracellular fluid and cells that is carried by the lymphatic system.

Lymph nodes A type of secondary lymphoid tissue found at many sites in the body where lymphatic vessels converge. Antigens are delivered by the lymph and presented to lymphocytes within the lymph node where adaptive immune responses are initiated.

Lymphatic vessels (lymphatics) Thin-walled vessels that carry lymph from tissues to secondary lymphoid tissues (with the exception of the spleen) and from secondary lymphoid tissues to the thoracic duct.

Lymphocyte function-associated antigen-1 (LFA-1) One of the leukocyte integrins that mediate the adhesion of lymphocytes, especially T cells, to endothelial cells and antigen-presenting cells.

Lymphocyte function-associated antigen-3 (LFA-3) Cell adhesion molecule of the immunoglobulin superfamily that is expressed on antigen-presenting cells (and other types of cell) and mediates their adhesion to T cells.

Lymphocytes A class of white blood cells that consist of small and large lymphocytes. The small lymphocytes bear variable cell-surface receptors for antigen and are responsible for adaptive immune responses. There are two main classes of small lymphocyte B lymphocytes (B cells) and T lymphocytes (T cells). Large granular lymphocytes are natural killer (NK) cells, lymphocytes of innate immunity.

Lymphoid Containing lymphocytes or pertaining to lymphocytes.

Lymphoid lineage All types of lymphocyte and the bone marrow cells that give rise to them.

Lymphoid organs (lymphoid tissues) Organized tissues that contain very large numbers of lymphocytes held in a nonlymphoid stroma. The primary lymphoid organs, where lymphocytes are generated, are the thymus and bone marrow. The main secondary lymphoid tissues, in which adaptive immune responses are initiated, are the lymph nodes, spleen, and mucosa-associated lymphoid tissues such as tonsils, Payer's patches, and the appendix.

Lymphoid progenitor Stem cell in bone marrow cell that gives rise to all lymphocytes.

Lymphokines Cytokines produced by lymphocytes.

Lymphomas Tumors of lymphocytes that grow in lymphoid and other tissues but do not enter the blood in large numbers.

Lymphotoxin (LT) A cytotoxic cytokine secreted by some CD4 T cells. Also known as tumor necrosis factor-13 (TNF-13).

Lytic granules Intracellular storage granules of cytotoxic T cells and NK cells that contain perforin and granzymes.

M cells Specialized cells in intestinal epithelium through which antigens and pathogens enter gut-associated lymphoid tissue from the intestines. Short for microfold cells.

Macrophage activation Stimulation of macrophages, which increases their phagocytic, antigen-presenting, and bacterial killing functions. It occurs in the course of infection.

Macrophages Large mononuclear phagocyte cells resident in most tissues. They are derived from blood monocytes and contribute to innate immunity and early nonadaptive phases of host defense. They function as professional antigen-presenting cells and as effector cells in humoral and cell-mediated immunity.

MAdCAM-1 Mucosal cell adhesion molecule-1, a mucosal addressin that is recognized by the lymphocyte surface proteins L-selectin and VLA-4. This interaction mediates the specific homing of lymphocytes to mucosal tissues.

Major basic protein A constituent of eosinophil granules that is released on eosinophil activation. It acts on mast cells to cause their degranulation.

Major histocompatibility complex (MHC) A cluster of genes on the short arm of human chromosome 6 that encodes a set of polymorphic membrane glycoproteins called the MHC molecules, which are involved in presenting peptide antigens to T cells.

Major histocompatibility complex (MHC) molecules *see* **MHC molecules**

Malignant transformation the changes that occur in a cell to make it cancerous.

Malignant tumors Tumors that are capable of uncontrolled and invasive growth.

Mannose-binding lectin (MBL) An acute phase protein in the blood that binds to mannose residues on pathogen surfaces and when bound activates the complement system. It is also known as **mannose-binding protein (MBP)** and **mannan-binding lectin.**

Mannose-binding protein pathway *see* **lectin-mediated pathway**

Mantle zone in lymphoid follicles, a rim of B lymphocytes that surrounds a follicle.

Mast cells Large bone marrow derived cells found resident in connective tissues throughout the body. They contain large granules that store a variety of chemical mediators including histamine. Mast cells have high-affinity Fee receptors (FceRI) that bind free IgE. Antigen binding to mast cell associated IgE triggers mast cell activation and degranulation, producing a local or systemic immediate hypersensitivity reaction. Mast cells have a crucial role in allergic reactions.

Mature B cells B cells that have IgM and IgD on their surface and are able to respond to antigen.

Mature dendritic cells Dendritic cells in secondary lymphoid tissues that express costimulatory molecules and other cell-surface molecules that enable them to present antigen to naive T cells and activate them.

Megakaryocytes Large cells of the erythroid lineage, produced in the bone marrow and resident there. They produce platelets.

Membrane cofactor protein (MCP) Complement regulatory protein on human cells that promotes the inactivation of C3b and C4b by factor I.

Membrane-attack complex The complex of terminal complement components that forms a pore in the membrane of the target cell, damaging the membrane and leading to cell lysis.

Memory B cells Long-lived antigen-specific B cells that are produced from activated naive B cells during the primary immune response to an antigen. On subsequent exposure to their specific antigen they are reactivated to differentiate into plasma cells as part of the secondary and subsequent immune responses.

Memory cells General term for lymphocytes that are responsible for the phenomenon of immunological memory and protective immunity.

Memory T cells Long-lived antigen-specific T cells that are activated in secondary and subsequent immune responses to an antigen.

Metastasis The spread of a tumor from its site of origin to other tissues. Some cells from the primary tumor invade other tissues and grow and divide to become secondary tumors.

Methotrexate Cytotoxic drug used to inhibit graft-versus-host reactions in bone marrow transplant recipients.

MHC class I molecules The class of MHC molecules that present peptides generated in the cytosol to CD8 T cells. They consist of a heterodimer of a class I heavy chain associated with 132-microglobulin.

MHC class II molecules The class of MHC molecules that present peptides generated in intracellular vesicles to CD4 T cells.

MHC class II transactivator (CIITA) A transcriptional activator of MHC class II genes. When defective it causes a type of bare lymphocyte syndrome.

MHC molecules Major histocompatibility complex molecules. Highly polymorphic glycoproteins encoded by the major histocompatibility complex (MHC). They form complexes with peptides and present peptide antigens to T cells. There are two classes MHC class I and MHC class II molecules with different roles in the immune response. They are also known as major histocompatibility antigens because they are the main alloantigens involved in the rejection of transplanted tissues.

MHC restriction The fact that a given T-cell receptor will recognize its peptide antigen only when the peptide is bound to a particular form of MHC molecule.

Minor histocompatibility antigens (minor H antigens) Peptides of polymorphic cellular proteins that can lead to graft rejection when they are bound by MHC molecules and recognized by T cells.

Minor histocompatibility loci The genes encoding proteins that can act as minor histocompatibility antigens.

Mixed lymphocyte reaction Cellular assay for detecting MHC differences between two individuals. The T cells from one individual proliferate in response to allogeneic MHC molecules on the cells of the other individual.

Molecular mimicry Antigenic similarity between a pathogen antigen and a cellular antigen, which results in the induction of antibodies or T cells that act against the pathogen but also cross-react with the self antigen.

Monoclonal antibodies Antibodies produced by a single clone of B lymphocytes and that are therefore identical in structure and antigen specificity.

Monocytes White blood cells with a bean-shaped nucleus. They are the precursors of tissue macrophages.

Monomorphic Having only one form. The term is used, for example, for genes that have only one allele.

Mucosa The mucus-secreting epithelia that line the respiratory, intestinal, and urogenital tracts. The conjunctiva of the eye and the mammary glands are also in this category.

Mucosa-associated lymphoid tissue (MALT) Aggregations of lymphoid cells in mucosal epithelia and in the lamina propria beneath. The main mucosa-associated lymphoid tissues are the gut-associated lymphoid tissues (GALT) and the bronchial-associated lymphoid tissues (BALT).

Mucosal surfaces *see* **mucosa**

Mucus Slimy protective secretion produced by many internal epithelia.

Multiple sclerosis A chronic progressive neurological disease characterized by patches of demyelination in the central nervous system and lymphocyte infiltration into the brain, it is believed to be an autoimmune disease.

Multivalent Having more than one binding site for the same or different ligands.

Mutagen Any agent, such as a chemical or radiation, which can cause a mutation.

Mutation An alteration in the DNA sequence of a gene.

Myasthenia gravis An autoimmune disease in which autoantibodies against the acetylcholine receptor on skeletal muscle cells cause a block of signal transmission from nerve to muscle at neuromuscular junctions, leading to progressive muscle weakness and eventually to death.

Myeloablative therapy A conditioning regime used before a bone marrow transplant. The recipient's immune system is destroyed with a combination of cytotoxic drugs and irradiation.

Myeloid lineage A subset of bone-marrow derived cells comprising granulocytes, monocytes, and macrophages.

Myeloid progenitors Stem cells in the bone marrow that give rise to granulocytes, monocytes, and macrophages.

Myelomas Tumors of plasma cells resident in bone marrow.

Myelopoiesis The production of monocytes and granulocytes in the bone marrow. N-nucleotides nucleotides added at the junctions between gene segments of T-cell receptor and immunoglobulin heavy-chain variable-region sequences during somatic recombination, which contribute to the diversity of these molecules. They are not encoded in the gene segments but are inserted by the enzyme terminal deoxynucleotidyltransferase (TdT).

Naive B cell A mature B cell that has left the bone marrow but has not yet encountered its specific antigen.

Naive T cell A mature T cell that has left the thymus but not yet encountered its specific antigen.

Natural cytotoxicity receptors (NCRs) A group of activating NK-cell receptors of the immunoglobulin superfamily.

Natural interferon-producing cells (NIPCs) *see* **interferon-producing cells**

Natural killer cells (NK cells) Large, granular, cytotoxic lymphocytes that circulate in the blood. NK cells are important in innate immunity to viruses and other intracellular pathogens and also kill certain tumor cells. They are the cytotoxic cells in antibody-dependent cell-mediated cytotoxicity (ADCC).

Necrosis the death of cells by lysis that results from chemical or physical injury. It leaves extensive cellular debris that must be removed by phagocytes. Neighboring tissue is also damaged by the molecules released from necrotic cells.

Negative selection Process in the thymus whereby developing T cells that recognize self antigens are induced to die by apoptosis.

Neoplasm A tumor, which may be benign or malignant.

Neutralization The mechanism by which antibodies binding to sites on pathogens prevent growth of the pathogen and/or its entry into cells. The toxicity of bacterial toxins can similarly be **neutralized** by bound antibody.

Neutropenia A deficiency of neutrophils in the blood.

Neutrophils Phagocytic white blood cells that enter infected tissues in large numbers. They contain granules that stain with neutral dyes. After their entry into infected tissues, neutrophils engulf and kill extracellular pathogens in large numbers. They are also known as neutrophilic polymorphonuclear leukocytes and are a type of granulocyte. The most abundant white blood cell.

NFAT (nuclear factor of activated T cells) A transcription factor that is activated as a result of signaling from the T-cell receptor. It functions as a complex of the NFAT protein with the dimer of Fos and Jun proteins known as AP-1.

NFKB Nuclear factor KB, a transcription factor that helps turn on the expression of many immune system genes.

NK-cell lectin-like receptors One of the two main structural classes of NK-cell receptors. They include both activating and inhibitory receptors.

Non-obese diabetic (NOD) mice A strain of mice in which diabetes arises spontaneously and has clinical and immunological characteristics similar to those in human insulin-dependent diabetes mellitus.

Oligomorphic Describes genes that have only a small number of different alleles in the population.

Oncogenes Genes involved in the control of cell growth. When these genes are defective in either structure or expression, they can cause cells to proliferate abnormally and form a tumor.

Oncogenic viruses Viruses that are involved in causing cancer.

Oncology the clinical discipline that deals with the study, diagnosis, and treatment of cancer.

Opportunistic pathogen A microorganism that causes disease only in individuals whose immune systems are in some way compromised.

Opsonins Antibodies and complement components that bind to pathogens and facilitate their phagocytosis by neutrophils or macrophages.

Opsonization The coating of the surface of a pathogen or other particle with any molecule that makes it more readily ingested by phagocytes. Antibody and complement opsonize extracellular bacteria for phagocytosis by neutrophils and macrophages because the phagocytic cells carry receptors for these molecules.

Oral tolerance The fact that harmless antigens, such as those in food, taken into the body by mouth do not usually cause an immune response.

Organ-specific autoimmune diseases Autoimmune diseases targeted at a particular organ, such as the thyroid in Graves' disease.

Original antigenic sin A bias seen in successive immune responses to structurally related antigens such as those on different strains of influenza virus. On infection for the second time with influenza, the antibody response is restricted to epitopes that the second strain shares with the first strain to which the person was exposed. Other highly immunogenic epitopes on the second and subsequent viruses are ignored.

P-nucleotides Nucleotides added into the junctions between gene segments during the somatic recombination that generates a rearranged variable-region sequence. They are an inverse repeat (a palindrome) of the nucleotide sequence at the end of the adjacent gene segment, which gives them their name of palindromic or P-nucleotides.

P-selectin *see* **selectins**

Pandemic Outbreak of an infectious disease that spreads worldwide.

Panel reactive antibody (PRA) A measure of the likelihood that a patient seeking a transplant is sensitized to potential donors. The patient's serum is tested against tissue from a representative panel of individuals for antibodies that would cause immediate hyperacute rejection of a graft. The PRA is the percentage of individuals in the panel whose cells react with the patient's antibodies.

Paracrine Term applied to a cytokine that is released from one type of cell and acts on other cells nearby.

Parasites The unicellular protozoa and multicellular worms that infect animals and humans and live within them.

Paroxysmal nocturnal hemoglobinuria (PNH) A disease in which the complement regulatory proteins CD59 and DAF are defective, so that complement activation leads to episodes of spontaneous hemolysis. The defect is in the attachment of CD59 and DAF to cell membranes via a glycolipid anchor.

Passive immunization The injection of specific antibodies to provide protection against a pathogen or toxin. The administered antibodies may derive from human blood donors, immunized animals or hybridoma cell lines.

Passive transfer of immunity Transfer of immunity to a nonimmune individual by the injection of specific antibody, immune serum, or T cells.

Pathogen an organism, most commonly a microorganism, which can cause disease.

Pathology the scientific study of disease or detectable damage to tissue caused by disease.

Pemphigus foliaceus and **pemphigus vulgaris** autoimmune diseases involving blistering of the skin.

Pentraxins A family of acute-phase proteins to which C-reactive protein belongs. They are formed of five identical subunits.

Peptide-binding motif of an MHC isoform, the combination of anchor residues that are common to the amino acid sequences of peptides that bind to the isoform.

Perforin One of the proteins released by cytotoxic T cells on contact with their target cells. It forms pores in the target cell membrane that contribute to cell killing.

Peripheral lymphoid tissues *see* **secondary lymphoid tissues**

Payer's patches Gut-associated lymphoid tissue present in the wall of the small intestine, especially the ileum.

Phagocyte A cell specialized to perform phagocytosis. The principal phagocytic cells in mammals are neutrophils and macrophages.

Phagocytosis Cellular internali7ation of particulate matter, such as bacteria, by means of endocytosis. Cells specialized in phagocytosis are known as phagocytes.

Phagolysosome Intracellular vesicle formed by fusion of a phagosome with a lysosome, in which the phagocytosed material is broken down by degradative lysosomal enzymes.

Phagosome Intracellular vesicle containing material taken up by phagocytosis.

Plasma cells Terminally differentiated B lymphocytes that secrete antibody.

Plasmablast An activated B cell differentiating within a lymphoid follicle at the stage at which it shows some features of a plasma cell.

Plasmacytoid dendritic cells (PDCs) Dendritic-like cells derived from interferon-producing cells cultured with microbial products and inflammatory cytokines.

Pluripotent hematopoietic stem cell Stem cell in bone marrow that gives rise to all the cellular elements of the blood.

PNH *see* paroxysmal **nocturnal hemoglobinuria**

Poly-Ig receptor A receptor present on the basolateral membrane of epithelial cells that binds polymeric immunoglobulins, especially dimeric IgA, and transports them across the epithelium by transcytosis.

Polymorphism The existence of different variants of a gene or trait in the population. Genetic polymorphism is defined as the existence of two or more forms (alleles) of a given gene within the population, with the variant alleles each occurring at a frequency greater than 1%.

Polymorphonuclear leukocytes *see* **granulocytes**

Polyspecificity The ability to bind to many different antigens, a property shown by some antibodies. It is also known as polyreactivity.

Positive selection a process in the thymus that selects immature T cells with receptors that recognize peptide antigens presented by self-MHC molecules. Only cells that are positively selected are allowed to continue their maturation.

Pre-B cells A stage in B-cell development at which the B cells have rearranged their heavy-chain genes but not their light-chain genes.

Pre-B-cell receptor Immunoglobulin-like receptor that is expressed on the surface of pre-B cells. It consists of *ILL* heavy chains in association with surrogate light chains. Its appearance signals the cessation of heavy-chain gene rearrangement.

Pre-T-cell receptor Receptor that is present on the surface of some immature thymocytes. It consists of a T-cell receptor 13 chain associated with a surrogate a chain called pTa.

Prednisolone The biologically active compound to which the immunosuppressive drug prednisone is converted *in vivo*.

Prednisone A synthetic steroid drug with potent anti-inflammatory and immunosuppressive activity. Prescribed to patients who have had organ transplants.

Primary immune response or primary response The adaptive immune response that follows a person's first exposure to an antigen.

Primary lymphoid follicles The name given to the B-cell areas of secondary lymphoid tissues in the absence of an immune response. They contain resting B lymphocytes.

Primary lymphoid tissues Anatomical sites of lymphocyte development. The bone marrow and the thymus gland.

Pro-B cells An early stage in B-cell development at which B-cell precursors express B-cell marker proteins and rearrange their heavy-chain genes.

Pro-drug Biologically inactive compound that is metabolized in the body to produce an active drug.

Productive rearrangements DNA rearrangements within immunoglobulin and T-cell receptor genes that lead to a gene that can direct the synthesis of a functional polypeptide chain.

Professional antigen-presenting cells Cells that can present antigen to naive T cells and activate them. A professional antigen-presenting cell not only displays peptide antigens bound to appropriate MHC molecules but also has costimulatory molecules on its surface that are needed to activate the T cell. Only dendritic cells, macrophages, and B cells can be professional antigen-presenting cells.

Programmed cell death *see* **apoptosis**

Properdin A blood protein that helps to activate the alternative pathway of complement activation. It binds to and stabilizes the alternative pathway C3 and C5 convertases on the surfaces of bacterial cells. It is also known as factor P.

Proteasome Large multisubunit protease present in the cytosol of all cells that degrades cytoplasmic proteins. It generates the peptides presented by MHC class I molecules.

Protective immunity The specific immunological resistance to a pathogen that follows either from specific vaccination or recovery from an infection with the pathogen.

Protein tyrosine kinases Enzymes that phosphorylate tyrosine residues on proteins. They are involved in signal transduction from many types of cell-surface receptor, including the antigen receptors on B cells and T cells.

Proto-oncogenes Cellular genes that regulate the control of cell growth and division. When mutated or aberrantly expressed, they contribute to the malignant transformation of cells, which leads to cancer.

Provirus The DNA form of a retrovirus when it is integrated into the host cell genome. In this state it can remain transcriptionally inactive for a long time.

Purine nucleotide phophorylase (PNP) enzyme involved in purine metabolism. Its deficiency results in the accumulation of purine nucleosides, which are toxic for developing T cells. This leads to severe combined immunodeficiency.

Pus Thick yellowish-white fluid that is formed in infected wounds. It is composed of dead and dying white blood cells (principally neutrophils), tissue debris, and dead microorganisms.

Pyogenic bacteria Extracellular encapsulated bacteria that cause the formation of pus at sites of infection.

RAG-1, RAG-2 *see* **recombination activation genes**

Rapamycin *see* **sirolimus**

Receptor editing A process in developing B cells that have generated a self-reactive receptor by which further rounds of light-chain gene rearrangement can produce a new light chain to replace the self-reactive one.

Recirculation of lymphocytes, their continual movement from blood to secondary lymphoid tissues to lymph and back to the blood. An exception to this pattern is traffic to the spleen; lymphocytes both enter and leave the spleen in the blood.

Recombination activation genes (RAG-1, RAG-2) Two genes whose expression is required for immunoglobulin and T-cell receptor gene rearrangement in B cells and T cells.

Recombination signal sequences (RSSs) Short stretches of DNA that flank the gene segments that are rearranged to generate V-region exons. They are the sites at which somatic recombination occurs.

Regulators of complement activation (RCA) Proteins that regulate the activity of complement and contain a particular structural motif called the CCP motif.

Regulatory CD4 T cells (TR) Antigen-specific CD4 T cells whose actions can suppress immune responses.

Respiratory burst Metabolic change accompanied by a transient increase in oxygen consumption that occurs in neutrophils and macrophages when they have taken up opsonized particles. It leads to the generation of toxic oxygen metabolites and other antibacterial substances that attack the phagocytosed material.

Respiratory syncytial virus (RSV) A paramyxovirus that is a common cause of severe chest infection in young children. Often associated with wheezing.

Rev Protein product of the rev gene of the human immunodeficiency virus (Fm). The protein promotes the passage of viral RNA from nucleus to cytoplasm during HIV replication.

Rheumatic fever Autoimmune disease involving inflammation of the heart, joints, and kidneys, which can follow 2-3 weeks after a throat infection with certain strains of *Streptococcus pyogenes*. It is due to antibodies made against bacterial antigens cross-reacting with components of heart tissue, and the continued deposition of immune complexes.

Rheumatoid arthritis A common inflammatory disease of joints that is due to an autoimmune response.

Rheumatoid factor An IgIVI antibody with specificity for human IgG that is produced in some people with rheumatoid arthritis.

RSS *see* **recombination signal sequences**

RSV *see* **respiratory syncytial virus**

Sarcoma A tumor that arises from a cell of connective tissue.

SE *see* **staphylococcal enterotoxins**

Secondary immune response or secondary **response** The adaptive immune response provoked by a second exposure to an antigen. It differs from the primary response by starting sooner and building more quickly.

Secondary lymphoid follicle The name given to the B-cell areas of secondary lymphoid tissues that are responding to antigen. They contain proliferating B cells.

Secondary lymphoid tissues The lymph nodes, spleen and mucosa-associated lymphoid tissues. These are the tissues in which immune responses are initiated. The more highly organized tissues such as lymph nodes and spleen are also often known as **secondary lymphoid organs.**

Secretory component (secretory piece) Fragment of the poly-Ig receptor left attached to dimeric IgA after its transport across epithelial cells.

Segmental exchange *see* **gene conversion**

Selectins Family of adhesion molecules present on the surfaces of leukocytes and endothelial cells. They are lectins and bind to sugar moieties on certain mucin-like glycoproteins.

Self antigens A term used to describe all the normal constituents of the body to which the immune system would respond were it not for the mechanisms of tolerance that destroy or inactivate self-reactive B and T cells.

Self-MHC A person's own MHC molecules.

Self-peptides Peptides produced from the body's own proteins. In the absence of infection these peptides occupy the peptide-binding sites of MHC molecules on cell surfaces.

Self-renewal The ability of a population of cells to renew itself.

Self-tolerance The normal situation whereby a person's immune system does not respond to constituents of the person's body.

Sensitization in connection with allergy, the first exposure to an allergen that elicits an IgE response. Allergic reactions occur only in individuals who have already been **sensitized.**

Sepsis The toxic effects of infection of the bloodstream. Usually caused by Gram-negative bacteria. *See also* **septic shock.**

Septic shock Shock syndrome that is frequently fatal, caused by the systemic release of the cytokine INF-a after bacterial infection of the bloodstream, usually with Gram-negative bacteria.

Septicemia Bacterial invasion of the blood.

Seroconversion The phase of an infection when antibodies against the infecting agent are first detectable in the blood.

Serotypes Antigenically different strains of a bacterium or other pathogen that can be distinguished by immunological means, for example by antibody-based detection tests. Also used to describe human alloantigens such as HLA and blood group antigens.

Serum sickness The collection of symptoms that follow the injection of large amounts of a foreign molecule (such as a serum protein) into a person. It is caused by the immune complexes formed between the injected protein and the antibodies that are made against it. Characterized by fever, arthralgias, and nephritis.

Severe combined immune deficiency (SCID) Immune deficiency disease in which neither antibody nor T-cell responses are made. It is usually the result of genetic defects that lead to T-cell deficiencies, and is fatal in childhood if not treated.

Single-positive thymocytes A late stage of T-cell development in the thymus characterized by the expression of either the CD4 or the CD8 coreceptor on the cell surface.

Sirolimus The proprietary name for the immunosuppressive drug rapamycin. Both names are in common use.

SLE *see* **systemic lupus erythematosus**

Small lymphocytes The general name for resting T and B lymphocytes as they recirculate.

Small pre-B cells Pre-B cells in which light-chain gene rearrangements are being made.

Somatic gene therapy A possible therapy for curing inherited immunodeficiency diseases. Stem cells isolated from the patient are transfected with a normal copy of the gene that is defective in the patient. The stem cells, which now express a good copy of the formerly defective gene, are reinfused into the patient's circulation.

Somatic hypermutation Mutation that occurs at high frequency in the rearranged variable-region DNA of immunoglobulin genes in activated B cells, resulting in the production of variant antibodies, some of which have a higher affinity for the antigen.

Somatic recombination DNA recombination that occurs between gene segments in the immunoglobulin genes and T-cell receptor genes in developing B cells and T cells respectively. It generates a complete exon that encodes the variable region of an immunoglobulin or T- cell receptor polypeptide chain.

Specificity The property of antibodies and other antigen-binding molecules for selective interaction with only one or a few types of molecule or cell.

Spleen Organ situated adjacent to the cardiac end of the stomach. One function of the spleen is to remove old or damaged red blood cells from the circulation; the other is as a secondary lymphoid organ that responds to blood-borne pathogens and antigens.

Staphylococcal enterotwdns (SEs) Toxins secreted by strains of staphylococcus that act on the gut and cause the symptoms of food poisoning. They are also superantigens.

STATs Signal transducers and activators of transcription. Proteins that are activated to become transcription factors through the Janus kinase signaling pathway from cytokine receptors.

Stromal cells Cells that provide the supporting framework of a tissue or organ.

Subunit vaccines Vaccines composed only of isolated antigenic components of a pathogen and not the pathogen itself, either alive or dead.

Superantigens Molecules that, by binding nonspecifically to MHC class II molecules and T-cell receptors, stimulate the polyclonal activation of T cells.

Suppressor CD4 T cells *see* regulatory CD4 **T cells**.

Surrogate light chain A protein that mimics an immunoglobulin light chain and made up of two subunits, VpreB and M. It is produced by pro-B cells and together with p. heavy chain forms the pre-B-cell receptor.

Switch regions (switch sequences) DNA sequences preceding heavy-chain constant-region genes at which somatic recombination occurs when B cells switch from producing one immunoglobulin isotype to another.

Sympathetic ophthalmia An autoimmune response that sometimes follows damage to an eye and affects both the damaged eye and the healthy eye.

Syngeneic genetically identical. A syngeneic tissue graft is one made between two genetically identical individuals. It does not provoke an immune response or a rejection reaction.

Systemic anaphylaxis A rapid-onset and potentially fatal form of IgE-mediated allergic reaction, in which antigen in the bloodstream triggers the activation of mast cells throughout the body, causing circulatory collapse and suffocation due to tracheal swelling.

Systemic autoimmune disease (systemic autoimmunity) Autoimmunity that involves reactions to common components of the body and whose effects are not confined to one particular organ.

Systemic lupus erythematosus A systemic autoimmune disease in which autoantibodies made against DNA, RNA, and nucleoprotein particles form immune complexes that damage small blood vessels.

T cells (T lymphocytes) Lymphocytes that develop in the thymus and are responsible for cell-mediated immunity. T cells include all T cells that recognize peptide antigen presented by MHC class I and II molecules. Their cell-surface antigen receptor is called the T-cell receptor.

T-cell activation The stimulation of mature naive T cells by antigen presented to them by professional antigen-presenting cells. It leads to their proliferation and differentiation into effector T cells.

T-cell areas parts of secondary lymphoid tissues where the lymphocytes are predominantly T cells.

T-cell priming The activation of mature naive T cells by antigen presented to them by professional antigen-presenting cells.

T-cell receptor a chain (TCRa) One of the two polypeptide chains that make up the most common form of T-cell receptor.

T-cell receptor 13 chain (TCRI3) One of the two polypeptide chains that make up the most common form of T-cell receptor.

T-cell receptor complex The complex of T-cell receptor a and 13 chains and the invariant CD3 and C chains that makes up a functional antigen receptor on the T-cell surface.

T-cell receptor The highly variable antigen receptor of T lymphocytes. On most T cells it is composed of a variable a chain and 131 chain and is known as the a:p T-cell receptor. On a minority of T cells, the variable chains are 7 and (5 chains, and this receptor is known as the y:8 T-cell receptor. Both types of receptor are present at the cell surface in association with the complex of invariant CD3 chains and chains, which have a signaling function.

T lymphocyte *see* **T cells**

Tacrolimus Immunosuppressive polypeptide drug that inactivates T cells by inhibiting signal transduction from the T-cell receptor. It is widely used to suppress transplant rejection. It is also known as FK506.

TAP *see* **transporter of antigen processing**

Tapasin TAP-associated protein, a chaperone protein involved in the assembly of peptide-MHC class I molecule complexes in the endoplasmic reticulum.

Target cell Any cell that is acted on directly by effector T cells, effector cells or molecules. For example, virus-infected cells are the targets of cytotoxic T cells, which kill them, and naive B cells are the targets of effector CD4 T cells, which help to stimulate them to produce antibodies.

Tat Protein product of the tat gene of the human immunodeficiency virus (HIV), which enhances the rate of transcription of viral RNA.

TD antigens *see* **thymus-dependent antigens**

Terminal deoxynucleotidyltransferase (TdT) Enzyme that inserts nontemplated nucleotides (N-nucleotides) into the junctions between gene segments during the rearrangement of T-cell receptor and immunoglobulin heavy-chain genes.

Tetanus toxin Protein neurotoxin produced by the bacterium *Clostridium tetani*. The cause of the disease tetanus.

TGF-13 *see* **transforming** growth factor-13

TH1 cells A subset of CD4 T cells that are characterized by the cytokines they produce. They are involved mainly in activating macrophages. Also called inflammatory T cells.

TH2 cells A subset of CD4 T cells that are characterized by the cytokines they produce. They are involved mainly in stimulating B cells to produce antibody. Also called helper T cells.

Thymectomy The surgical removal of the thymus gland.

Thymic anlage The tissue from which the thymic stroma develops during embryogenesis.

Thymic stroma The reticular epithelial cells and connective tissue of the thymus, which form the essential microenvironment for T-cell development.

Thymocytes Developing T cells in the thymus.

Thymus A lymphoepithelial organ in the upper part of the middle of the chest, just behind the breastbone. It is the site of T-cell development.

Thymus-dependent antigens (TD antigens) Antigens for which the elicitation of an antibody response on immunization or vaccination is dependent upon help provided by antigen-specific T cells. Most protein antigens are of this type.

Thymus-dependent lymphocyte *see* **T cells**

Thymus-independent antigens (TI antigens) Antigens that can elicit antibody production in the absence of T cells. There are two types of TI antigen: TI-1 antigens, which have intrinsic B-cell activating activity, and TI-2 antigens, which have multiple identical epitopes that cross-link B-cell receptors.

TI- l antigens, TI-2 antigens *see* **thymus-independent antigens**

Tangible body macrophages Phagocytic cells that are seen in histological sections engulfing apoptotic B cells in germinal centers.

TNF-a *see* **tumor necrosis factor-a TNF-I3** *see* **lymphotoxin**

Tolerance When the immune system of a person does not or cannot respond to an antigen. In such cases the individual is said to be tolerant of the antigen.

Tonsils large aggregates of lymphoid cells lying on each side of the pharynx.

Toxic shock Syndrome a systemic toxic reaction caused by the over-production of cytokines by CD4 T cells activated by the bacterial superantigen **toxic shock syndrome toxin-1 (TSST-1),** which is secreted by *Staphylococcus aureus.*

Toxoids Toxins that have been deliberately inactivated by heat or chemical treatment so that they are no longer toxic but can still provoke a protective immune response on vaccination.

Toxoplasmosis The disease caused by the protozoan parasite *Toxoplasma gondii.*

Transcytosis The transport of molecules from one side of an epithelium to the other by endocytosis into vesicles within the epithelial cells at one face of the

Transforming growth factor-I3 (TGF-I3) A multifunctional cytokine produced by TH2 cells and other cell types.

Transfusion effect Improved outcome of transplantation if the recipient has been given prior blood transfusions from people who share an HLA-DR allotype with the organ with which the patient is subsequently transplanted.

Translocation A chromosomal abnormality in which a piece of one chromosome has become joined to another chromosome. The rear-ranging genes of B and T cells are often the sites of translocation in B-cell and T-cell tumors.

Transplant rejection Immune reaction that is directed towards transplanted tissue and leads to death of the graft.

Transplantation The grafting of organs or tissues from one individual to another.

Transporter associated with antigen processing (TAP) An ATP-binding protein in the endoplasmic reticulum membrane that transports peptides from the cytosol to the endoplasmic reticulum lumen. It is composed of two subunits, TAP-1 and TAP-2. It supplies MHC class I molecules with peptides.

Tuberculin test Clinical test to detect exposure to *Mycobacterium tuberculosis*, the causal agent of tuberculosis. Subcutaneous injection of purified protein derivative (PPD) of M. *tuberculosis* elicits a delayed-type hypersensitivity reaction in individuals who have had tuberculosis or have been immunized against it.

Tumor A growth arising from uncontrolled cell proliferation. It may be benign and self-limiting, or malignant and invasive.

Tumor antigens Cell-surface components of tumor cells that can elicit an immune response in the affected individuals. *See also* **tumor-associated antigens; tumor-specific antigens**.

Tumor-associated antigens Antigens characteristic of certain tumor cells that are also present on some types of normal cells.

Tumor necrosis factor-a (TNF-a) A cytokine produced by macrophages and T cells that has several functions in the immune response and is the prototype of the TNF family of cytolcines . These cytokines function as cell-associated or secreted proteins that interact with receptors of the tumor necrosis factor receptor (TNFR)

Tumor-specific antigens Antigens that are characteristic of tumor cells and are not expressed by normal cells.

Tumor suppressor genes Genes for cellular proteins that function to prevent cells from becoming cancerous.

Type I, type II, type III, type IV hypersensitivity reactions *see* **hyper-sensitivity reactions**

Type I interferon Cytokines (interferons-α and -13) produced by virus-infected cells that interfere with viral replication by the infected cell, and also signal neighboring uninfected cells to prepare for infection.

Unproductive rearrangements DNA rearrangements of immunoglobulin and T-cell receptor genes that produce a gene that cannot make a functional polypeptide chain.

Urticaria The technical term for hives, which are red, itchy skin welts usually brought on by an allergic reaction.

V domain *see* **variable domain**

V gene segment *see* **variable (V) gene segment**

V(D)J recombinase The set of enzymes needed to recombine V, D, and J segments.

V region *see* **variable region.**

Vaccination The deliberate induction of protective immunity to a pathogen by the administration of killed or nonpathogenic forms of the pathogen, or its antigens, to induce an immune response.

Vaccine Any preparation made from a pathogen that is used for vaccination and provides protective immunity against infection with the pathogen.

Vaccinia The cowpox virus. It causes a limited infection in humans that leads to immunity to the human smallpox virus. Was used as a vaccine against smallpox.

Variable domain (V domain) The amino-terminal domain of immunoglobulin and T-cell receptor polypeptide chains. Paired variable domains make up the antigen-binding site.

Variable (V) gene segment DNA sequence in the immunoglobulin or T-cell receptor genes that encodes the first 95 or so amino acids of the V domain.

Variable region (V region) The part of an immunoglobulin or T-cell receptor, or of its constituent polypeptide chains, that varies in amino acid sequence between isoforms having different antigenic specificities. It is responsible for determining antigen specificity.

Variable surface glycoproteins (VSGs) Glycoproteins that form the surface coat of African trypanosomes. The trypanosome can repeatedly change its glycoprotein coat by expressing different glycoprotein genes using a process akin to gene conversion.

Variola Name given to both the smallpox virus and the disease it causes: smallpox.

Variolation Historical procedure for immunization against smallpox in which a small amount of live smallpox virus was introduced through scarification of the skin.

Vascular addressins Mucin-like cell adhesion molecules on endothelial cells to which some leukocyte adhesion molecules bind. They determine the selective homing of leukocytes to particular sites in the body.

Viruses Submicroscopic pathogens composed of a nucleic acid genome enclosed in a protein coat. They replicate only in a living cell because they do not possess all the metabolic machinery required for independent life. A viral particle is called a virion.

VLA-4 Integrin present on the surface of T lymphocytes that binds to mucosal cell adhesion molecules.

Weibel-Palade bodies Granules containing P-selectin, which are present inside endothelial cells.

Wheal-and-flare reaction The reaction observed when small amounts of allergen are injected into the dermis of an individual who is allergic to the antigen. It consists of a raised area of skin containing fluid (the wheal) with a spreading, red, itchy reaction around it (the flare).

Wiskott-Aldrich syndrome A genetic disease in which interactions of T cells and B cells are defective. Antibody responses against polysaccharide antigens are deficient, and patients are susceptible to infection with pyogenic bacteria .

X-linked aganirnaglobulinemia (XLA) A genetic disorder in which B-cell development is arrested at the pre-B-cell stage and neither mature B cells or antibodies are formed. The disease is due to a defect in the gene encoding the protein tyrosine kinase Btk.

X-linked hyper-IgM syndrome *see* **hyper IgM syndrome**

X-linked lymphoproliferative syndrome Immunodeficiency due to a defect in the SH2D1A gene on the X chromosome, resulting in an inability to control EBV infections.

Xenoantibodies Antibodies produced in one species against the antigens of another species.

Xenoantigens Antigens on the tissues of one species that provoke an immune response in members of another species.

Xenogeneic Coming from a different species.

Xenograft An organ from one species transplanted into another species.

Xenotransplantation The transplantation of organs from one species into another. It is being explored as a possible solution to the shortage of human organs for clinical transplantation.

ZAP-70 A cytoplasmic tyrosine kinase in T cells that forms part of the signal transduction pathway from T-cell receptors.

Zymogen The inactive form in which some enzymes are synthesized. Active enzyme is usually produced by proteolytic cleavage of the zymogen.

INDEX

A

B

C

D

E

F

G

H

I

J

K

L

M

N

O

P

R

S

T

U

V

W

X

Y

Z